KU-286-043

369 0246333

MONKLANDS HOSPITAL
LIBRARY
MONKSCOURT AVENUE
AIRDRIE ML60JS
☎01236712005

Fundamentals of
Revision Hip Arthroplasty
Diagnosis, Evaluation, and Treatment

Fundamentals of
Revision Hip Arthroplasty
Diagnosis, Evaluation, and Treatment

EDITED BY

David J. Jacofsky, MD
Chairman
The CORE Institute
Center for Orthopedic Research and Education
Phoenix, Arizona

Anthony K. Hedley, MD, FRCS
Arizona Institute for Bone & Joint Disorders
Phoenix, Arizona

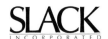

3690246333

WE312 JAC
£109.25

MONKLANDS HOSPITAL
LIBRARY
MONKSCOURT AVENUE
AIRDRIE ML60JS
☎ 01236712005

www.Healio.com/books

ISBN: 978-1-55642-952-1

Copyright © 2013 by SLACK Incorporated

All rights reserved. No part of this book may be reproduced, stored in a retrieval system or transmitted in any form or by any means, electronic, mechanical, photocopying, recording or otherwise, without written permission from the publisher, except for brief quotations embodied in critical articles and reviews.

The procedures and practices described in this publication should be implemented in a manner consistent with the professional standards set for the circumstances that apply in each specific situation. Every effort has been made to confirm the accuracy of the information presented and to correctly relate generally accepted practices. The authors, editors, and publisher cannot accept responsibility for errors or exclusions or for the outcome of the material presented herein. There is no expressed or implied warranty of this book or information imparted by it. Care has been taken to ensure that drug selection and dosages are in accordance with currently accepted/recommended practice. Off-label uses of drugs may be discussed. Due to continuing research, changes in government policy and regulations, and various effects of drug reactions and interactions, it is recommended that the reader carefully review all materials and literature provided for each drug, especially those that are new or not frequently used. Some drugs or devices in this publication have clearance for use in a restricted research setting by the Food and Drug and Administration or FDA. Each professional should determine the FDA status of any drug or device prior to use in their practice.

Any review or mention of specific companies or products is not intended as an endorsement by the author or publisher.

SLACK Incorporated uses a review process to evaluate submitted material. Prior to publication, educators or clinicians provide important feedback on the content that we publish. We welcome feedback on this work.

Published by: SLACK Incorporated
                  6900 Grove Road
                  Thorofare, NJ 08086 USA
                  Telephone: 856-848-1000
                  Fax: 856-848-6091
                  www.Healio.com/books

Contact SLACK Incorporated for more information about other books in this field or about the availability of our books from distributors outside the United States.

Library of Congress Cataloging-in-Publication Data

Jacofsky, David J.
  Fundamentals of revision hip arthroplasty : diagnosis, evaluation, and treatment / edited by David J. Jacofsky, Anthony K. Hedley.
       p. ; cm.
  Includes bibliographical references and index.
  ISBN 978-1-55642-952-1 (alk. paper)
  I. Hedley, Anthony K. II. Title.
  [DNLM: 1. Arthroplasty, Replacement, Hip--adverse effects. 2. Hip Joint--surgery. 3. Hip Prosthesis. 4. Postoperative Complications--surgery. 5. Reoperation--methods. WE 860]

  617.5'810592--dc23
                        2012024447

For permission to reprint material in another publication, contact SLACK Incorporated. Authorization to photocopy items for internal, personal, or academic use is granted by SLACK Incorporated provided that the appropriate fee is paid directly to Copyright Clearance Center. Prior to photocopying items, please contact the Copyright Clearance Center at 222 Rosewood Drive, Danvers, MA 01923 USA; phone: 978-750-8400; website: www.copyright.com; email: info@copyright.com

Printed in the United States of America.

Last digit is print number: 10   9   8   7   6   5   4   3   2   1

DEDICATION

To my mentors... you know who you are.
David J. Jacofsky, MD

To my fellows, past and present.
Anthony K. Hedley, MD, FRCS

CONTENTS

ABOUT THE EDITORS

David J. Jacofsky, MD was born in Long Island, New York and is an international authority on adult reconstruction of the hip and knee. He received his residency training at the Mayo Clinic in Rochester, Minnesota and did his fellowship training at Johns Hopkins University in Baltimore, Maryland, during which time he was awarded the Mayo Scholar's Award and the Joe Janes' Humanitarian award. Dr. Jacofsky started his career as an attending at the Mayo Clinic and subsequently moved to Phoenix, Arizona where he founded The Center for Orthopedic Research and Education (CORE) Institute. Dr. Jacofsky has published over 40 articles and 20 book chapters and has lectured around the world. He has a keen interest in health care reform, cost containment, improved outcomes, and the changing demographics of arthroplasty. Dr. Jacofsky is an avid martial artist and enjoys weight-lifting and running.

Anthony K. Hedley, MD, FRCS is a fellow of the Royal College of Surgeons of Edinburgh and an acclaimed orthopedic surgeon, author, researcher, and educator specializing in joint reconstruction.

After graduating from medical school in South Africa, Dr. Hedley completed his general and orthopedic residency training at Natalspruit Hospital in Johannesburg. He then sat for the exams and was named a Fellow of The Royal College of Surgeons of Edinburgh. Dr. Hedley returned to South Africa to complete an orthopedic residency at Johannesburg General Hospital. After, having registered as a Specialist Orthopedic Surgeon with the South African boards, he traveled to London and did a brief sojourn with the late, world-famous teacher and author Alan Apley at St. Thomas Hospital. Dr. Hedley came to the University of California, Los Angeles (UCLA) in 1977 to start a fellowship in Orthopedic Bioengineering with Dr. Harlan Amstutz of the Division of Orthopedic Surgery at UCLA. This was followed by 4 years in the Junior Professor ranks as an Assistant Professor.

Dr. Hedley left UCLA at the end of 1982 and moved to Phoenix, Arizona to join a private practice partnership. He served as the Chairman of the Department of Orthopedics at St. Luke's Hospital from 1987 to 2005. He became an inventor with Howmedica in 1982. He is currently an inventor and consultant with Stryker Orthopaedics and is involved in several clinical research projects.

Dr. Hedley is well known in the arthroplasty world for his various contributions both from the podium and in referee journals. He has headed a joint replacement fellowship since 1983 and continues to do so. From this, he is now associated with 45 fellows who have gone out into the community to continue their work as hip or knee arthroplasty surgeons.

MONKLANDS HOSPITAL
LIBRARY
MONKSCOURT AVENUE
AIRDRIE ML60JS
☎ 01236712005

CONTRIBUTING AUTHORS

Wael K. Barsoum, MD (Chapter 8)
Surgical Operations Chairman
Department of Orthopaedic Surgery
Cleveland Clinic
Cleveland, Ohio

Christopher P. Beauchamp, MD (Chapter 13)
Associate Professor of Orthopedic Surgery
Mayo Clinic College of Medicine
Phoenix, Arizona

Michael R. Bloomfield, MD (Chapter 8)
Department of Orthopaedic Surgery
Cleveland Clinic
Cleveland, Ohio

Justin Brothers, MD (Chapter 11)
Geisinger Medical Center
Danville, Pennsylvania

James Cashman, MD (Chapter 11)
Arthroplasty Fellow
Rothman Institute
Philadelphia, Pennsylvania

Robert M. Cercek, MD (Chapter 4)
Orthopedic Surgeon
The Center for Orthopedic Research and
    Education
Sun City West, Arizona

Craig J. Della Valle, MD (Chapter 6)
Associate Professor of Orthopedic Surgery
Director
Adult Reconstructive Fellowship
RUSH University Medical Center
Chicago, Illinois

Douglas A. Dennis, MD (Chapter 10)
Adjunct Professor
Department of Biomedical Engineering
University of Tennessee
Knoxville, Tennessee
Adjunct Professor of Bioengineering
University of Denver
Director
Rocky Mountain Musculoskeletal Research
    Laboratory
Denver, Colorado

Jared R. H. Foran, MD (Chapter 6)
Orthopedic Surgeon
Panorama Orthopedics and Spine Center
Golden, Colorado
OrthoColorado Hospital
Lakewood, Colorado

Gregory J. Golladay, MD (Chapter 9)
Orthopaedic Associates of Michigan, PC
Clinical Assistant Professor
Michigan State University
Lansing, Michigan
Clinical Advisor for Joint Replacement
Spectrum Health
Grand Rapids, Michigan

Ian M. Gradisar, MD (Chapter 5)
Clinical Instructor Orthopedic Surgery
Northeast Ohio Medical University
Summa Health System
Crystal Clinic Orthopaedic Center
Akron, Ohio

Kenneth A. Greene, MD (Chapter 5)
Professor of Orthopedic Surgery
Northeast Ohio Medical University
Staff Orthopedic Surgeon
Cleveland Clinic
Cleveland, Ohio

Carlos A. Higuera, MD (Chapter 8)
Orthopedic Surgery Clinical Fellow,
    Adult Reconstruction
Rothman Institute
Philadelphia, Pennsylvania

David E. Jaffe, MD (Chapter 2)
Resident
University of Maryland Medical System
Department of Orthopedics
Baltimore, Maryland

Aaron J. Johnson, MD (Chapter 2)
Fellow
Rubin Institute for Advanced Orthopedics
Center for Joint Preservation and
    Reconstruction
Sinai Hospital of Baltimore
Baltimore, Maryland

Raymond H. Kim, MD (Chapter 10)
Colorado Joint Replacement
Adjunct Associate Professor of Bioengineering
Department of Mechanical and Materials
  Engineering
University of Denver
Denver, Colorado

Viktor E. Krebs, MD (Chapter 5)
Director
Center for Adult Reconstructive Surgery &
  General Orthopaedics
Cleveland Clinic
Cleveland, Ohio

Steven M. Kurtz, PhD (Chapter 12)
Exponent Inc
Philadelphia, Pennsylvania

Michael T. Manley, FRSA, PhD (Chapter 12)
Academic Director
Homer Stryker Center for Orthopaedic
  Education and Research
Mahwah, New Jersey
Visiting Professor
Department of Biomechanics
University of Bath
Bath, United Kingdom

David C. Markel, MD (Chapter 9)
Chairman
Detroit Medical Center/Providence Hospital
  Orthopedic Surgery Residency Program
Chair, Orthopedic Surgery
Providence Hospital
Detroit, Michigan

Andrew Michael, MD (Chapter 3)
Medical Researcher
Midwest Orthopedics
Chicago, Illinois

Michael A. Mont, MD (Chapter 2)
Director
Center for Joint Preservation and
  Reconstruction
Rubin Institute for Advanced Orthopedics
Sinai Hospital of Baltimore
Assistant Professor
Department of Orthopedic Surgery
The Johns Hopkins Medical Institutions
Baltimore, Maryland

Steven L. Myerthall, MD, FRCS(C) (Chapter 1)
The Center for Orthopedic Research and
  Education
Division of Orthopedic Surgery
Mercy Gilbert Medical Center
Phoenix, Arizona

Kevin L. Ong, PhD (Chapter 12)
Senior Managing Engineer
Exponent Inc
Philadelphia, Pennsylvania

Javad Parvizi, MD, FRCS (Chapter 11)
Professor of Orthopedics
Thomas Jefferson University
Director of Clinical Research
Rothman Institute
Philadelphia, Pennsylvania

Michael D. Ries, MD (Chapter 7)
Professor of Orthopedic Surgery
Chief of Arthroplasty
University of California, San Francisco
Department of Orthopedic Surgery
San Francisco, California

Adam J. Schwartz, MD (Chapter 13)
Assistant Professor of Orthopedic Surgery
Mayo Clinic College of Medicine
Phoenix, Arizona

Scott Sporer, MD (Chapter 3)
Associate Professor Orthopaedic Surgery
RUSH University Medical Center
Chicago, Illinois

Bryan D. Springer, MD (Chapter 10)
OrthoCarolina Hip and Knee Center
Adult Reconstruction Fellowship Director
Charlotte, North Carolina

Creighton C. Tubb, MD (Chapter 5)
Adjunct Assistant Professor of Surgery
Uniformed Services University of
  the Health Sciences
Bethesda, Maryland
Orthopaedic Surgery Service
Madigan Healthcare System
Tacoma, Washington

Jonathan M. Vigdorchik, MD (Chapter 9)
Chief Resident
Detroit Medical Center/Providence Hospital
  Orthopedic Surgery Residency Program
Detroit, Michigan

Antonia Woehnl, MD (Chapter 2)
Fellow
Rubin Institute for Advanced Orthopedics
Center for Joint Preservation and
  Reconstruction
Sinai Hospital of Baltimore
Baltimore, Maryland

INTRODUCTION

This book is designed for surgeons who are not necessarily in the academic field, but who are encountering revisions more commonly in their practice and are capable of managing simpler revision cases. Unlike most texts in the revision arena, this text does not focus on the most difficult and challenging of cases to be tackled by experienced and high-volume revision surgeons. Rather, it is intended to guide the surgeon in the evaluation of the painful total joint replacement, review the basic tenants and principles of revision arthroplasty, and help the surgeon determine whether a given case is one he or she is competent and capable of managing, or whether it might best be managed via referral to a tertiary orthopedic center. As the number of these cases exponentially increases, this book is designed to serve as a concise resource to turn to for guidance.

This book is aimed at the orthopedic surgeon's formative years, namely residency, fellowship, and the early years of practice. The chapters have been contributed by well-known orthopedic surgeons who have expertise in the field of hip arthroplasty; their expertise is brought to the forefront with their contributions.

1

Evaluation of the Painful Total Hip Arthroplasty

Steven L. Myerthall, MD, FRCS(C)

In the decades since its introduction, total hip arthroplasty (THA) has proven to be a reliable and reproducible surgical procedure for relieving pain and improving function in patients with symptomatic hip arthritis. As with all surgical procedures, appropriate patient selection and surgical indications will minimize poor outcomes. Nonetheless, despite clinical success rates approaching 95% at the 10-year follow-up,[1-3] a small percentage of patients will continue to experience symptoms of pain and impaired function even after THA.

Hip, groin, or anterior thigh pain after THA can result from a multitude of etiologies. In general, when trying to establish the diagnosis, it is helpful to divide the possible causes into 2 broad categories: those that are directly related to the hip prosthesis (ie, intrinsic or intra-articular), and those that are not related to the hip replacement (ie, extrinsic or extra-articular). Furthermore, the importance of a systematic approach to identifying the possible causes cannot be overlooked. Evaluation must begin with a thorough history and physical examination; afterwards, laboratory tests, plain radiographs, arthrocentesis, and additional imaging analysis can provide additional information. Only after the diagnosis has been established should treatment be initiated.

The most important principles in the management of patients with pain after THA must be to avoid any form of surgical intervention until a definitive diagnosis has been made. A systematic approach to the evaluation of patients with pain and impaired function after THA is presented in this chapter.

DIFFERENTIAL DIAGNOSIS

Many things can lead to pain and decreased function after THA. These can be broadly categorized into factors that are intrinsic to the hip joint and factors that are extrinsic to the hip joint. The extrinsic factors can be further divided into those factors that are local to the hip but are extra-articular, and those that are remote from the hip joint itself (Tables 1-1 to 1-3).

The intrinsic causes of a painful THA are extensive and include loosening, infection, instability, impingement, particulate synovitis, and modulus of elasticity mismatch. A THA that is painful at rest must be evaluated with a high index of suspicion for infection. Early, acute

Jacofsky DJ, Hedley AK.
*Fundamentals of Revision Hip Arthroplasty:
Diagnosis, Evaluation, and Treatment (pp 1-10).*
© 2013 SLACK Incorporated.

TABLE 1-1. DIFFERENTIAL DIAGNOSIS OF THE PAINFUL TOTAL HIP ARTHROPLASTY: INTRINSIC FACTORS

- Loosening
- Infection
- Instability
- Impingement
- Particulate synovitis
- Modulus mismatch

TABLE 1-2. DIFFERENTIAL DIAGNOSIS OF THE PAINFUL TOTAL HIP ARTHROPLASTY: LOCAL EXTRINSIC FACTORS

- Bursitis (trochanteric, iliopsoas, iliopectineal)
- Tendinitis (piriformis, iliopsoas, hamstring)
- Heterotopic ossification
- Greater trochanteric/abductor avulsion fracture
- Stress fracture (pubic rami, sacral, femoral shaft)

TABLE 1-3. DIFFERENTIAL DIAGNOSIS OF THE PAINFUL TOTAL HIP ARTHROPLASTY: REMOTE EXTRINSIC FACTORS

- Spinal pathology (radiculopathy, stenosis, facet disease)
- Neuropathy/nerve palsy (femoral, sciatic, obturator)
- Nerve entrapment (meralgia paresthetica, ilioinguinal, genitofemoral)
- Peripheral vascular disease/claudication (femoral, iliac, gluteal)
- Osteitis pubis/pubic symphysitis
- Hernia (inguinal, femoral, obturator)
- Quadriceps/fascia lata herniation
- Intra-abdominal pathology
- Tumor

infection is easily diagnosed. Chronic infections are more common, but more difficult to diagnose. Persistent, unexplained pain; erythema; prolonged wound drainage; or failure of primary wound healing should raise suspicions of deep wound infection. The diagnosis of infection should always be in the foreground of the differential diagnosis for patients presenting with pain related to THA.

Of the remote extrinsic factors, degenerative disc disease of the lumbar spine, neurogenic problems, and peripheral vascular disease are frequently comorbidities in patients who undergo THA. Common disorders that can produce hip pain include spinal stenosis, neurogenic claudication, lumbar radiculopathy, and vascular claudication. These problems usually are easily confirmed with the appropriate tests. Although they may develop after hip replacement surgery, unfortunately in some cases, these problems were not initially considered by the surgeon prior to undertaking the index surgical procedure.

HISTORY

The first step in making the diagnosis is to establish the chief problem. Although patients usually present with pain, its relationship to instability, stiffness, or weakness must be considered. A pain scale is often useful for characterizing the level of the presenting pain and any response to treatment. The temporal relationship, location, and nature of the pain should be evaluated in order to establish the characteristics of the pain.

It is necessary to determine if the symptoms that the patient was experiencing prior to the index THA began early in the postoperative period or if it occurred after a long period of pain relief. The potential causes of early postoperative pain include acute infection, impingement or instability, the formation of heterotopic bone, or misdiagnosis of the initial presenting complaint. In contrast, delayed onset of pain is more characteristic of prosthesis loosening. Other potential causes of late onset pain include late or chronic infection, bursitis or tendinitis, stress fracture, or particulate synovitis.

The location of the patient's pain can assist in determining the source of the problem. Pain located in the groin is usually related to acetabular component loosening, erosion of the acetabular cartilage that may occur after hemiarthroplasty, iliopsoas impingement, or tendinitis, while buttock pain is related to sacroiliitis or lower back issues. Pain located in the anterior thigh is most often related to femoral component loosening or modulus mismatch. Pain located in the distal thigh is often related to knee pathology, but may also be associated with femoral loosening. Pain located at the superficial level of the lateral thigh is usually neurologic in nature, while deep lateral hip or thigh pain can be related to trochanteric bursitis, gluteal tendinitis, or femoral component loosening.

Mechanical pain usually occurs with activity and tends to be sharp, whereas pain at rest usually is not mechanical. Pain after activity is characteristic of synovial irritation or tendinitis. Radiating pain may indicate extra-articular sources such as the sacroiliac joint or the spine. Night or rest pain should raise concerns about infection or neurogenic pain. Also, the persistence of the symptoms that the patient was experiencing prior to THA would suggest misdiagnosis prior to surgery and the possibility of an extra-articular source of pain.

As with any patient encounter, a complete history should include a list of the patient's other medical, psychiatric, and surgical problems. Vascular, neurologic, or psychiatric disorders may be responsible for the hip pain. The patient's use of medications, most importantly narcotics, should be established. The possibility of alternate or secondary gains must be considered especially in cases where long-term narcotic usage was present prior to THA. Furthermore, the use of specific medications such as beta-blockers or anxiolytics may suggest comorbid conditions such as peripheral vascular disease or neurogenic pain as the source. Finally, an accurate review of systems should be undertaken and may identify important etiological clues. Bursitis is not uncommon in fibromyalgia and systemic symptoms such as fever, chills, night sweats, or lethargy may accompany infection.

PHYSICAL EXAMINATION

The physical examination should always begin with inspection. Asymmetry in the patient's posture may indicate scoliosis, pelvic obliquity, or leg length discrepancy. Asymmetry of posture necessitates a thorough examination of the spine and pelvis as well as the measurement of the true and apparent leg lengths. Assessment of gait for either a Trendelenburg or antalgic pattern must be undertaken. The Trendelenburg gait pattern is usually indicative of muscle weakness about the hip and is positive when the patient's center of gravity shifts toward the stance leg during the single leg stance phase of gait. This may also be seen in patients guarding the hip with this lurch to decrease the joint reactive force. In contrast, an antalgic gait pattern is indicative of pain and is manifested by a temporally short stance phase on the affected side as well as the patient's center of gravity moving away from the stance leg during the single leg stance phase of gait. Excessive internal or external rotation of the foot during gait or at rest may be indicative of malpositioning of the femoral component. External rotation and shortening is typical of femoral component loosening with subsidence. The presence and location of scars about the hip should also be noted. Marked erythema or visible discharge should raise concerns about possible infection. Skin changes over the hip, thigh, or lower leg may rarely be associated with complex regional pain syndrome but are commonly associated with peripheral vascular disease.

Groin pain with flexion of the hip against resistance in the seated position is highly indicative of psoas irritation and may indicate malposition of the acetabulum or impingement with a large head. Occasionally stressing the hip in the "figure 4" position will also elicit pain.

Palpation of the hip should be performed in a systematic manner and include a careful evaluation of all painful areas identified by the patient. Tenderness over the bony prominences indicates underlying pathology, specifically at the sacroiliac joint or greater trochanter. Surrounding hip musculature should also be examined for snapping or crepitation. Finally, careful palpation of the wound may identify neuromas or underlying fascial dehiscence.

Joint stability and range of motion of the hip also should be assessed. A positive Stinchfield or FABER (Flexion ABduction External Rotation) test may be indicative of muscle tightness but is usually more likely with intra-articular problems. Apprehension on the patient's part may be noted with flexion, adduction, and internal rotation in hips that are unstable and prone to sublux or dislocate. Pain with any active or passive motion is usually related to synovitis or infection, while pain at the extremes of motion is usually related to instability or component loosening.

A complete and thorough hip examination should also include a neurovascular examination of the lower extremities as well as an examination of the lumbar spine and ipsilateral knee. More specifically, the spine should be assessed for root tension signs with the straight leg raise and femoral nerve stretch tests. Also, an examination of the abdomen for inguinal hernia, aneurysm, and visceral pathology should be undertaken.

RADIOGRAPHIC ANALYSIS

High quality x-rays provide an important role in the evaluation of the painful THA and should be the first imaging study obtained. Often, any problems associated with the implant can be determined from these radiographs alone. The standard series should include an anterior-posterior (AP) view of the pelvis as well as an AP and cross-table lateral view of the hip in question. Although an AP and frog-leg lateral view of the hip provides orthogonal views of the femur, it does not do so for the acetabulum. Therefore, the frog-leg lateral should not be considered part of the routine follow-up x-rays after THA.

If acetabular malposition is suspected, a cross-table lateral x-ray is indicated and will clearly illustrate the problem.

Radiographs should be utilized to evaluate component positioning and sizing, as well as for implant loosening, lucencies at the implant/cement-bone interface, osteolysis, polyethylene wear and component, cement mantle, or periprosthetic fracture. Furthermore, the importance of serial radiographs cannot be overemphasized, especially in assessing for loosening of the implants (Figure 1-1).

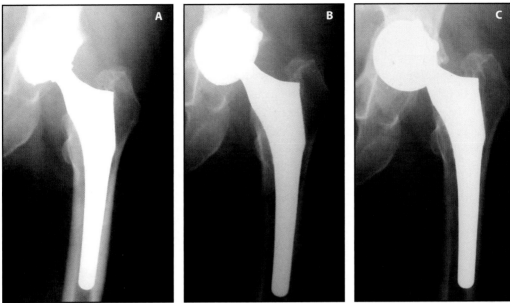

Figure 1-1. Serial radiographs of an uncemented left THA. (A) Represents the immediate postoperative radiograph. (B) Represents 2-year follow-up and (C) 4-year follow-up. When viewed in isolation, (B) does not provide significant concerns. However, when viewed in comparison to (A), this radiograph clearly shows position change of both the femoral and acetabular components indicative of loosening. Unfortunately, no revision procedure was undertaken until failure of the acetabular component occurred 4 years post index procedure.

When using radiographs to assess for evidence of loosening of cemented components, it is necessary to look for lucencies that occur at the cement-bone interface, for fractures that occur in the cement mantle, or for component migration. Hodgkinson et al[4] reported on the comparison of acetabular radiolucent lines at the bone-cement interface and operative findings of loosening in 200 Charnley low-friction arthroplasties. Acetabular components that showed no radiolucencies were found to be solidly fixed. Seven percent of components that showed radiolucencies in DeLee zone I were loose, and when zones I and II showed lucencies, 71% of sockets were loose. Ninety-four percent of the sockets that showed lucencies in all 3 zones were loose, and all acetabular components that showed either implant migration or cement mantle fracture were found to be loose at the time of revision. On the femoral side, Harris et al[5] in 1982 reported on 171 cemented femoral components with an average follow-up of 3.3 years. Three categories of loosening were defined in this study. Definite loosening required radiographic evidence of migration of the component or cement or fracture of the component or cement mantle. Probable loosening required evidence of a complete radiolucent zone around the cement mantle on one or more radiograph. Possible loosening required a radiolucent zone in more than 50% but less than 100% of the cement-bone interface.

When assessing uncemented components in THA, Udomkiat et al[6] reported on the fixation of porous-coated sockets in 52 revision total hip replacements and compared the findings to sequential radiographic findings in the same patients. The results showed the following to be indicative of loosening:

- Radiolucent lines that initially appeared 2 or more years after primary surgery
- Progression of radiolucent lines after 2 years
- Radiolucent lines in all 3 DeLee zones
- Radiolucent lines of greater than 2 mm in any zone
- Migration

The sensitivity of these criteria was 94%, and the specificity was 100%. Utilizing serial radiographs to assess for loosening in uncemented femoral components generally depends on the following factors:

- Complete radiolucent lines around the ingrowth portion of the stem
- Progressive migration, subsidence, or varus tilt of the stem
- Divergent radiolucent lines that are more widely spaced from the stem at its extremes
- Hypertrophy of the bone at either the calcar or distal to the stem (pedestal)[7]

With proximally porous-coated implants, changes at the distal stem can be highly indicative of loosening. Bone formation alone does not necessarily mean loosening of the component. If a fine (1 to 2 mm) lucency exists between the end of the stem and the consolidated bone, the component is most likely not loose. If, however, there is no lucency and the stem appears to be directly in contact with the pedestal, the component is probably loose.

LABORATORY TESTS

The standard laboratory screening tests for a painful THA include a complete blood count (CBC), the erythrocyte sedimentation rate (ESR), and C-reactive protein (CRP). The ESR is a measurement of erythrocyte rouleaux formation and is usually elevated when an inflammatory condition is present. CRP is an acute-phase protein that is synthesized in the liver. The CRP level is also increased in many inflammatory, infectious, and some neoplastic conditions. Unfortunately, the results of these tests tend to be nonspecific for infection and are controversial.[8]

Obtaining a white blood cell count, as a part of the CBC, is an investigation that is of little or no diagnostic value in the work-up of the painful THA. Spangehl et al[9] evaluated the diagnostic accuracy of an elevated white blood cell count in predicting infection in the hip. A value of greater than 11.0×10^9 WBC/L was considered to be positive for infection. They found the sensitivity to be 0.20 and a specificity of 0.96. However, the positive predictive value was only 0.54 and the negative predictive value was 0.85. Similarly, Di Cesare et al[10] prospectively studied 58 patients undergoing revision total joint arthroplasty. In their study, the sensitivity of an elevated white cell count was found to be 0.47 and the specificity to be 1.00. The positive predictive value was 1.00 and the negative 0.82. It would seem, based on this evidence, that an elevated white cell count is only of value when the pretest probability is high.

The elevation of the ESR in isolation is extremely poor at predicting infection. Feldman et al[11] reported the results of the ESR in 32 patients undergoing revision total joint arthroplasty (23 hips and 9 knees). The mean ESR was 73 for the infected group (range: 14 to 118) and 28 for the noninfected group (range: 4 to 116). An ESR of greater than 50 showed a sensitivity of 0.78 and a specificity 0.79 with an accuracy of 0.81 in detecting infection. Spangehl et al[9] showed similar results when an ESR of greater than 30 was used to predict infection. The sensitivity was found to be 0.82 and the specificity 0.85. Furthermore, Canner et al[12] studied 52 cases of infection at the site of a prosthetic hip replacement and found that only 54% of the patients had a preoperative ESR of greater than 30.

While the elevation of the CRP levels taken in isolation appears to be more reliable than the ESR, it also provides limited value. Spangehl and colleagues[9] found the sensitivity of predicting infection to be 0.96 and the specificity to be 0.92, while Di Cesare and coworkers[10] found the sensitivity to be 0.95 and the specificity to be 0.76.

It would appear that combining the results of the ESR and CRP provides the greatest value in determining the presence or absence of infection after total joint replacement. Once again, Spangehl et al,[9] using a cut-off value of 30 mm/hr for the ESR and 10 mg/L for the CRP, showed that if both tests were negative then the probability of infection was 0 and if both tests were positive the probability was 0.83. Similarly, Greidanus et al[13] evaluated 145 revision total knee replacement patients. This study found the sensitivity of an elevated ESR to be 0.93 in predicting infection and an elevated CRP to be 0.91. However, combining these 2 tests increased the overall sensitivity to 0.95 for the diagnosis of infection. Furthermore, this study found the optimal cut-off point to be 22.5 mm/hr for the ESR and 13.5 mg/L for the CRP.

ARTHROCENTESIS

In addition to the evaluation of the previously-mentioned laboratory tests, the work-up of a suspected acute or chronic infection after THA should also include arthrocentesis. Any joint fluid that is collected should be sent for a complete cell count with differential as well as aerobic and anaerobic cultures.

Historically, greater than 25,000 WBC/mm^3 or greater than 75% polymorphonuclear leukocytes was highly suggestive of infection.[14] However, a recent study by Schinsky et al[15] suggests that these values, at much lower levels, should be concerning for the presence of infected THA. In this study, 201 revision THAs were assessed with intraoperative synovial fluid collection and preoperative measurements of the ESR and CRP. Of this sample, 55 were considered to be infected based on 2 of the following 3 criteria:

1. A positive intraoperative culture
2. Gross purulence at the time of revision
3. Positive histopathological findings

No hip was found to be infected if the preoperative ESR was less than 30 mm/hr and the CRP less than 10 mg/dL. Analysis of the synovial fluid showed a white cell count of greater than 4200 WBC/mL and a differential of greater than 80% neutrophils was indicative of infection. Furthermore, when combined with an elevated ESR and CRP, the optimal cut-off point for synovial fluid cell count was greater than 3,000 WBC/mL. This combination yielded the highest specificity, sensitivity, positive predictive value, negative predictive value, and accuracy of the tests.

To minimize the potential of a false-negative result, all antibiotics should be discontinued for a period of 2 weeks prior to aspiration.[15] Also, in patients where infection is highly suspected, if the initial aspiration after a 2-week hiatus from antibiotics is negative, a second aspiration should be undertaken after a 4-week period without antibiotics.

IMAGING STUDIES

Radionuclide scans are often a necessary component in the evaluation of a painful THA. The most frequently utilized tests are the 3-phase technetium bone scan, the indium-labeled white blood cell bone scan, and the sulfur-colloid marrow scan. To differentiate between infection, aseptic loosening, and periprosthetic fractures, these 3 scans should be ordered together.

The 3-phase bone scan can be helpful in evaluating for suspected component loosening. Unlike after total knee arthroplasty in which increased activity can persist indefinitely,[16,17] in THA the bone scan typically returns to normal by 6 to 24 months postoperatively.[18] Unfortunately, although the bone scan shows a very high sensitivity, the specificity is low in the diagnosis of deep infection of the hip, and therefore, this test should not be performed alone in the evaluation of the painful THA. Magnuson et al[19] compared 50 patients undergoing revision THA for infection, as diagnosed by culture or histologic results, with 48 patients undergoing revision without infection. Technetium-99 scans showed a sensitivity of 100%, but a specificity for infection of only 18% and an accuracy of 53%. On the other hand, the Indium[111] labeled white blood cell scan showed a sensitivity of 88% with a specificity and accuracy of 73% and 81% respectively.[19] Furthermore, when Indium[111] labeled leukocyte scans are used in conjunction with sulphur-colloid marrow scans of the knee, the sensitivity, specificity, and accuracy are reported to be 100%, 97%, and 98%.[20]

Computed tomography (CT) scans can help determine the extent of osteolysis and component rotational position better than conventional radiographs. Also, although difficult to interpret and rarely utilized, dynamic CT scans have been utilized to assess for femoral loosening.

Miscellaneous Diagnostic Studies

When all other potential etiologies of the painful THA have been eliminated, remote causes for the pain must be evaluated. As well as undertaking a thorough history and physical examination pertaining to the spine, a magnetic resonance imaging scan of the lumbar spine must be obtained. Furthermore, in order to rule out radiculopathy secondary to spinal pathology, electromyography and nerve conduction studies should also be considered.

Summary

Despite high success rates following primary THA, a small percentage of patients will complain of pain and decreased function. In evaluating these patients a thorough history and physical examination is extremely important. Often, a complete work-up will require laboratory studies such as ESR, CRP, and joint aspiration, as well as diagnostic imaging including serial radiographs and possibly nuclear imaging studies. The presence or absence of an extra-articular cause for hip pain needs to be determined. Once an intra-articular etiology has been established, appropriate treatment may include revision total hip replacement. However, it must be emphasized that revision THA performed for unexplained hip pain is often associated with a poor outcome.

References

1. Mahomed NN, Barrett JA, Katz JN, et al. Rates and outcomes of primary and revision total hip replacement in the United States Medicare population. *J Bone Joint Surg Am.* 2003;85:27-32.
2. Barrett JA, Losina E, Baron JA, et al. Survival following total hip replacement. *J Bone Joint Surg Am.* 2005;87:1965-1971.
3. McLaughlin JR, Lee KR. Total hip arthroplasty with an uncemented tapered femoral component. *J Bone Joint Surg Am.* 2008;90:1290-1296.
4. Hodgkinson JP, Shelley P, Wroblewski BM. The correlation between the roentgenographic appearance and operative findings at the bone-cement junction of the socket in Charnley low friction arthroplasties. *Clin Orthop.* 1988;228:105-109.
5. Harris WH, McCarthy JC, O'Neill DA. Femoral component loosening using contemporary techniques of femoral cement fixation. *J Bone Joint Surg Am.* 1982;64:1063-1067.
6. Udomkiat P, Wan Z, Dorr LD. Comparison of preoperative radiographs and intraoperative findings of fixation of hemispheric porous-coated sockets. *J Bone Joint Surg Am.* 2001;83:1865-1870.
7. Engh CA, Bobyn DJ. The influence of stem size and extent of porous coating on femoral bone resorption after primary cementless hip arthroplasty. *Clin Orthop.* 1988;231:7-28.
8. Duff GP, Lachiewicz PF, Kelley SS. Aspiration of the knee joint before revision arthroplasty. *Clin Orthop.* 1996;331:132-139.
9. Spangehl MJ, Masri BA, O'Connell JX, et al. Prospective analysis of preoperative and intraoperative investigations for the diagnosis of infection at the sites of two hundred and two revision total hip arthroplasties. *J Bone Joint Surg Am.* 1999;81:672-682.
10. Di Cesare PE, Chang E, Preston CF, et al. Serum interleukin-6 as a marker of periprosthetic infection following total hip and knee arthroplasty. *J Bone Joint Surg Am.* 2005;87:1921-1927.
11. Feldman DS, Lonner JH, Desai P, Zuckerman JD. The role of frozen section in revision total joint arthroplasty. *J Bone Joint Surg Am.* 1995;77:1807-1813.
12. Canner GC, Steinberg ME, Heppenstall RB, Balderston R. The infected hip after total hip arthroplasty. *J Bone Joint Surg Am.* 1984;66:1393-1399.

13. Greidanus NV, Masri BA, Gaebuz DS, et al. Use of erythrocyte sedimentation rate and C-reactive protein level to diagnose infection before revision total knee arthroplasty. A prospective evaluation. *J Bone Joint Surg Am*. 2007;89:1409-1416.

14. Windsor RE, Bono JV. Infected total knee replacements. *J Am Acad Orthop Surg*. 1994;2:44-53.

15. Schinsky MF, Della Valle CJ, Sporer SM, Paprosky WG. Perioperative testing for joint infection in patients undergoing revision total hip arthroplasty. *J Bone Joint Surg Am*. 2008;90:1869-1875.

16. Barrack RL, Jennings RW, Wolfe MW, Bertot AJ. The value of preoperative aspiration before total knee revision. *Clin Orthop*. 1997;345:8-16.

17. Rosenthall L, Lepanto L, Raymond F. Radiophosphate uptake in asymptomatic knee arthroplasty. *J Nucl Med*. 1987;28:1546-1549.

18. Utz JA, Lull RJ, Galvin EG. Asymptomatic total hip prosthesis: natural history determined using Tc-99m MDP bone scans. *Radiology*. 1986;161:509-512.

19. Magnuson JE, Brown ML, Hauser MF, et al. In-111-labelled leukocyte scintigraphy in suspected orthopedic prosthesis infection: comparison with other imaging modalities. *Radiology*. 1988;168:235-239.

20. Palestro CJ, Swyer AJ, Kim CK, Goldsmith SJ. Infected knee prosthesis: diagnosis with In-111 leukocyte, Tc-99m sulfur colloid, and Tc-99m MDP imaging. *Radiology*. 1991;179:645-648.

Modes of Failure in Total Hip Arthroplasty

2

David E. Jaffe, MD; Antonia Woehnl, MD; Michael A. Mont, MD;
and Aaron J. Johnson, MD

The rate of primary total hip arthroplasties (THAs) in the United States has increased over the past decade by approximately 50%, and it is estimated to rise by 174% in the next 20 years.[1,2] It is estimated that by 2030 there will be nearly 100,000 revision hip procedures for any reason performed per year in the United States.[2] Causes of failure leading to the need for revision include hardware infection, joint instability, component loosening, and periprosthetic fracture. In a nationwide database review, Bozic et al evaluated the mechanisms of failure after THA in the United States performed within 15 consecutive months between 2005 and 2006.[3] The most common causes for revision hip arthroplasties were instability and dislocation (accounting for 22.5%), followed by aseptic loosening (19.7%) and periprosthetic infection (18.4%).[3] Similar numbers were reported in a retrospective study assessing the causes for implant failure in total hip replacement.[4] According to this study, instability contributed to 35%, aseptic loosening to 30%, osteolysis and wear to 12%, infection to 12%, and periprosthetic fracture to 2% of revisions.[4] The purpose of this chapter is to describe the failure mechanisms in these most prevalent causes of revision THA.

INFECTION

Introduction

Periprosthetic hip infection remains the most devastating complication after THA, due to its association with high morbidity and cost. With improvements in the operating room environment (ie, body exhaust systems, laminar air flow, minimal operating room traffic) and the use of antibiotic prophylaxis, the overall incidence of infection has decreased over the past 20 years.[5-7] However, in the past decade Dale et al have documented a small but increasing infection rate (in this study, the relative risk of revision due to infection was 3.0 for patients who underwent THA between 2003 and 2007, when compared with those who were implanted between 1987 and 1992).[8] Although the exact reasons for this are unknown, this might reflect an increased awareness or surveillance for periprosthetic infections in recent years.

Jacofsky DJ, Hedley AK.
Fundamentals of Revision Hip Arthroplasty:
Diagnosis, Evaluation, and Treatment (pp 11-30).

© 2013 SLACK Incorporated.

It has been estimated that infected THAs make up 15% of all revision procedures.[3,9,10] A database review of patients undergoing total hip surgery in the United States has revealed an acute postoperative prosthetic hip infection rate of 0.2% after primary total hip replacement and 1.1% after revision THA for aseptic reasons.[9] Other studies have found an incidence of periprosthetic hip infection after total hip replacement of 0.7% to 1.63% in the first 1 to 2 postoperative years and 0.59% to 1.4% between 2 and 20 years after surgery.[11-13] These rates are similar to infection rates reported at long-term follow-up between 0.57% and 2.2% after primary THA.[7,14,15]

When a patient presents with a painful THA, a thorough history should always be performed in order to identify any potential risk factors for postoperative infection. These include rheumatoid arthritis, diabetes mellitus, sickle cell disease, malignancy, immunodeficient states (including AIDS and chronic corticosteroid use), concurrent infections like urinary tract or skin infections, obesity, hypokalemia, malnutrition, and low socioeconomic status.[13,16-20] In addition to these predisposing factors, the infection risk can be increased if the patient has undergone previous hip surgery, if the duration of the surgical procedure was prolonged, if the patient had an extended hospital stay, or if the patient developed a urinary tract infection after postoperative bladder catheterization.[17]

Etiology

Infections following THA are classified into 3 categories: acute (early), chronic (late), and acute hematogenous. Acute periprosthetic infection is defined as an early postoperative infection that is attributed to an intraoperative contamination. It usually occurs within 4 to 6 weeks postoperatively, however, some authors have extended this time up to 12 weeks.[21] After this time, an infection is defined as a chronic or delayed infection. These are also attributed to intraoperative contamination, but usually there is a low virulence or an insufficient number of bacteria present to cause an early acute, clinically significant infection. Acute hematogenous infection refers to an infected prosthesis that may be the result of seeding from a blood borne pathogen into the joint. This type of infection involves a specific infection source (ie, urinary tract infection, phlebitis from intravenous line placement, antecedent febrile illness). Controversy exists regarding dental procedures increasing the risk of prosthetic hip infections.[22,23] Although previous reports have suggested that they may be a risk factor, a prospective case-control study performed between 2001 and 2006 by Berbari et al demonstrated that dental procedures do not appear to be a risk factor for developing infection after total joint arthroplasty and that antibiotic prophylaxis prior to dental procedures did not decrease the risk of subsequent prosthetic joint infection.[23] In addition to these 3 categories (ie, acute, chronic, and acute hematogenous), a fourth type of infection was described by Segawa et al, wherein patients who are undergoing aseptic revision surgery have positive intraoperative cultures. This scenario occurred in 5 of the 133 revision knee arthroplasties (4%) on which the authors reported. All of these patients were treated with single stage revision (due to lack of concern for infection at the time of revision); upon return of positive cultures during the postoperative period, patients were administered 6 weeks of appropriate intravenous antibiotic therapy and did not require any subsequent revision procedures.[24]

Presentation and Diagnosis

An infected hip joint can present with either quite vague symptoms, such as malaise or decreased function of the affected joint, or it can show characteristic signs of infection, such as fever, pain, tenderness, swelling, or erythema.[25] Pain appears to be one of the most frequent complaints in patients with an infected hip prosthesis.[26,27] For early diagnosis and intervention it is crucial to perform a physical exam and obtain a detailed history and radiographic images at each follow-up appointment. In their history, the patient may complain of delayed wound healing or a draining sinus tract. The clinician should question the use of antibiotics around the time of the patient's index procedure, as this may give clues to the presence of superficial

TABLE 2-1. INFECTION CRITERIA OF A PROSTHETIC JOINT

CRITERIA	DESCRIPTION
1	Evidence of the same organism in 2 or more cultures of specimens obtained by joint aspiration or deep-tissue samples obtained intraoperatively
2	Acute inflammation found on histopathologic analysis of intra-articular tissue
3	Gross purulence detected during surgery
4	Actively discharging sinus tract

Adapted from Leone JM, Hanssen AD. Management of infection at the site of a total knee arthroplasty. *J Bone Joint Surg Am.* 2005;87(10):2335-2348.

perioperative infection. It is important to understand whether the patient experiences pain at rest or with weight bearing, and if he or she has had any other infections, such as a urinary tract or skin infection, that preceded his or her current complaints. If there is any suspicion of a possible joint infection a complete blood count (CBC), including differential and erythrocyte sedimentation rate (ESR) or C-reactive protein (CRP), should be obtained. Recent American Academy of Orthopaedic Surgeons (AAOS) guidelines have recommended this blood screening on all painful joints.[28] Although these parameters are nonspecific, they can assist in the diagnosis or serve as follow-up when an infection is treated.[26] Radiographic images should be analyzed for evidence of soft tissue swelling, femoral component subsidence, or signs of loosening. Radiolucencies of 2 mm or more in width at the cement-bone interface or a lacy pattern of new bone formation are suspicious of infection. These signs do not distinguish between septic and aseptic component loosening. Additionally, early infections may not be detected by radiographic analysis since it takes several weeks for an infection to induce visible bone destruction. According to recent AAOS guidelines for the work-up of patients who are suspected to have periprosthetic joint infections, aspirations should be performed following a positive screening test (either ESR or Westergren CRP) to further help with diagnosis by assessing cell count and differential.[28] Although reports vary, aspiration results are typically considered positive if there are greater than 1,100 leukocytes per microliter, along with greater than 65% neutrophils.[29,30] If the results of the aspiration are negative in a patient with suspected infection, the guidelines recommend performing a nuclear imaging study combined with some form of radionucleotide labeled leukocyte imaging with either technetium or indium.

Leone and Hanssen described 4 criteria to diagnose an infection after total knee arthroplasty, which are also applicable in the detection of an infected prosthetic THA (Table 2-1).[31] According to these criteria, which may be less useful preoperatively, the diagnosis of an infection is made if at least one of the following is present:

- Evidence of the same organism in 2 or more cultures of either specimen obtained by joint aspiration or deep-tissue samples obtained intraoperatively
- Acute inflammation found on histopathologic analysis of intra-articular tissue
- Gross purulence detected during surgery
- An actively discharging sinus tract[31]

Management

Options for management of an infected hip prosthesis are dependent on the time between infection and diagnosis and on the severity of the infection. A hip aspirate can help determine the responsible organism in the joint fluid. In general, antibiotic therapy should not be initiated preoperatively and subsequent surgical interventions consist of incision and drainage, débridement, and one- or two-stage revision THA. Detailed techniques will be discussed in a later chapter.

During revision THA frozen sections should be performed intraoperatively on multiple tissue samples to ensure successful elimination of the infection in the periprosthetic tissue or to distinguish between septic and aseptic implant failure in questionable cases. The sensitivity and specificity of frozen sections have been reported between 18% and 50% and between 89% and 98%, respectively.[32-38] Controversy exists regarding how many polymorphonuclear leukocytes (PMNs) per high power field are sufficient to classify acute infection in the tissue sample. However, between 5 and 10 PMNs per high power field appear to be sufficient.[34,39]

To minimize the occurrence of a prosthetic hip infection, preventive measures should be taken intraoperatively by giving antibiotic therapy and, depending on the risk factors for the individual patient, these antibiotics should be continued for a specific time postoperatively.[40-42]

Summary

Prosthetic hip infections remain one of the most devastating complications of THA. Therefore, it is important to minimize the incidence of infection through antibiotic prophylaxis, avoiding extended operative time and hospital stay, and avoiding prolonged use of urinary catheters. A thorough exam at each follow-up visit is crucial for early diagnosis and early intervention. Deep joint infections often require multiple surgical revisions to completely eradicate the infection and regain functionality. Several studies have demonstrated that early surgical treatment once an infection is suspected after THA helps to eliminate the infection more efficiently than delayed treatment.[43,44] In acute postoperative infections and acute hematogenous prosthetic hip infections, it may be possible to save the implant if early intervention with meticulous débridement and systemic antibiotic therapy is initiated within the first 2 weeks of symptom onset.[45]

INSTABILITY

Introduction

Instability following THA is another common mode of implant failure and a frequent cause of surgical revision.[46-50] A sample database of revision THAs performed within a time period of 15 months across the United States was evaluated by Bozic et al in a retrospective study to analyze mechanisms of failures and types of revisions after total hip replacement.[3]

Implant instability and dislocation were found to be the most common cause for failure, contributing to 22.5% of revisions.[3] Instability following THA can be divided into 2 subtypes: dislocation and subluxation. While subluxation refers to a partial separation of the femoral head from the acetabular component, dislocation refers to a complete separation of the 2 components.

Different mechanisms can lead to dislocations, resulting in either a posterior, anterior, or lateral dissociation. Posterior dislocations are the most common. In a series of 5167 THAs, Cobb et al reported 70% of the 111 radiographically determined dislocations were posterior, while anterior and lateral comprised 21% and 9%, respectively.[51] Dislocated THAs can additionally be temporally divided as either early or late depending on the time after index arthroplasty. A late dislocation is defined as having occurred a minimum of 5 years following primary arthroplasty. Although late dislocations are not uncommon, patients are at greatest risk for dislocation immediately after the operation.[52] However, the cumulative risk of first time dislocation increases as time progresses from the date of primary arthroplasty.[53-55] According to Berry et al, the risk of initial dislocation was 1% at 1 month and 1.9% at 1 year in a series of 5459 primary THAs. It then increased at a constant rate of approximately 1% every 5 years until reaching 7% at 25 years.[56] Despite an increased risk in the early postoperative period, late dislocations still comprise nearly one-third of all dislocations.[50] Because of this, dislocation remains a concern in patients many years after index arthroplasty, regardless of whether there was a history of prior dislocation. Though surgical revision may not always be necessary, instability remains a common mode of failure of THA.

Etiology and Biomechanics

The etiology of both early and late prosthetic hip instability is multifactorial. Various factors, from component positioning, design specifications, and surgical approach to patient noncompliance, soft-tissue laxity, and anatomic abnormalities, have been associated with increased risk for instability and dislocation. Risk factors for early dislocation include female gender, increased age, baseline neurologic and/or cognitive impairment, osteonecrosis of the femoral head, preoperative femoral neck fracture, and inflammatory arthritis.[47,48,53,56,57] Late dislocation risk factors include female gender, younger age, new onset of neurologic or cognitive impairment, severe hip trauma, previous subluxations, acetabular protrusio, and weak abductor muscles. Excessive consumption of alcohol has also been associated with an increased risk of dislocation.[57,58]

The most common reason for instability is a direct result of the placement of the components. This typically occurs by using an improper femoral neck length or malpositioning of the acetabular component. Lewinnek et al reported a "safe zone" for appropriate version of the acetabulum. This zone was described as having acetabular inclination of 40 ± 10 degrees, and anteversion of 15 ± 10 degrees. If the acetabulum was placed with increased anteversion, there was a significantly higher rate of anterior dislocation (1.5% versus 6.1%).[59] Also, implant design and surgical technique can result in different rates of instability. For example, the use of a high-walled acetabular liner has been reported to reduce the risk of dislocation from 3.8% to 2.2%.[51] Appropriately used larger femoral head sizes have been shown to result in lower dislocation rates.[60] The effect of surgical approach has been studied in depth regarding its effect on dislocation risk. Historically, a posterior approach to the hip has been associated with significantly higher rates of dislocation. A 1982 study of greater than 3,000 hip arthroplasty procedures reported less dislocations in anterior approached hips (2.3%, 3.1%, and 5.8% in anterolateral, lateral transtrochanteric, and posterior approach, respectively).[61] Berry similarly reported dislocation rates of 3.1%, 3.4%, and 6.9% over 10 years for anterolateral, lateral transtrochanteric, and posterior approach, respectively.[62] Many further studies have consistently quoted higher dislocation rates after a posterior approach in THA.[57,63-65] Repair of the posterior capsule may minimize dislocation when the posterior approach is used.

Patient noncompliance is another factor thought to be associated with dislocation. If the prosthetic recommended range of motion is exceeded, dislocation can result. Properly selected and inserted components have limitations that require optimal patient compliance with range of motion restrictions. These restrictions are dependent on the approach used. In posteriorly approached hips, patients are taught to avoid flexion past 90 degrees and to minimize adduction and internal rotation movements. To functionally adhere to these restrictions, patients are typically instructed to utilize an abduction pillow, to sit only in elevated seats (including elevated toilet seats), and to use caution when traveling in an automobile (entering and exiting automobiles involves excessive flexion and rotation of the hip). If the hip is approached anteriorly, dislocations instead occur in extension, adduction, and external rotation. The value of these restrictions is dependent on the approach. In anteriorly approached hips, Peak et al found no difference in dislocation frequency in patients who had strict postoperative restrictions versus a control group with no restrictions.[66] However, in posteriorly approached hips, poor compliance with these precautions could lead to dislocation.

Soft tissue laxity is another factor that plays a role in dislocation. Shortening in either the horizontal or vertical direction (decreased offset) can lead to soft tissue imbalance resulting in dislocation. Gradual stretching of the pseudocapsule can cause laxity of the joint and lead to late dislocations. In addition, gradual wear over time on the polyethylene component can lead to late dislocation.[47,50]

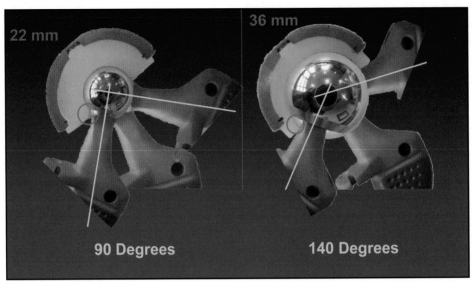

Figure 2-1. Note how a larger femoral head with the same femoral and acetabular implant design allows for greater range of motion prior to impingement.

Impingement can be responsible for instability of a prosthetic hip, leading to dislocation.[51,67-71] Impingement occurs with contact between the artificial femoral neck and implanted cup or bone-on-bone contact between the greater trochanter and the pelvis. The degree of impingement is dependent on the femoral head-neck ratio. A decreased ratio leads to cam impingement. Pincer impingement occurs with placement of a small femoral head in a large cup, use of a hooded liner, or failure to remove anterior acetabular osteophytes. When impingement occurs there is sliding between the femoral head and the polyethylene liner, with the polyethylene providing resistance to maintain stability. However, if the external loading forces that created the impingement are great enough, dislocation will result.[69]

Whether due to shorter femoral offset distances, smaller femoral component sizes, or effects of the patient's anatomy, the femoral head component must displace a certain lateral distance before it can completely dislocate out of the acetabular component. This distance is termed the *jump distance*. Smaller jump distances carry larger theoretical risk for dislocation.[72] Larger femoral heads increase this distance and therefore increase stability. Accordingly, larger femoral heads have been associated with lower rates of dislocation.[62,73] This concept is illustrated in Figure 2-1.

Presentation and Diagnosis

Instability must be suspected when a patient with a THA presents with pain or a feeling of instability. Instability may develop in the early postoperative period, but can develop at any point after the surgery. A thorough history should be obtained in order to identify any potential risk factors for instability. The typical complaint is an incredibly painful popping sensation. Many times the patient will recall a sudden vigorous movement or trauma, but other times there may not be a discrete precipitating event. The patient will typically have pain at rest that increases greatly with any movement. The date of the original surgery should be noted, and it is also important to determine if the patient has any prior history of dislocation.

Next, a physical exam should be performed. Any signs of infection should be noted. These include fever, chills, erythema at the surgical site, or a purulent draining sinus tract. Even if no signs of infection are obvious, unless there is a clear mechanical reason for the dislocation, infection must be ruled out. If a posterior dislocation has occurred, the hip may be in extension with internal rotation. If an anterior dislocation has occurred, the hip is usually externally rotated.

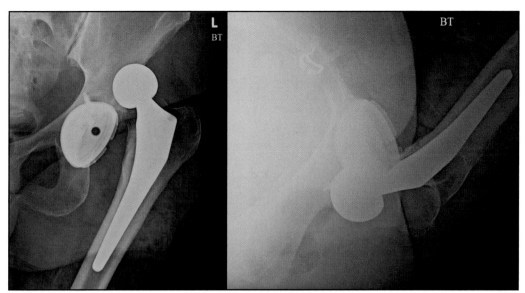

Figure 2-2. Two radiographic views of a superoposterior hip dislocation.

Note the location of the patient's scar to indicate the surgical approach that was used. An accurate neurovascular exam should be documented, with special attention to any sensory, motor, or vascular deficits on the affected limb. Also note limb lengths, range of motion, and joint stability. Appropriate laboratory studies (eg, ESR, Westergren CRP, leukocyte count, and joint aspiration with leukocyte count and differential) should be performed if there is any clinical concern for infection.

Following the history and physical, radiographic evaluation should be conducted. The position of the components should be evaluated for proper placement and dislocation. Figure 2-2 demonstrates a superoposterior dislocation. A thorough inspection for periprosthetic fracture is indicated, as the presence of such an injury would alter management. Sometimes the components may appear in good position on radiographs. If this is the case but suspicion is high for dislocation, soft tissue laxity could be the cause of the patient's instability. Direct examination under fluoroscopy is useful in these situations to determine the cause of instability.

Management

The timing and etiology of the patient's first dislocation determines his or her subsequent treatment. Simple closed reduction with a course of postreduction bracing is an ideal treatment and is often successful in early dislocations. Surgical revision may be required in severe, multiple, or late dislocations and may consist of revision of one or all components. Bozic et al observed an all-component revision in 41.1% of 51,345 total hip revisions conducted within 15 consecutive months across the United States.[3] Various surgical options are discussed in depth in a later chapter.

Summary

As dislocations are relatively common complications of THA, prevention of such events is crucial. Proper performance of a surgical technique is a key element in reducing the frequency of unstable prosthetic joints. Patient education should be clear and thorough to ensure adherence to range of motion restrictions. Identifying any preoperative risk factors can help prevent future dislocations. Despite undertaking these necessary precautions, dislocations may occur following primary THA.

Unfortunately, simple closed reduction is often not a definitive treatment for an unstable prosthetic hip. Frequently, operative revision is required to correct total hip instability. A 1999 study by Li et al examined the frequency and timing of posterior dislocations of THAs performed over a 4-year period. More than 1000 primary THAs were evaluated, and 3.9% had posterior dislocations. Fifty-eight percent of the dislocations suffered redislocation, and 40% of the hips required surgical revision.[52] Though dislocations will inevitably occur with some frequency, the THA remains an overwhelmingly successful procedure as treatment for this complication does have successful long-term outcomes.

COMPONENT LOOSENING

Introduction

Component loosening represents the second most frequent long-term complication after total hip replacement that contributes to 19.7% of revision hip arthroplasties.[3] The diagnosis is made by clinical assessment and radiographic evaluation. Roentgenographic evidence of aseptic loosening can be present with either intact or diminished clinical function (Figures 2-3 and 2-4). Also, component loosening may be diagnosed by clinical presentation alone. In general, radiolucent zones of 2 mm or more in width at the cement-bone, cement-component, or component-bone interface define the diagnosis of loosening on radiographic analysis. However, a failure of the implant is only indicated if these radiolucent lines are progressive and the patient presents with pain.[74,75] Component migration and cement mantle fracture are definite signs of loosening as well.

With the introduction of improved materials (advanced bearing materials), implant design, and surgical techniques, the incidence of aseptic loosening has decreased over the past decade.[76,77] Recent studies have demonstrated improved wear and longevity of newer implants and materials.[77,78] The long-term outcome and benefit of these advanced technologies is still in the process of evaluation in prospective studies and only short- and midterm data are currently available.[78-81]

Etiology

Component loosening is a multifactorial process. The contributing variables can be categorized into patient-specific factors, implant-specific factors, and surgical factors.[82] Patient-specific factors include the activity level of the patient, body mass index, gait mechanics, preoperative diagnosis, comorbidities, and revision versus primary surgery. Implant-specific factors consist of material (metallic alloy, ceramic, highly cross-linked polyethylene, ultrahigh molecular weight polyethylene [UHMWPE]), bearing couple (highly cross-linked polyethylene-on-metal, UHMWPE-on-metal, UHMWPE-on-ceramic, metal-on-metal, ceramic-on-ceramic), and implant design (fixation, component thickness). Surgical factors include component composition, reconstruction of the joint mechanics, component fixation and initial stability, and the surgeon's experience.

The activity level and the body mass index of the patient have a high impact on the development of osteolysis. Increased load and magnitude of force in general leads to increased wear and osteolysis. However, a survey of the American Association for Hip and Knee Surgeons demonstrated a wide range of recommendations for the optimal activity level after THA.[83] More than 95% of the 139 participating surgeons recommended low-impact activities such as level surface walking, stair climbing, level surface bicycling, or swimming. Since the development of component loosening is a multifactorial process and insufficient data are available to support clear guidelines on physical activities after THA, all recommendations in this survey were based on the surgeon's experience and expectations on patient performance postoperatively rather than on scientific evidence.[83] Active lifestyle as well as a higher body mass index means greater force and higher load to the joint, which then leads to increased wear and osteolysis in a patient post THA. However,

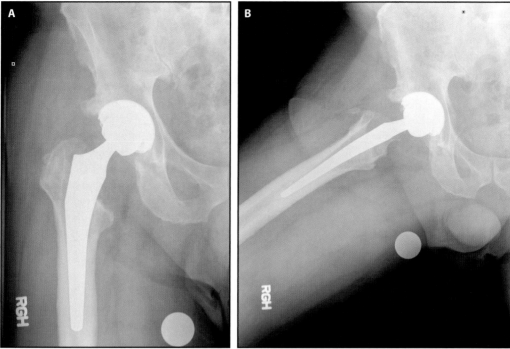

Figure 2-3. (A) Anteroposterior and (B) lateral radiographs of a 51-year-old male who had undergone a THA, showing signs of loosening and a migrated stem. Of note is the radiolucency around proximal porous surface of the femoral component. (Reprinted with permission from Sinai Hospital of Baltimore, Inc.)

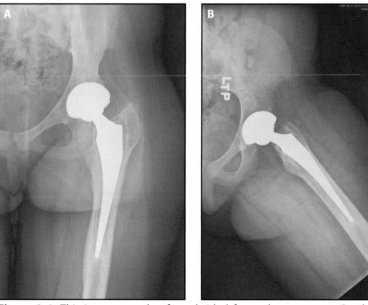

Figure 2-4. This is an example of a subsided femoral component. On the (A) anteroposterior and (B) lateral views proximal radiolucencies can be seen, and distally there is evidence of increased cortical thickness at the stem tip seen in the anteroposterior view, indicating poor fit and nonuniform load sharing. (Reprinted with permission from Sinai Hospital of Baltimore, Inc.)

activity and body mass index often interact and may counterbalance each other in some patients.[82] Frequently, a high body mass index, which itself would be expected to cause increased osteolysis, is counterbalanced by a sedentary lifestyle, and therefore this patient may be less likely to develop early component loosening.[84]

Other patient-related factors influencing component loosening after THA include the patient's preoperative diagnosis and comorbidities. Certain etiologies, such as osteonecrosis and post-traumatic arthritis, have been associated with a higher incidence of osteolysis following hip arthroplasty than osteoarthritis.[82,85]

Multiple prospective studies have compared highly cross-linked polyethylene with conventional UHMWPE in THAs.[78-81] While long-term results are currently unavailable, midterm results have shown improved wear resistance and longevity of the implant with highly cross-linked polyethylene. Despite a higher incidence of breakage with increased contact stress in the joint, highly cross-linked polyethylene appears to be the favorable material of choice in hip arthroplasties. Highly cross-linked polyethylene may be more prone to failure as contact stresses in the joint increase. Since contact stress in the hip joint is not as high as in the knee, for example, fatigue wear mechanisms occur less frequently in THAs.[86,87] Additionally, alternative bearing surfaces such as metal-on-metal, highly cross-linked polyethylene-on-metal, and ceramic-on-ceramic bearings in THA have been associated with improved wear characteristics and minimal evidence of osteolysis in currently available midterm data.[77]

Surgical techniques have an impact on the joint mechanics and may therefore contribute to component loosening after THAs. Increased contact stress and focal load on the joint that predispose to osteolysis can be caused by malalignment or malrotation of the components. Resection of residual bone chips or debris, cementing technique, choice of implant size, technical execution of stabilizing the implant, and achieving optimal soft-tissue balance are all decisive for the longevity of the implant in THAs. Computerized instrumentation systems that may improve the surgical outcome by providing intraoperative kinematic data are currently evolving.[82]

Component loosening after THA is caused by a complex process of interactions between patient factors, implant design, and surgical technique. Joint loads, kinematics, and wear resistance are directly or indirectly affected by all of these variables, and may lead to different modes of implant failure.

Mechanisms Leading to Failure

Mechanisms leading to component loosening after THA are categorized into modes of failure of femoral versus acetabular loosening. Failures can then be further categorized into cemented and noncemented implants.

Gruen et al classified modes of failure in cemented femoral stems by analysis of mechanics and radiographic evaluation (Table 2-2).[88] Mode I describes pistoning behavior. Mode IA explains loosening of the stem within the cement, caused by loss of proximal medial support through axial load and insufficient midlateral fixation that leads to distal stem displacement. Therefore, a Mode IA failure produces a radiolucent zone between stem and cement in the proximal lateral aspect of the stem and is frequently accompanied by a punch-out fracture at the same location. Mode IB describes loosening of the stem with the cement component within the bone, caused by stresses at the cement-bone interface leading to subsidence of the stem and the cement mantle within the femur. In this case, a radiolucent zone is often seen around the entire cement mantle, frequently with a thin line of sclerotic bone "halo" reaction. Mode II describes the medial stem pivot. The underlying mechanism is a medial migration of the proximal stem combined with a lateral migration of the distal stem. It is caused by insufficient proximal medial and distal lateral support of the cement component, and may result in a fracture of the sclerotic bone lateral to the stem tip or a fracture of the cement mantle in the midstem region. Mode III describes the calcar pivot. It is characterized by medial and lateral toggle of the stem tip, which is caused by inadequate distal stem support, leading to sclerotic bone reaction at the stem tip. The rotational axis of this mode

TABLE 2-2. MODES OF FAILURE IN CEMENTED FEMORAL STEMS

MODE OF FAILURE	DESCRIPTION	MECHANISM
Mode IA	Pistoning behavior	Loosening of stem within cement mantle
Mode IB	Pistoning behavior	Loosening of stem and cement within the bone
Mode II	Medial stem pivot	Medial migration of proximal stem combined with lateral migration of distal stem
Mode III	Calcar pivot	Medial and lateral toggle of stem tip, "windshield wiper"-type distal stem loosening
Mode IV	Cantilever-bending	Loss of proximal stem support with remaining fixed distal stem

Adapted from Gruen TA, McNeice GM, Amstutz HC. "Modes of failure" of cemented stem-type femoral components: a radiographic analysis of loosening. *Clin Orthop Relat Res*. 1979(141):17-27.

of failure is located in the proximal stem, and this mechanism results in a "windshield wiper"-type of loosening in the distal stem. Mode IV describes cantilever-bending fatigue. This is caused by loss of proximal stem support while the distal stem remains fixed in the cement mantle. Since the load transfer to the proximal femur is lost, the stem subsequently undergoes deformation and medial migration. Radiolucent zones in this mechanism of failure are seen proximally, medial, and lateral to the stem.

In contrast to femoral loosening, acetabular loosening rarely occurs at the cup-cement interface (if the cup has been cemented), and it appears to be a biological rather than a mechanical process.[75,89] DeLee and Charnley classified acetabular component loosening in total hip replacement by describing radiographic demarcation at the cement-bone interface and migration of the entire acetabular cement component.[75] Demarcation was categorized into 4 different groups of width and into 3 circumferential zones (Types I, II, and III) where the demarcation occurred. Sixty-nine percent of the patients in this study developed demarcation at various degrees, and 13% of those progressed to migration after several years. Progressive migration of the cement socket was observed in 9.2% of all participating patients. Analysis of comorbidities of the patients and possible problems in surgical techniques revealed that acetabular component loosening appears to occur mainly due to biological changes and not due to mechanical failure of the implant.[75]

Multiple attempts have been made to classify noncemented femoral and acetabular loosening. Femoral component loosening in noncemented implants, for example, is explained based on different types of fixation of the implant, classified as bone ingrowth, stable fibrous, or unstable fixation.[90] Engh et al have reported on the radiographic ability to determine these classifications. Bone ingrowth is defined as an implant with no subsidence and minimal or no radio-opaque lines around the stem. Stable fibrous fixation is characterized by an implant with no progressive migration, but with extensive radio-opaque lines. These lines are typically parallel and separated from the implant by a small radiolucent space. Unstable fixation is defined as components with definite migration or subsidence (see Figure 2-3), as well as diverging radio-opaque lines. It may also be possible to see increased cortical thickness at the stem tip (see Figure 2-4), indicating poor fit and nonuniform load sharing.[91]

To minimize the incidence of femoral or acetabular component loosening, technical factors that contribute to failure of the implant should always be considered. For cemented components, the surgical factors include a cement mantle that is too thin or failure to pressurize the cement adequately. In cementless components, surgical factors include inadequate removal of soft cancellous bone in the femoral neck, component undersizing, missed occult fracture, and component malpositioning.

Presentation and Diagnosis

In the symptomatic patient, component loosening after THA usually presents with pain with weight bearing, localized to the thigh (femoral component) or groin (acetabular component). Rotation of the hip will aggravate the pain, and the pain is relieved by rest. In extreme cases with component migration, the patient may also complain of a shortened and externally rotated leg. On physical exam, a Trendelenburg or antalgic gait may be observed. Most patients experience an asymptomatic postoperative period but in some cases the patient will have pain shortly after surgery. In this case it is especially important to rule out an infectious cause of the patient's complaint. In general, a comprehensive history and physical should be performed, and each patient should be evaluated for possible infection. In the symptomatic patient, the diagnosis of aseptic component loosening is usually made if the radiographic evaluation reveals a radiolucent zone of 2 mm or more in width around the implant. In an asymptomatic patient, it is crucial to obtain serial radiographs to evaluate for progressive changes of the radiolucent zones. Radiographic changes frequently occur before the onset of symptoms, and not all radiolucent zones imply component loosening. They could, for example, be produced by age-related femoral expansion of the femoral canal, which thins the cortex and may appear radiographically as progressive radiolucency around the implant.[92] Subsequently, the diagnosis of component loosening is based on multiple criteria. A detailed history and physical is necessary to obtain information on possible surgical complications or comorbidities and to exclude infection. The patient should be evaluated for these signs and symptoms, and additionally, serial radiographs should be followed for progressive loosening of 2 mm or more around the implant.

Management

The management of component loosening after THA is mainly determined by the patient's symptoms and functional impairment on presentation. If loosening is only diagnosed on radiographic images it may be observed and followed up with serial radiographic evaluations. However, once a progressive process of aseptic loosening is detected on radiographic images and the patient has pain or diminished function in the affected hip joint, a surgical revision is frequently necessary. Detailed surgical techniques are discussed in a later chapter.

Summary

Aseptic component loosening is a multifactorial process based on patient-specific factors, implant design, and surgical techniques, and it remains one of the most frequent complications of THA.[3,4] To minimize the incidence of loosening, surgical techniques should be optimized to avoid common technical causes that predispose for component failure. While advanced implant design and surgical techniques are still undergoing evaluation in prospective long-term studies, midterm data that are currently available have shown improved longevity and wear rates.[77,78] Joshi et al have demonstrated in a retrospective study evaluating the outcome of Charnley primary low-friction arthroplasties with a follow-up of 10 years that improved surgical techniques can decrease the incidence of osteolysis.[93] The overall incidence of component loosening was 14.9% but when criteria for optimized surgical techniques were met the incidence decreased to 5.2%.[93]

PERIPROSTHETIC FRACTURE

Introduction

As the population ages, the number of THAs performed increases. Compared to when THA was first developed, more patients are selected for arthroplasty including those who are younger, heavier, and have more preoperative bone loss.[94] With patients now decades removed from primary arthroplasty, the number of patients with subsequent bone loss around their prostheses has increased. With this in consideration, the rate of periprosthetic fracture will most likely increase. Periprosthetic fractures can be a devastating injury that ultimately leads to failure of the arthroplasty. Fractures can occur at different stages of arthroplasty. The injury can either occur intraoperatively or in the postoperative period. An intraoperative fracture may or may not be detected at the time of surgery.

The exact frequency of periprosthetic fracture has been difficult to determine. Multiple studies have reported the incidence of these injuries at their institutions with rates being broadly reported between 0.1% and 18% with most rates reported between 1% to 4%.[95-100] This broad number attempts to approximate their frequency, but is clearly not a precise measure of their incidence. Though their exact rate can only be approximated, recognition of definite risk factors in order to identify patients at increased risk for periprosthetic fracture would decrease the frequency of such injuries. As this complication carries significant morbidity and mortality (a reported fatality rate of 4% in men of at least 80 years of age), all means necessary must be taken to avoid them.[101]

Etiology

There are numerous risk factors for sustaining a periprosthetic fracture. General risks are female gender, increased age, history of trauma (especially falls), osteoporosis, previous hip fracture or surgery, rheumatoid arthritis, Paget's disease, osteogenesis imperfecta, and a cementless prostheses. Intraoperative and early postoperative fracture risks include any stress risers on the femur including cortical windows or perforations (ie, penetrating the anterior femoral cortex with reamers). Risks for late fracture include component loosening, osteolysis, infection, and proximal femoral bone loss.[100,102,103]

The greatest risk factor for periprosthetic fracture is a history of trauma. In 1996, Beals and Tower reported 92% of 93 periprosthetic fractures occurred as a result of a definitive traumatic event. The vast majority of these traumatic events were falls.[104] Accordingly, risk factors for falls should also be considered as risk factors for fractures. Fall risks include lower limb dysfunction, neurologic conditions, barbiturate use, and visual impairment.[105] Conditions that lead to bone loss provide additional risk for fracture with minimal trauma (ie, falling from standing). Decreased bone minimal density is directly linearly related to the minimal force needed to fracture the femur,[106] and thus, poor bone quality around a previously operated arthroplasty site leads to the threat of periprosthetic fracture with minimal trauma.

Johannsen et al reported the single most important risk factor for incurring an intraoperative fracture was prior hip surgery. Their study described 22 patients who suffered an intraoperative periprosthetic hip fracture, all having previous hip surgery. If any defect in the femoral cortex is created (perhaps by use of a cortical window for cement removal or by erosion caused by loose components), there is greater intraoperative risk.[107]

Differing surgical techniques and varying prostheses portend different inherent risk for periprosthetic fracture. In particular, the use of cemented components has been shown to influence fracture risk. A cadaver study concluded that cementation of components increases femoral stability and reduces risk of periprosthetic fracture. Ten cementless prostheses and 10 cemented prostheses were inserted into cadaveric femurs. Force was applied to the different groups. All 10 femora in the cementless group fractured at a median 2625 N. Only 5 cemented femora fractured (at a median 9,127 N) and 5 did not fracture at the maximum applied force of 10,000 N.[108] Berend et al examined 2551 hips over a 16-year period and found that cementless femoral fixation was associated with an increased risk of periprosthetic fracture.[109] Similarly, Hailer et al retrospectively reviewed over 170,000 THAs and found that uncemented arthroplasty was associated with lower component survival. The predominant reason for their failure was femoral fracture in the first 2 years.[110] Thus, cementless techniques have been correlated with an increased risk of periprosthetic fracture.

Presentation and Diagnosis

Periprosthetic fractures typically present with typical signs and symptoms of fracture. These fractures may occur intraoperatively, but may not be noted until later in the postoperative period. Postoperative periprosthetic fractures will present with pain, inability to use the limb, swelling, deformity, and/or instability. A history of a traumatic event acutely precipitating the pain is typical, but the trauma can be quite minimal and patients may not remember such an event. Though unlikely, it is possible for fractures to occur without definitive trauma.[104] A complete history should be obtained to identify any of the previously discussed risk factors (including an in-depth past medical, past surgical, and family histories). The history should elicit any symptoms of infection. The operative note should be reviewed for a description of the procedure to identify any difficulties encountered during the operation and to note which prostheses were implanted.

A physical examination should be performed. The limb should be examined for any obvious deformity, its position at rest, and for any limb length inequality. Tenderness will be noted at the fracture site. If able, assess the stability of the joint. Any signs of infection (including fever, erythema, and purulence draining) should be noted. An accurate neurovascular exam should be documented, with special attention to any sensory, motor, or vascular deficits on the affected limb. Appropriate laboratory studies (eg, ESR, Westergren CRP, leukocyte count, and joint aspiration with leukocyte count and differential) should be performed if there is any clinical concern for infection.

Following the history and physical, radiographic evaluation should be conducted. The bone quality should be noted as a thorough scan for any fracture is conducted. The position of the components should be evaluated for proper placement and dislocation. The location and character of periprosthetic fracture should be described, allowing appropriate classification. Correct classification of periprosthetic fractures is critical as it helps to determine the treatment algorithm.

Classification

Development of a consistent classification of periprosthetic fractures has been a priority in order to establish consistent and successful management plans. Several systems have been devised based on the location of the periprosthetic fracture. The first such location-based system was developed from 9 patient cases by Parrish and Jones in 1964.[111] Subsequent schemes were developed by various authors.[107,112-115] As new schemes have been developed, it has been difficult to maintain consistent labels and therefore have consistent treatment plans for periprosthetic hip fractures. Recently there has been increasing acceptance of the Vancouver classification scheme in order to achieve such consistency. The Vancouver classification system was first described by Duncan and Masri in 1995. The system aimed to create a system that incorporated multiple aspects of a periprosthetic fracture to provide a rational treatment protocol. It integrates the location of the fracture, status of stem fixation, and the quality of bone stock available.[116-118]

The first aspect considered by the Vancouver system is the fracture location. Type A fractures are trochanteric. Type B fractures are around the stem. Type C fractures are distal to the stem. Both Types A and B are further divided into subtypes. Type A fractures can be further separated as AG or AL depending on involvement of either the greater (G) or lesser (L) trochanter. Type B fractures are divided into B1, B2, or B3 based on bone stock and component stability. B1 and B2

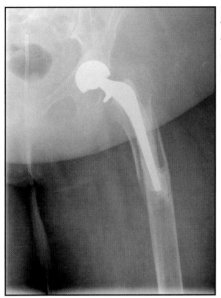

Figure 2-5. Anteroposterior radiograph of a THA with a Vancouver type B2 periprosthetic femur fracture. The fracture is around the stem; however, the implant is not stable. (Reprinted with permission from Sinai Hospital of Baltimore, Inc.)

fractures both have adequate bone stock, but are classified by prosthetic stability. If the prosthesis is stable, the fracture is defined as B1. Loose component fractures are Type B2 (Figure 2-5). B3 fractures are periprosthetic fractures that have inadequate bone stock. Type B fractures are the most commonly seen, composing greater than 85% of periprosthetic hip fractures.[116-118]

The purpose of this system was to delineate treatment options. Most of these fractures require operative fixation. Type AL fractures frequently do not require operative fixation, while Type AG fractures more often require surgery. Type B fractures all require surgery unless the fracture has minimal displacement and the components are stable. Operative treatments include biplanar fixation, long stem revision with bone grafting, and proximal femoral replacement. Type C fractures are managed as a typical femoral fracture.[119] The techniques and strategies for managing these fractures will be discussed in detail in a later chapter.

The validity of this system has been recently tested. Brady et al assessed its reliability by statistically analyzing interobserver agreement and tested its validity by comparing radiographic classification to intraoperative classification. They concluded substantial agreements and asserted their system's validity and reliability.[120] A European study sought to provide an unbiased report on the system's validity and reliability. Experienced surgeons, training surgeons, and medical students were asked to classify periprosthetic fractures using the Vancouver system. Interobserver reliability was statistically analyzed and there was significant agreement among the experience levels.[121] Accordingly, this system has gained global acceptance for classification of periprosthetic hip fractures.

Management

The treatment of periprosthetic fractures requires adherence to basic principles of any fracture. Biomechanical integrity of the bone and joint must be restored in order to ultimately regain functionality. Surgical intervention is often required to accomplish this. The surgical treatment is dependent on the individual fracture pattern and can be guided by an accurate classification. Nonsurgical treatment may be offered in stable, nondisplaced fractures. Such treatment includes protective nonweightbearing status and immobilization with a cast or brace. Treatment plans will be discussed in detail in a later chapter.

Summary

The complication of periprosthetic fracture is a common mode of failure for THA. As the population ages and the frequency of arthroplasty increases, so will the occurrence of periprosthetic fractures. An understanding of the risk factors and etiology of periprosthetic fractures could reduce their incidence. Despite taking precautions to reduce fracture frequency, arthroplasty failure due to periprosthetic fracture is inevitable.

Functional outcomes following a periprosthetic fracture are generally poor and have high associated mortality rates.[101,122-124] A Swedish retrospective review compared mortality rates of more than 27,000 primary THAs to 736 patients who were identified to have periprosthetic hip fractures. The fracture patients had significantly greater short-term and long-term mortality rates.[101] A New Zealand study of 232 periprosthetic fracture hip revisions concluded that these patients had a higher mortality rate compared to revisions for loose components (7.3% versus 0.9%). They also found higher rerevision rates (7.3% versus 2.6%) and lower functional outcome scores.[124] Bhattacharyya et al reported an 11% 1-year mortality rate following surgical intervention for periprosthetic hip fractures, which was comparable to the mortality rate of surgical intervention for native hip fracture (16.5%).[122] Appropriately managing these injuries with efficient, timely diagnosis that utilizes a universal, reliable classification system will allow the best possible outcome for a potentially devastating, dangerous injury.

REFERENCES

1. Kurtz S, Mowat F, Ong K, Chan N, Lau E, Halpern M. Prevalence of primary and revision total hip and knee arthroplasty in the United States from 1990 through 2002. *J Bone Joint Surg Am.* 2005;87(7):1487-1497.
2. Kurtz S, Ong K, Lau E, Mowat F, Halpern M. Projections of primary and revision hip and knee arthroplasty in the United States from 2005 to 2030. *J Bone Joint Surg Am.* 2007;89(4):780-785.
3. Bozic KJ, Kurtz SM, Lau E, Ong K, Vail TP, Berry DJ. The epidemiology of revision total hip arthroplasty in the United States. *J Bone Joint Surg Am.* 2009;91(1):128-133.
4. Springer BD, Fehring TK, Griffin WL, Odum SM, Masonis JL. Why revision total hip arthroplasty fails. *Clin Orthop Relat Res.* 2009;467(1):166-173.
5. Charnley J. Postoperative infection after total hip replacement with special reference to air contamination in the operating room. *Clin Orthop Relat Res.* 1972;87:167-187.
6. Gaine WJ, Ramamohan NA, Hussein NA, Hullin MG, McCreath SW. Wound infection in hip and knee arthroplasty. *J Bone Joint Surg Br.* 2000;82(4):561-565.
7. Kurtz SM, Lau E, Schmier J, Ong KL, Zhao K, Parvizi J. Infection burden for hip and knee arthroplasty in the United States. *J Arthroplasty.* 2008;23(7):984-991.
8. Dale H, Hallan G, Espehaug B, Havelin LI, Engesaeter LB. Increasing risk of revision due to deep infection after hip arthroplasty. *Acta Orthop.* 2009;80(6):639-645.
9. Phillips CB, Barrett JA, Losina E, et al. Incidence rates of dislocation, pulmonary embolism, and deep infection during the first six months after elective total hip replacement. *J Bone Joint Surg Am.* 2003;85-A(1):20-26.
10. Mahomed NN, Barrett JA, Katz JN, et al. Rates and outcomes of primary and revision total hip replacement in the United States medicare population. *J Bone Joint Surg Am.* 2003;85-A(1):27-32.
11. Hamilton H, Jamieson J. Deep infection in total hip arthroplasty. *Can J Surg.* 2008;51(2):111-117.
12. Pulido L, Ghanem E, Joshi A, Purtill JJ, Parvizi J. Periprosthetic joint infection: the incidence, timing, and predisposing factors. *Clin Orthop Relat Res.* 2008;466(7):1710-1715.
13. Ong KL, Kurtz SM, Lau E, Bozic KJ, Berry DJ, Parvizi J. Prosthetic joint infection risk after total hip arthroplasty in the Medicare population. *J Arthroplasty.* 2009;24(6 Suppl):105-109.
14. Ridgeway S, Wilson J, Charlet A, Kafatos G, Pearson A, Coello R. Infection of the surgical site after arthroplasty of the hip. *J Bone Joint Surg Br.* 2005;87(6):844-850.
15. Phillips JE, Crane TP, Noy M, Elliott TS, Grimer RJ. The incidence of deep prosthetic infections in a specialist orthopaedic hospital: a 15-year prospective survey. *J Bone Joint Surg Br.* 2006;88(7):943-948.
16. Bongartz T, Halligan CS, Osmon DR, et al. Incidence and risk factors of prosthetic joint infection after total hip or knee replacement in patients with rheumatoid arthritis. *Arthritis Rheum.* 2008;59(12):1713-1720.

17. Cordero-Ampuero J, de Dios M. What are the risk factors for infection in hemiarthroplasties and total hip arthroplasties? *Clin Orthop Relat Res*. 2010;468(12):3268–3277.

18. Malinzak RA, Ritter MA, Berend ME, Meding JB, Olberding EM, Davis KE. Morbidly obese, diabetic, younger, and unilateral joint arthroplasty patients have elevated total joint arthroplasty infection rates. *J Arthroplasty*. 2009;24(6 Suppl):84-88.

19. Soohoo NF, Farng E, Lieberman JR, Chambers L, Zingmond DS. Factors that predict short-term complication rates after total hip arthroplasty. *Clin Orthop Relat Res*. 2010;468(9):2363-2371.

20. Webb BG, Lichtman DM, Wagner RA. Risk factors in total joint arthroplasty: comparison of infection rates in patients with different socioeconomic backgrounds. *Orthopedics*. 2008;31(5):445.

21. Anagnostakos K, Schmid NV, Kelm J, Grun U, Jung J. Classification of hip joint infections. *Int J Med Sci*. 2009;6(5):227-233.

22. LaPorte DM, Waldman BJ, Mont MA, Hungerford DS. Infections associated with dental procedures in total hip arthroplasty. *J Bone Joint Surg Br*. 1999;81(1):56-59.

23. Berbari EF, Osmon DR, Carr A, et al. Dental procedures as risk factors for prosthetic hip or knee infection: a hospital-based prospective case-control study. *Clin Infect Dis*. 2010;50(1):8-16.

24. Segawa H, Tsukayama DT, Kyle RF, Becker DA, Gustilo RB. Infection after total knee arthroplasty. A retrospective study of the treatment of eighty-one infections. *J Bone Joint Surg Am*. 1999;81(10):1434-1445.

25. Trampuz A, Zimmerli W. Prosthetic joint infections: update in diagnosis and treatment. *Swiss Med Wkly*. 2005;135(17-18):243-251.

26. Muller M, Morawietz L, Hasart O, Strube P, Perka C, Tohtz S. Diagnosis of periprosthetic infection following total hip arthroplasty: evaluation of the diagnostic values of pre- and intraoperative parameters and the associated strategy to preoperatively select patients with a high probability of joint infection. *J Orthop Surg Res*. 2008;3:31.

27. Bozic KJ, Rubash HE. The painful total hip replacement. *Clin Orthop Relat Res*. 2004(420):18-25.

28. Parvizi J, Della Valle CJ. AAOS clinical practice guideline: diagnosis and treatment of periprosthetic joint infections of the hip and knee. *J Am Acad Orthop Surg*. 18(12):771-772.

29. Della Valle CJ, Sporer SM, Jacobs JJ, Berger RA, Rosenberg AG, Paprosky WG. Preoperative testing for sepsis before revision total knee arthroplasty. *J Arthroplasty*. 2007;22(6 Suppl 2):90-93.

30. Ghanem E, Houssock C, Pulido L, Han S, Jaberi FM, Parvizi J. Determining "true" leukocytosis in bloody joint aspiration. *J Arthroplasty*. 2008;23(2):182-187.

31. Leone JM, Hanssen AD. Management of infection at the site of a total knee arthroplasty. *J Bone Joint Surg Am*. 2005;87(10):2335-2348.

32. Musso AD, Mohanty K, Spencer-Jones R. Role of frozen section histology in diagnosis of infection during revision arthroplasty. *Postgrad Med J*. 2003;79(936):590-593.

33. Fehring TK, McAlister JA, Jr. Frozen histologic section as a guide to sepsis in revision joint arthroplasty. *Clin Orthop Relat Res*. 1994(304):229-237.

34. Banit DM, Kaufer H, Hartford JM. Intraoperative frozen section analysis in revision total joint arthroplasty. *Clin Orthop Relat Res*. 2002(401):230-238.

35. Della Valle CJ, Bogner E, Desai P, et al. Analysis of frozen sections of intraoperative specimens obtained at the time of reoperation after hip or knee resection arthroplasty for the treatment of infection. *J Bone Joint Surg Am*. 1999;81(5):684-689.

36. Lonner JH, Desai P, Dicesare PE, Steiner G, Zuckerman JD. The reliability of analysis of intraoperative frozen sections for identifying active infection during revision hip or knee arthroplasty. *J Bone Joint Surg Am*. 1996;78(10):1553-1558.

37. Feldman DS, Lonner JH, Desai P, Zuckerman JD. The role of intraoperative frozen sections in revision total joint arthroplasty. *J Bone Joint Surg Am*. 1995;77(12):1807-1813.

38. Tohtz SW, Muller M, Morawietz L, Winkler T, Perka C. Validity of frozen sections for analysis of periprosthetic loosening membranes. *Clin Orthop Relat Res*. 468(3):762-768.

39. Bori G, Soriano A, Garcia S, Mallofre C, Riba J, Mensa J. Usefulness of histological analysis for predicting the presence of microorganisms at the time of reimplantation after hip resection arthroplasty for the treatment of infection. *J Bone Joint Surg Am*. 2007;89(6):1232-1237.

40. Meehan J, Jamali AA, Nguyen H. Prophylactic antibiotics in hip and knee arthroplasty. *J Bone Joint Surg Am*. 2009;91(10):2480-2490.

41. Walenkamp GH. Joint prosthetic infections: a success story or a continuous concern? *Acta Orthop*. 2009; 80(6):629-632.

42. AlBuhairan B, Hind D, Hutchinson A. Antibiotic prophylaxis for wound infections in total joint arthroplasty: a systematic review. *J Bone Joint Surg Br*. 2008;90(7):915-919.

43. Hernigou P, Flouzat-Lachianette CH, Jalil R, Uirassu Batista S, Guissou I, Poignard A. Treatment of infected hip arthroplasty. *Open Orthop J.* 2010;4:126-131.

44. Ure KJ, Amstutz HC, Nasser S, Schmalzried TP. Direct-exchange arthroplasty for the treatment of infection after total hip replacement. An average ten-year follow-up. *J Bone Joint Surg Am.* 1998;80(7):961-968.

45. Crockarell JR, Hanssen AD, Osmon DR, Morrey BF. Treatment of infection with débridement and retention of the components following hip arthroplasty. *J Bone Joint Surg Am.* 1998;80(9):1306-1313.

46. Fackler CD, Poss R. Dislocation in total hip arthroplasties. *Clin Orthop Relat Res.* 1980;151:169-178.

47. Pulido L, Camilo R, Parvizi J. Late instability following total hip arthroplasty. *Clin Med Res.* 2007;5(2):139-142.

48. Morrey BF. Instability after total hip arthroplasty. *Anglais.* 1992;2:237-248.

49. Parvizi J, Picinic E, Sharkey PF. Revision total hip arthroplasty for instability: surgical techniques and principles. *J Bone Joint Surg Am.* 2008;90(5):1134-1142.

50. von Knoch M, Berry DJ, Harmsen WS, Morrey BF. Late dislocation after total hip arthroplasty. *J Bone Joint Surg Am.* 2002;84(11):1949-1953.

51. Cobb TK, Morrey BF, Ilstrup DM. The elevated-rim acetabular liner in total hip arthroplasty: relationship to postoperative dislocation. *J Bone Joint Surg Am.* 1996;78(1):80-86.

52. Li E, Meding JB, Ritter MA, Keating EM, Faris PM. The natural history of a posteriorly dislocated total hip replacement. *J Arthroplasty.* 1999;14(8):964-968.

53. Ali Khan MA, Brakenbury PH, Reynolds IS. Dislocation following total hip replacement. *J Bone Joint Surg Br.* 1981;63-B(2):214-218.

54. Lindberg HkO, Carlsson ÅkS, Gentz C-F, Pettersson H. Recurrent and non-recurrent dislocation following total hip arthroplasty. *Acta Orthopaedica Scandinavica.* 1982;53(6):947-952.

55. Williams JF, Gottesman MJ, Mallory TH. Dislocation after total hip arthroplasty: treatment with an above-knee hip spica cast. *Clin Orthop Relat Res.* 1982;171:53-58.

56. Berry DJ, von Knoch M, Schleck CD, Harmsen WS. The cumulative long-term risk of dislocation after primary Charnley total hip arthroplasty. *J Bone Joint Surg Am.* 2004;86(1):9-14.

57. Woolson ST, Rahimtoola ZO. Risk factors for dislocation during the first 3 months after primary total hip replacement. *J Arthroplasty.* 1999;14(6):662-668.

58. Paterno SA, Lachiewicz PF, Kelley SS. The influence of patient-related factors and the position of the acetabular component on the rate of dislocation after total hip replacement. *J Bone Joint Surg Am.* 1997;79(8):1202-1210.

59. Lewinnek GE, Lewis JL, Tarr R, Compere CL, Zimmerman JR. Dislocations after total hip-replacement arthroplasties. *J Bone Joint Surg Am.* 1978;60(2):217-220.

60. Kelley SS, Lachiewicz PF, Hickman JM, Paterno SM. Relationship of femoral head and acetabular size to the prevalence of dislocation. *Clin Orthop Relat Res.* 1998;355:163-170.

61. Woo RY, Morrey BF. Dislocations after total hip arthroplasty. *J Bone Joint Surg Am.* 1982;64(9):1295-1306.

62. Berry DJ, von Knoch M, Schleck CD, Harmsen WS. Effect of femoral head diameter and operative approach on risk of dislocation after primary total hip arthroplasty. *J Bone Joint Surg Am.* 2005;87(11):2456-2463.

63. Bauer R, Kerschbaumer F, Poisel S, Oberthaler W. The transgluteal approach to the hip joint. *Arch Orthop Trauma Surg.* 1979;95(1):47-49.

64. Dall D. Exposure of the hip by anterior osteotomy of the greater trochanter. A modified anterolateral approach. *J Bone Joint Surg Br.* 1986;68(3):382-386.

65. Dorr LD, Wan Z. Causes of and treatment protocol for instability of total hip replacement. *Clin Orthop Relat Res.* 1998;355:144-151.

66. Peak EL, Parvizi J, Ciminiello M, et al. The role of patient restrictions in reducing the prevalence of early dislocation following total hip arthroplasty. A randomized, prospective study. *J Bone Joint Surg Am.* 2005;87(2):247-253.

67. Barrack RL, Butler RA, Laster DR, Andrews P. Stem design and dislocation after revision total hip arthroplasty: clinical results and computer modeling. *J Arthroplasty.* 2001;16(8):8-12.

68. Hedlundh U, Carlsson AS. Increased risk of dislocation with collar reinforced modular heads of the Lubinus SP-2 hip prosthesis. *Acta Orthop Scand.* 1996;67:2.

69. Malik A, Maheshwari A, Dorr LD. Impingement with total hip replacement. *J Bone Joint Surg Am.* 2007;89(8):1832-1842.

70. McCollum DE, Gray WJ. Dislocation after total hip arthroplasty causes and prevention. *Clin Orthop Relat Res.* 1990;261:159-170.

71. Padgett DE, Lipman J, Robie B, Nestor BJ. Influence of total hip design on dislocation: a computer model and clinical analysis. *Clin Orthop Relat Res.* 2006;447:48-52.

72. Sariali E, Lazennec JY, Khiami F, Catonne Y. Mathematical evaluation of jumping distance in total hip arthroplasty: influence of abduction angle, femoral head offset, and head diameter. *Acta Orthop.* 2009;80(3):277-282.

73. Learmonth ID. Total hip replacement and the law of diminishing returns. *J Bone Joint Surg Am.* 2006;88(7):1664-1673.

74. Bergstrom B, Lidgren L, Lindberg L. Radiographic abnormalities caused by postoperative infection following total hip arthroplasty. *Clin Orthop Relat Res.* 1974(99):95-102.

75. DeLee JG, Charnley J. Radiological demarcation of cemented sockets in total hip replacement. *Clin Orthop Relat Res.* 1976;(121):20-32.

76. Bragdon CR, Kwon YM, Geller JA, et al. Minimum 6-year followup of highly cross-linked polyethylene in THA. *Clin Orthop Relat Res.* 2007;465:122-127.

77. Callaghan JJ, Cuckler JM, Huddleston JI, Galante JO. How have alternative bearings (such as metal-on-metal, highly cross-linked polyethylene, and ceramic-on-ceramic) affected the prevention and treatment of osteolysis? *J Am Acad Orthop Surg.* 2008;16(Suppl 1):S33-S38.

78. Geller JA, Malchau H, Bragdon C, Greene M, Harris WH, Freiberg AA. Large diameter femoral heads on highly cross-linked polyethylene: minimum 3-year results. *Clin Orthop Relat Res.* 2006;447:53-59.

79. Bragdon CR, Barrett S, Martell JM, Greene ME, Malchau H, Harris WH. Steady-state penetration rates of electron beam-irradiated, highly cross-linked polyethylene at an average 45-month follow-up. *J Arthroplasty.* 2006;21(7):935-943.

80. Digas G, Karrholm J, Thanner J, Malchau H, Herberts P. Highly cross-linked polyethylene in cemented THA: randomized study of 61 hips. *Clin Orthop Relat Res.* 2003(417):126-138.

81. Digas G, Karrholm J, Thanner J, Malchau H, Herberts P. The Otto Aufranc Award. Highly cross-linked polyethylene in total hip arthroplasty: randomized evaluation of penetration rate in cemented and uncemented sockets using radiostereometric analysis. *Clin Orthop Relat Res.* 2004;(429):6-16.

82. Tsao AK, Jones LC, Lewallen DG. What patient and surgical factors contribute to implant wear and osteolysis in total joint arthroplasty? *J Am Acad Orthop Surg.* 2008;16(Suppl 1):S7-S13.

83. Swanson EA, Schmalzried TP, Dorey FJ. Activity recommendations after total hip and knee arthroplasty: a survey of the American Association for Hip and Knee Surgeons. *J Arthroplasty.* 2009;24(6 Suppl):120-126.

84. McClung CD, Zahiri CA, Higa JK, Amstutz HC, Schmalzried TP. Relationship between body mass index and activity in hip or knee arthroplasty patients. *J Orthop Res.* 2000;18(1):35-39.

85. Min BW, Song KS, Bae KC, Cho CH, Lee KJ, Kim HJ. Second-generation cementless total hip arthroplasty in patients with osteonecrosis of the femoral head. *J Arthroplasty.* 2008;23(6):902-910.

86. Ries MD. Highly cross-linked polyethylene: the debate is over—in opposition. *J Arthroplasty.* 2005;20(4 Suppl 2):59-62.

87. Beksac B, Salas A, Gonzalez Della Valle A, Salvati EA. Wear is reduced in THA performed with highly cross-linked polyethylene. *Clin Orthop Relat Res.* 2009;467(7):1765-1772.

88. Gruen TA, McNeice GM, Amstutz HC. "Modes of failure" of cemented stem-type femoral components: a radiographic analysis of loosening. *Clin Orthop Relat Res.* 1979(141):17-27.

89. Schmalzried TP, Kwong LM, Jasty M, et al. The mechanism of loosening of cemented acetabular components in total hip arthroplasty. Analysis of specimens retrieved at autopsy. *Clin Orthop Relat Res.* 1992(274):60-78.

90. Engh CA, Bobyn JD. Principles, techniques, results, and complications with a porous-coated sintered metal system. *Instr Course Lect.* 1986;35:169-183.

91. Engh CA, Bobyn JD, Glassman AH. Porous-coated hip replacement. The factors governing bone ingrowth, stress shielding, and clinical results. *J Bone Joint Surg Br.* 1987;69(1):45-55.

92. Poss R, Staehlin P, Larson M. Femoral expansion in total hip arthroplasty. *J Arthroplasty.* 1987;2(4):259-264.

93. Joshi RP, Eftekhar NS, McMahon DJ, Nercessian OA. Osteolysis after Charnley primary low-friction arthroplasty. A comparison of two matched paired groups. *J Bone Joint Surg Br.* 1998;80(4):585-590.

94. NIH Consensus Development Panel on Total Hip Replacement. Total hip replacement. *JAMA.* 1995;273(24):1950-1956.

95. Lewallen DG, Berry DJ. Periprosthetic fracture of the femur after total hip arthroplasty: treatment and results to date. *Instr Course Lect.* 1998;47:243-249.

96. Sarvilinna R, Huhtala HS, Sovelius RT, Halonen PJ, Nevalainen JK, Pajamaki KJ. Factors predisposing to periprosthetic fracture after hip arthroplasty: a case (n = 31)-control study. *Acta Orthop Scand.* 2004;75(1):16-20.

97. Schwartz JT Jr, Mayer JG, Engh CA. Femoral fracture during non-cemented total hip arthroplasty. *J Bone Joint Surg Am.* 1989;71(8):1135-1142.

98. Tower SS, Beals RK. Fractures of the femur after hip replacement: the Oregon experience. *Orthop Clin North Am*. 1999;30(2):235-247.

99. Cook RE, Jenkins PJ, Walmsley PJ, Patton JT, Robinson CM. Risk factors for periprosthetic fractures of the hip: a survivorship analysis. *Clin Orthop Relat Res*. 2008;466(7):1652-1656.

100. Fredin HO, Lindberg H, Carlsson AS. Femoral fracture following hip arthroplasty. *Acta Orthop Scand*. 1987;58(1):20-22.

101. Lindahl H, Oden A, Garellick G, Malchau H. The excess mortality due to periprosthetic femur fracture. A study from the Swedish national hip arthroplasty register. *Bone*. 2007;40(5):1294-1298.

102. McElfresh EC, Coventry MB. Femoral and pelvic fractures after total hip arthroplasty. *J Bone Joint Surg Am*. 1974;56(3):483-492.

103. Sarvilinna R, Huhtala H, Pajamaki J. Young age and wedge stem design are risk factors for periprosthetic fracture after arthroplasty due to hip fracture. A case-control study. *Acta Orthop*. 2005;76(1):56-60.

104. Beals RK, Tower SS. Periprosthetic fractures of the femur. An analysis of 93 fractures. *Clin Orthop Relat Res*. 1996(327):238-246.

105. Grisso JA, Kelsey JL, Strom BL, et al. Risk factors for falls as a cause of hip fracture in women. The Northeast Hip Fracture Study Group. *N Engl J Med*. 1991;324(19):1326-1331.

106. Leichter I, Margulies JY, Weinreb A, et al. The relationship between bone density, mineral content, and mechanical strength in the femoral neck. *Clin Orthop Relat Res*. 1982(163):272-281.

107. Johansson JE, McBroom R, Barrington TW, Hunter GA. Fracture of the ipsilateral femur in patients wih total hip replacement. *J Bone Joint Surg Am*. 1981;63(9):1435-1442.

108. Thomsen MN, Jakubowitz E, Seeger JB, Lee C, Kretzer JP, Clarius M. Fracture load for periprosthetic femoral fractures in cemented versus uncemented hip stems: an experimental in vitro study. *Orthopedics*. 2008;31(7):653.

109. Berend ME, Smith A, Meding JB, Ritter MA, Lynch T, Davis K. Long-term outcome and risk factors of proximal femoral fracture in uncemented and cemented total hip arthroplasty in 2551 hips. *J Arthroplasty*. 2006;21(6 Suppl 2):53-59.

110. Hailer NP, Garellick G, Karrholm J. Uncemented and cemented primary total hip arthroplasty in the Swedish Hip Arthroplasty Register. *Acta Orthop*. 81(1):34-41.

111. Parrish TF, Jones JR. Fracture of the femur following prosthetic arthroplasty of the hip. Report of nine cases. *J Bone Joint Surg Am*. 1964;46:241-248.

112. Bethea JS 3rd, DeAndrade JR, Fleming LL, Lindenbaum SD, Welch RB. Proximal femoral fractures following total hip arthroplasty. *Clin Orthop Relat Res*. 1982(170):95-106.

113. Whittaker RP, Sotos LN, Ralston EL. Fractures of the femur about femoral endoprostheses. *J Trauma*. 1974;14(8):675-694.

114. Ninan TM, Costa ML, Krikler SJ. Classification of femoral periprosthetic fractures. *Injury*. 2007;38(6):661-668.

115. Mont MA, Maar DC. Fractures of the ipsilateral femur after hip arthroplasty. A statistical analysis of outcome based on 487 patients. *J Arthroplasty*. 1994;9(5):511-519.

116. Duncan CP, Masri BA. Fractures of the femur after hip replacement. *Instr Course Lect*. 1995;44:293-304.

117. Brady OH, Kerry R, Masri BA, Garbuz DS, Duncan CP. The Vancouver classification of periprosthetic fractures of the hip: a rational approach to treatment. *Techn Orthop*. 1999;14(2):107-114.

118. Brady OH, Garbuz DS, Masri BA, Duncan CP. Classification of the hip. *Orthop Clin North Am*. 1999;30(2):215-220.

119. Parvizi J, Rapuri VR, Purtill JJ, Sharkey PF, Rothman RH, Hozack WJ. Treatment protocol for proximal femoral periprosthetic fractures. *J Bone Joint Surg Am*. 2004;86-A(Suppl 2):8-16.

120. Brady OH, Garbuz DS, Masri BA, Duncan CP. The reliability and validity of the Vancouver classification of femoral fractures after hip replacement. *J Arthroplasty*. 2000;15(1):59-62.

121. Rayan F, Dodd M, Haddad FS. European validation of the Vancouver classification of periprosthetic proximal femoral fractures. *J Bone Joint Surg Br*. 2008;90(12):1576-1579.

122. Bhattacharyya T, Chang D, Meigs JB, Estok DM 2nd, Malchau H. Mortality after periprosthetic fracture of the femur. *J Bone Joint Surg Am*. 2007;89(12):2658-2662.

123. Higgins GA, Davis ET, Revell M, Porter K. The management and treatment of peri-prosthetic fractures around both total hip and hemiarthroplasty. *Trauma*. 2009;11(1):49-61.

124. Young SW, Walker CG, Pitto RP. Functional outcome of femoral peri prosthetic fracture and revision hip arthroplasty: a matched-pair study from the New Zealand Registry. *Acta Orthop*. 2008;79(4):483-488.

Preoperative Planning for Revision Total Hip Arthroplasty

Andrew Michael, MD and Scott Sporer, MD

Total hip arthroplasty (THA) is in growing demand in the United States and around the world. More than 300,000 total and partial hip arthroplasties and 36,000 revision THAs are performed every year.[1] As the indication for primary hip arthroplasties expand into younger and more active patients, the number of total hip revisions have increased and is estimated to grow significantly in the next 2 decades.[2,3] With this increasing demand for revision THAs, it is increasingly important for the total joint surgeon to properly diagnose and treat the revision patient. The components of a proper assessment and treatment of the revision patient includes a thorough patient history, physical exam, imaging, laboratory tests, and proper preoperative templating. Careful preoperative planning will prepare the surgeon for any foreseeable intraoperative complications that may require equipment not normally available during surgery. Poor preparation can lead to increased operative time and inadequate instrumentation and available prostheses, which can result in poor patient outcomes and increased intra- and postoperative complications such as fracture, infection, instability, loosening, or pain.

PATIENT HISTORY

Evaluation of any orthopedic patient should begin with a detailed patient history in reference to the chief complaint. Pain is the most common presenting complaint following a failed primary THA. The physician must first determine the onset of the patient's pain, including the presence or absence of any improvement in his or her preoperative pain following the primary THA. If the patient never experienced pain relief following the primary THA, the original diagnosis should be revisited. If the patient experienced improvement of his or her pain following his or her primary THA, the focus on the history should be on acute events that could have triggered the patient's new onset of pain including trauma, recent medical or dental procedures, or any recent illness. Specific inquiries of recent pulmonary, urinary, and systemic infections could raise suspicion of infectious causes of new onset hip pain. Once the onset of the pain has been established, the location of the pain can often yield clues to the correct diagnosis. Complaints of deep groin or buttock pain often point to the acetabulum as the source, while thigh pain may direct the

Jacofsky DJ, Hedley AK.
Fundamentals of Revision Hip Arthroplasty:
Diagnosis, Evaluation, and Treatment (pp 31-50).
© 2013 SLACK Incorporated.

surgeon to closely examine the femoral component. The chronicity and nature of the pain often differs between 2 major revision causes: aseptic loosening and infection. Aseptic loosening is the most common cause of revision surgery in long-term follow-up and often yields pain with load bearing and movement. Initial "start-up" pain is common, which will frequently improve slightly during the day only to intensify later in the day or with prolonged walking.[4] Pain caused by an infected hip arthroplasty often exists at rest, and patients may rarely have associated night sweats and fevers. Alternatively, patients with an infected hip may only complain of a dull persistent ache. As a result, infection should be considered in all patients with pain following total hip replacement and screening baseline inflammatory markers (ie, erythrocyte sedimentation rate [ESR] and C-reactive protein [CRP]) are advised in all patients with persistent pain following joint replacement.

Recurrent hip instability remains a common reason for revision surgery.[5,6] A detailed history of the patient's dislocations and any premorbid associated symptoms, such as snapping or popping of the hip, should be elucidated. The activity or position causing the dislocation should be elucidated as this will help identify the direction of instability. Activities causing the hip to be in a flexed and internally rotated position result in posterior dislocation, while activities that place the leg in an extended and externally rotated position result in anterior instability.

Once details of the patient's present complaints are obtained, a full past medical and surgical history is necessary to determine medical comorbidities that might place the patient at increased risk. A complete history of previous surgeries with a focus on previous surgery to the affected hip should be obtained. A proper history, including the patient's ambulatory and pain status prior to the primary hip arthroplasty, as well as subsequent need of revisions to the hip may assist in diagnosing the etiology of ongoing pain. Efforts should be made to obtain operative reports and implant stickers used during the primary procedure. Knowledge of the current implant is especially important if only one side of the joint is being revised to ensure adequate liner and femoral head options are available intraoperatively. A history of trauma and nonarthroplasty procedures to the affected limb should also be obtained as prior surgical procedures and approaches may result in altered pelvic anatomy. Similarly, the details of retained pelvic or femoral hardware should be known, as many fracture fixation implants required specialized extraction tools. Any complications of previous surgeries such as persistent drainage, residual pain, or postoperative dislocations should be noted. Also, any perioperative medical complications such as venous thromboembolism, systemic infection, myocardial infarction, cerebrovascular accident, or arrhythmia should direct the surgeon to order a thorough preoperative medical work-up prior to hip revision surgery. Preoperative measures such as a vena caval filter for venous thromboembolism may need to be employed to decrease operative morbidity and mortality in patients with a history of previous pulmonary embolism or recurrent or chronic deep vein thrombosis.

A complete past medical history of the patient is also used to risk stratify the patient for surgery and anesthesia. Perioperative morbidity and mortality is significantly increased by certain conditions such as congestive heart failure, chronic renal failure, chronic obstructive pulmonary disease, and cancer with bone metastases.[7] Some studies suggest in cancer patients a history of treatment with a focus on recent irradiation of the pelvis may guide the surgeon toward cemented polyethylene acetabular components instead of porous-coated implants.[8,9]

All extrinsic factors of hip pain must be explored before attributing the pain to the hip prosthesis. This includes spinal etiologies such as stenosis and disk herniation, musculotendinous etiologies such as iliopsoas tendonitis and muscle strain, occult pelvic fractures, and bursitis. Rarely, hip and buttock pain can arise from nonorthopedic conditions such as inguinal and femoral hernias and vascular claudication.

It is helpful during the initial hip evaluation to establish a functional score of the patient's current clinical status. A preoperative Harris hip score can be useful in comparing pre- and post-primary hip arthroplasty and pre- and post-revision hip arthroplasty improvement. This metric helps develop an objective reference point for clinically based outcomes for the patient.

PHYSICAL EXAMINATION

The physical exam is critical in establishing the diagnosis of the revision total hip patient. In conjunction with radiographic exam, the diagnosis can often be made in most cases. The physical exam should include examination of the affected limb as well as the contralateral limb and lumbar spine. The exam may begin with examining the patient's gait. This is important in patients who have undergone hip arthroplasty to assess the continuity and strength of the hip abductors. Adductor weakness will cause the patient to lurch to the unaffected side during stance phase of the affected limb, otherwise known as a Trendelenburg gait pattern. This test can be augmented by the Trendelenburg test; during single leg stance on the affected side, the pelvis tilts to the contralateral side. A positive test is indicative of abductor deficiency on the affected limb. If the patient's history includes recurrent hip instability, a weak or absent abductor can contribute to the cause. In a patient with a marked Trendelenburg gait and a history of instability, constrained liners and large femoral heads should be available even if component malposition exists and revision surgery is planned in order to decrease the risk of dislocation following surgery. Poor abductor strength, inadequate abductor repair, and inappropriately reduced offset leading to poor abductor tension can all present with a Trendelenburg gait. Trochanteric nonunion can be diagnosed radiologically and can also present with a Trendelenburg gait. If trochanteric nonunion is diagnosed, proper hardware for fixation of the trochanter should be available at the time of surgery.

The surgical scar must always be examined. A surgical incision may indicate previous surgeries that the patient may have failed to mention. The skin should be examined for any erythema, dehiscence, or discharge from the wound as this is indicative of an infection. Although the subcutaneous vascularity around the hip is more robust than the knee, the original scar should be used at the time of revision surgery if possible. A second incision parallel to the first one can disrupt the blood supply to the skin flap and compromise healing. Cutaneous sensation around the hip should be assessed as branches of the lateral femoral cutaneous nerve can be compromised during revision and primary surgery resulting in paresthesias and numbness on at the anterolateral thigh.

A thorough examination of the spine and lower extremity should be performed. Evaluation of the lower limb should include examination of leg length discrepancy and strength, sensation, and range of motion examinations. Full range of motion and strength tests of the hip can further evaluate abductor competence, bony impingement, and presence of contractures. The Thomas test can be performed by flexing the contralateral hip and knee and looking for involuntary flexion of the examined hip indicating a flexion contracture. Limited passive range of motion can be caused by contractures or bony impingement, and limited active range of motion can indicate weakness or disruption of the motor unit insertion such as in trochanteric malunion or avulsion. Muscle strength testing of the leg can reveal muscle disruption, nerve palsy, or poor hip mechanics as seen in cases with inappropriately reduced offset. Peripheral sensation should be tested preoperatively to evaluate for nerve palsy as well. Bilateral pulses should be recorded and the vascular status of the limb should be assessed. If there is suspicion of poor vascular supply to the affected limb, preoperative assessment by a vascular surgeon may be warranted. Furthermore, extra intraoperative measures can be taken during surgery in such high-risk patients to minimize manipulation of the vascular supply to the leg such as avoiding hyperflexion or extreme internal rotation.[10]

Leg lengthening is common in revision total hip procedures. Preoperative leg lengths should be measured and recorded. The most common way to assess leg lengths is measuring from the anterior superior iliac spine to the medial malleolus. Alternative methods include placing blocks under the patient's shorter leg until the pelvis no longer has any tilt and recording the block height measuring the difference in leg length. Scanograms can be used if the patient has moderate to severe scoliosis or other deformities that make leg lengths difficult to measure. Proper measurement of leg lengths is important for both patient education and anticipation of surgical complications. Patients should also be counseled about expectations of leg lengths. Often perceived (apparent) leg lengths and actual leg lengths are different, and patient education can improve patient satisfaction postoperatively. If the operative hip will experience a leg length increase of 2.7 cm or more, the patient is at risk of sciatic nerve palsy.[11] A peroneal nerve traction injury is the most common neurologic deficit seen postoperatively. In a majority of these cases, full function returns.[11] Once identified, the patient's hip should be extended and his or her knee flexed in order to minimize tension on the nerve.

A lumbar spine examination should be done to rule out any spinal pathology contributing to the patient's complaints. Often radicular pain can radiate into the buttocks and mimic hip pain. If spinal pathology is suspected, a work-up should be pursued to determine the etiology including imaging studies as well as directed injections. If the patient has spinal pathology such as a disc herniation or spinal stenosis, he or she is predisposed to postoperative nerve palsy through the "double crush phenomenon" and should have his or her neurologic status monitored closely postoperatively should he or she require revision surgery.[3]

RADIOGRAPHIC EVALUATION AND IMAGING

Radiographic evaluation provides invaluable information regarding the patient's bony anatomy and information about the current hip prosthesis. A routine radiographic examination of the revision patient should include a low anteroposterior (AP) view of the pelvis, AP view of the affected hip, a frog-leg lateral view of the affected hip, and a shoot through lateral view of the affected hip.

The AP of the pelvis can be taken with the patient supine or standing with the feet 15 degrees internally rotated. Care should be taken to point the central beam to the mid-pelvis minimizing rotation. The AP pelvis radiograph can augment the physical exam in assessing leg lengths by comparing the interischial line with a fixed point on each femur such as the lesser trochanter. It is important to remember that this radiographic technique will only assess leg length differences at the level of the hip joint; any abnormalities distally may contribute to leg length inequality and should be assessed at the time of the physical examination.

Similar to the AP of the pelvis, the AP of the femur can be taken supine or standing with the foot rotated 15 degrees internally. The beam should be centered at the tip of the greater trochanter perpendicular to the table. If the patient and x-ray are properly positioned, it will facilitate proper diagnosis and templating. If the leg is externally rotated or if the x-ray is not taken perpendicular to the femoral neck, it could lead to underestimation of offset and improper preoperative templating. The radiograph should show all components from the acetabular implant to the distal femoral stem and cement mantle to anticipate any difficulties that may be encountered when attempting cement removal.

The lateral radiograph should also encompass the entire hip prosthesis and the cement mantle. A shoot through lateral is performed with the patient lying supine with the hip to be studied extended. The contralateral hip and knee are flexed to move it away from the x-ray beam. The x-ray is centered at the femoral head and directed parallel to the table at a 20-degree cephalic angle to align it perpendicular to the femoral neck. The film cassette is then placed along the lateral hip. This view is the best plain radiograph for assessing acetabular version and in conjunction with other lateral views can aid in determining the anterior bow of the femur. An exam showing a retroverted cup in a patient with recurrent dislocations often confirms suspicion of component malalignment as the cause. A frog-leg lateral is taken with the patient supine, the hips maximally abducted, and the plantar surfaces of the feet touching. The beam is directed to the hip center with a 15-degree cephalic angle. The frog-leg lateral should not be performed in the revision patient suspected of having an anterior dislocation. The best lateral view for assessing femoral bow is the table down or Lowenstein lateral. This is performed with the patient's affected limb entirely in contact with the table with the hip and knee flexed. The x-ray is then focused on the proximal femur. This view is especially important in femoral revisions necessitating a long-stem prosthesis.

If any femoral hardware such as plates, screws, or the femoral component of a knee arthroplasty is present, a full-length AP view of the femur should be ordered. This is also necessary in addition

TABLE 3-1. ENGH CLASSIFICATION OF
UNCEMENTED EXTENSIVELY-COATED FEMORAL STEMS

- Stable bony ingrowth
  - Spot welds at the end of the porous coating
  - Absence of a radiolucent line next to the porous coating—
    may have radiolucent line next to nonporous coated areas
  - Calcar atrophy secondary to stress shielding
- Stable fibrous ingrowth
  - Parallel sclerotic lines or radiolucent line around porous coating
  - No component migration
- Unstable fibrous ingrowth
  - Component migration
  - Divergent radiolucent lines
  - Pedestal formation at stem tip

to the Lowenstein lateral view to prepare and plan for implantation of a long-stem prosthesis if necessary. Full-length femoral views can distort the femoral canal diameter due to magnification; therefore, avoid templating the femoral component using this view. Judet views can be employed to visualize the acetabular component interface as well as acetabular bone stock. This is accomplished by having a supine patient anteriorly or posteriorly rotate the side to be studied 45 degrees. The beam should be directed perpendicular to the table at the affected hip.

Once obtained, the imaging studies can provide necessary diagnostic and implant information. If the implant type is not already known, it should be identified from previous hospital records in the event that well-fixed hardware will be retained. Revising a hip implant without knowledge of the previous hardware can lead to a more extensive surgery if compatible components are not available in the operating room. If the stem is a monoblock design, radiographs can help identify the head size so that in the case of an isolated acetabular revision, the proper polyethylene liner sizes can be available. More commonly, the implant will be of a modular design, and in a case where the stem is being retained, modular heads should be available if the implanted head needs to be replaced. Again it is important to know the specific manufacturer as well as design as multiple orthopedic manufacturers have similar-looking implants and individual manufacturers often have several taper designs.

The radiographs should be examined carefully for signs of femoral or acetabular loosening. If available, all current radiographs should be compared to previous films to assess implant migration. Cementless femoral stems should be examined for absence of changes indicative of bony ingrowth to the implant. The Engh criteria are a helpful tool for assessing whether a femoral stem is well fixed (Table 3-1). A score from -31 to 27 is assigned using appearance of lines or lucencies at both the porous and smooth surfaces, as well as the presence or absence of spot welds, pedestals, calcar modeling, migration, and particle shedding. Revisions on stems with a score of less than -10 usually have gross stem instability, and those with a score between -10 and 0 often have suboptimal fixation such as fibrous ingrowth. The presence of spot welding and bony bridging from the cancellous surface and the porous surface indicate a well-fixed stem.[12] If the spot weld is found distal to an area of stress shielding, it strongly suggests that the stem is well fixed. This is caused by load transfer onto the distal portion of the stem causing relative unloading of the proximal stem. If the stem is not well fixed, there may be pedestal formation at the distal stem tip. This can be incomplete (not spanning from cortex to cortex) or complete (spanning the cortices). This is caused by cancellous hypertrophy at the stem tip trying to provide support to compensate for a lack of stem

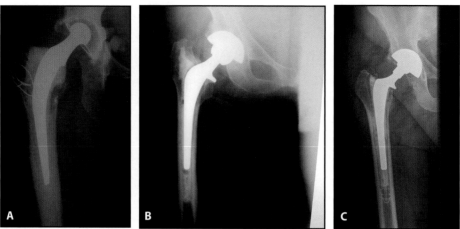

Figure 3-1. (A) Possibly loose cemented stem showing radiolucent lines are present at greater than 50% of the cement-bone interface. (B) Probably loose cemented stem showing radiolucent lines spanning the entire bone-cement interface. (C) Definitely loose cemented stem showing gross stem migration.

fixation. The pedestal may or may not be preceded by a radiolucent line along the stem that also indicates a loosened implant. Cemented femoral stems can be classified radiographically into 3 categories.[13] The most subtle is possible loosening in which radiolucent lines are present at 50% to 100% of the bone-cement interface on either the AP or lateral radiograph. Probable loosening is designated by radiolucent lines spanning the entire bone-cement interface in both the AP and lateral radiograph. Definite loosening can be diagnosed with stem migration, stem fracture, or cement mantle fracture (Figure 3-1).

Loosening of cementless acetabular components is best determined by examining serial radiographs for migration of the cup. Moore et al found that the absence of radiolucent lines, medial bone stress shielding, radial trabeculae, and presence of a superolateral inferomedial buttress were shown to be radiographically significant factors of good acetabular fixation.[14] Gross hardware failure such as fractures of the screws or the cup itself as well as the presence of radiolucent lines is indicative of loosening.

Cemented acetabular components can be classified similarly to cemented femoral stems. Possible loosening is defined by a radiolucency of 50% to 100% of the cement-bone interface; probable loosening features a continuous radiolucent line greater than 2 mm thick, and definite loosening is characterized by cup migration over 5 mm or a crack in the cement mantle. A continuous radiolucent line at the cement-bone interface of a cemented acetabular component predicted a 94% failure rate.[15]

Polyethylene wear and osteolysis can also be diagnosed radiographically. Osteolysis is a macrophage mediated foreign body reaction caused by particulate polyethylene, metal, or polymethylmethacrylate debris. The degree of osteolysis is thought to be related to its contact with a bony surface. Some studies have shown that cemented THAs have a slower rate and lesser risk of osteolysis because the cement acts as a good barrier to the polyethylene debris.[16] When osteolysis does occur, it can be diagnosed radiographically. However, a computed tomography (CT) scan may diagnose osteolysis at a much earlier time, as plain radiographs frequently underestimate the degree of acetabular bone loss. When osteolysis does occur in cemented components, the fibrous layer between the cement and the host bone allows for a linear passage of the particulate debris leading to a linear osteolytic pattern.[17] In cementless components, osteolysis tends to be more focal in nature.[17] Some studies also suggest that circumferential pressed fit stems offer better protection because the porous coating might act as a barrier to debris.[18] Polyethylene wear is difficult to diagnose through radiographs until the wear becomes eccentric, but it should always be suspected in patients with signs of osteolysis.

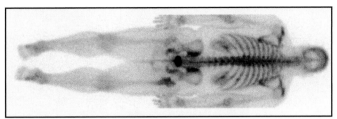

Figure 3-2. A "hot" technetium bone scan in the left hip of this patient increases suspicion for a joint infection.

Infection is not a radiographic diagnosis; however, its diagnosis can be aided by the presence of a lacy periosteal reaction, loss of subchondral sclerosis superior to the acetabular component, and unusual osteolytic lesions. Presence of these signs should increase suspicion of infection, which should be diagnosed by physical exam and laboratory testing.

Other entities that should be noted if present during radiographic examination are heterotopic ossification (HO) and malpositioned hardware. The presence of HO may necessitate adjunctive therapies either pre- or postoperatively from the revision surgery. Minimizing recurrent HO can be accomplished with prophylactic radiation or nonsteroidal anti-inflammatory drugs (NSAIDs). A systemic review of perioperative NSAID use found them to reduce the occurrence of HO by 59% (95% CI 54% to 64%).[19] Radiotherapy was generally more effective perioperatively in preventing HO but had a dose dependant relationship with 6 gy of radiotherapy being equal to NSAIDs and additional doses adding to the efficacy.[20] Once graded, if irradiation is deemed necessary, care must be taken to shield any cementless components and trochanteric osteotomes to prevent loosening and nonunion.[21-23] Intrapelvic screws or acetabular component migration should be noted. If any components violate Kohler's line, further imaging such as a CT scan, angiogram, or magnetic resonance angiography should be considered to determine the hardware proximity to major blood vessels and nervous structures.

CT scans can be important and useful adjunctive tests in the preparation for a revision THA. In cases of recurrent hip instability, one study showed CT imaging to have an intraobserver reliability between 96.8 and 99.9 in determining both acetabular and femoral version and is preferred when precise version is needed in preparation for revision surgery.[24] A clear idea of component version is important in the unstable hip in order to make a decision on which components need to be revised in order to properly treat the patient. In addition, CT scans can assist in quantifying bone loss and identify a pelvic discontinuity. In bone defects suspicious for a pelvic discontinuity on radiograph, CT scans can be used to better quantify the defect and reveal the discontinuity. Internal and external rotation CT scans of the hip can also be employed to detect femoral loosening with good sensitivity and specificity if loosening is not clear on radiographic examination.[25] Soft tissue findings of joint infection such as edema in perimuscular fat and joint distention have good sensitivity and specificity on CT scanning. A study by Cyteval et al found that fluid collections in the perimuscular fat had 100% predictive value and absence of joint distention had a 96% negative predictive value for infection.[26]

In cases where the differentiation between infection and aseptic loosening is not clear, radioisotope scanning can assist in clarifying the diagnosis. Indium[111] tagged white blood cell uptake is sensitive but not specific for infection. Since uptake of Indium[111] also occurs in noninfectious bony remodeling, such as aseptic loosening, it can be combined with technetium-99m scintigraphy. Technetium-99m labeled white blood cells are not taken up in aseptic loosening but are taken up in cases of an infected prosthesis. Combining these studies increases the specificity of the test for diagnosis of infection to 97%.[27,28] If there is no uptake on a technetium-99m scan, a positive Indium[111] scan can lead the physician to be suspicious for aseptic loosening. These 2 nuclear studies together provide a powerful adjunct to radiographs and lab testing to assess aseptic loosening and joint infection (Figure 3-2).

Figure 3-3. The 4 radiographic criteria discussed by Paprosky are superior hip center migration, ischial osteolysis, teardrop osteolysis, and implant position relative to Kohler's line.

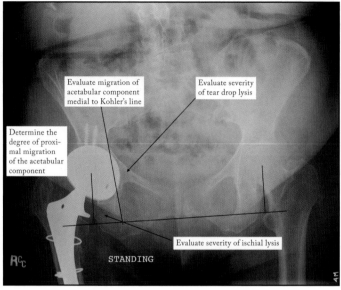

Evaluate migration of acetabular component medial to Kohler's line

Evaluate severity of tear drop lysis

Determine the degree of proximal migration of the acetabular component

Evaluate severity of ischial lysis

R^C_C STANDING

Lab Testing

Laboratory testing plays both a diagnostic and risk stratification role prior to revision hip surgery. Basic lab testing such as hemoglobin, hematocrit, blood chemistries, and total protein and albumin levels are used preoperatively to diagnose anemia, electrolyte imbalances, and nutritional status, all of which are important in the operative patient, and should be corrected prior to any operative intervention.[29-34] Additional preoperative laboratory screening should be patient dependent according to his or her comorbidities and risk factors (ie, blood glucose monitoring in a diabetic). Adjunctive lab tests can be helpful in confirming the diagnosis of an infected hip arthroplasty. Serum white blood cell counts are unreliable in diagnosing infection as it may or may not be elevated.[35,36] ESR and CRP are a relatively inexpensive and effective way to reliably diagnose septic THA and should be used liberally in the preoperative work-up prior to a revision total hip. An ESR greater than 30 mm/hr with a CRP greater than 10 mg/L is a frequently used cut-off for diagnosing infection in a patient suspected of having a septic hip arthroplasty.[37] Using these cut-offs, CRP has a sensitivity of 94% and a specificity of 71%. ESR alone has a sensitivity of 97% and a specificity of 39%. If the ESR and CRP are elevated in a patient with a history and physical consistent with infection, a hip aspiration should be performed, as a synovial white blood cell count offers better sensitivity and specificity over ESR and CRP alone. This should be done under fluoroscopic guidance whenever possible to increase the probability of getting diagnostic fluid. A synovial fluid white blood cell count greater than 3,000 in addition to positive CRP and ESR values increase sensitivity to 90% and specificity to 91% for joint infection.[37]

Management of Bone Loss

Bone deficiency should be thoroughly assessed during the radiographic examination. The surgeon must be prepared with augments, bone grafts, or allograft bone if needed in the revision surgery. For acetabular defects, major classifications include Paprosky, Gross, and American Academy of Orthopaedic Surgeons (AAOS). The Paprosky classification is specifically used for assessing bone loss following previous hip arthroplasty.[38] The 4 radiographic criteria discussed by Paprosky are superior hip center migration, ischial osteolysis, teardrop osteolysis, and implant position relative to Kohler's line (Figure 3-3). Type I defects have an intact rim with no

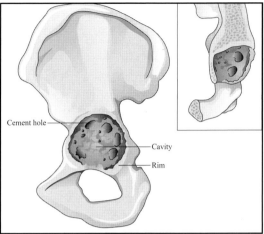

Figure 3-4. Paprosky type I acetabular defect.

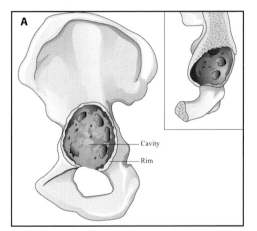

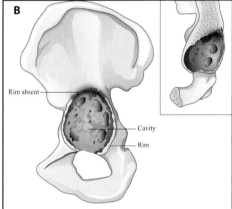

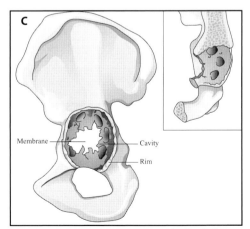

Figure 3-5. Paprosky type II acetabular defect.

distortion and the acetabular component has not migrated. There may be some focal bone loss but the implant is well supported almost entirely with native bone (Figure 3-4). Type II defects are marked by superior cup migration of up to 2 cm and are split into 3 subdivisions (Figure 3-5).

Figure 3-6. Radiograph of Paprosky type IIC acetabular defect.

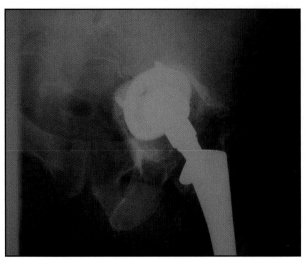

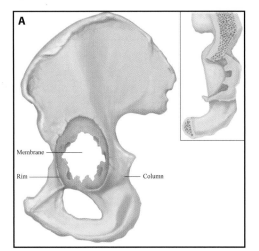
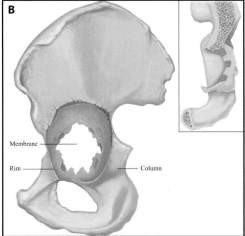

Figure 3-7. Paprosky type III acetabular defect. Note the superior and medial migration of the cup with violation of Kohler's line.

Type IIA defects have a superior and medial pattern of bone loss. The superior rim is intact; however, the component migrates medially into the defect. Type IIB defects have a superior and lateral pattern of bone loss, with less than one-third of the superior rim deficient. In type IIC defects, there is a medial defect and the implant violates Kohler's line with an intact acetabular rim (Figure 3-6). Type III defects have more than 2 cm of cup migration and an unstable acetabular rim, ischial lysis, and teardrop lysis (Figure 3-7). Type IIIA defects have an intact anteromedial wall and adequate host bone for biologic fixation (40% to 60% host bone contact). The defect is between one-third and one-half of the rim and usually located between the 10 o'clock and 2 o'clock positions. The component in a type IIIA defect migrates superiorly and laterally (Figure 3-8). Type IIIB defects lack the adequate host bone required for biologic fixation and stability and more than half of the acetabular rim is deficient. Patients with a type IIIB defect usually have complete destruction of the teardrop, extensive ischial lysis, migration medial to Kohler's line, and are at risk for pelvic discontinuity. The component in a type IIIB defect migrates superiorly and medially (Figure 3-9). Type III defects require the use of allograft, wedges, rings, or cages to achieve adequate intraoperative stability. Planning for such is therefore required and these cases may be among those best suited for referral to an experienced revision specialist.

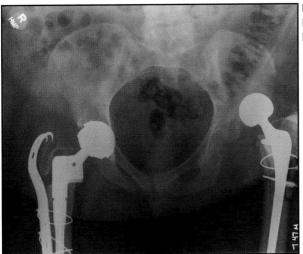

Figure 3-8. Radiograph of Paprosky type IIIA acetabular defect. Note the superior and lateral migration of the cup.

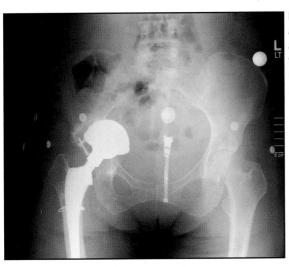

Figure 3-9. Radiograph of Paprosky type IIIB acetabular defect. Note the superior and medial migration of the cup with destruction of the teardrop, extensive ischial lysis, and migration medial to Kohler's line. These patients are at risk for pelvic discontinuity.

The Gross classification is a simple system that may be used to quantify acetabular bone loss as well. Type I is a cavitary or contained defect in which the acetabular walls and columns can still support fixation of a cup or ring. Type II defects are uncontained and involve the acetabular rim and are further quantified into IIA and IIB. Type IIA defects affect no more than 50% of the acetabulum in addition to loss of part of the rim and corresponding wall. Type IIB defects affect more than 50% of the acetabulum including loss of one column and corresponding wall. Type IIB may also be associated with a pelvic discontinuity.

The AAOS classification is divided into 5 categories.[39] Segmental deficiencies (type I) are described as complete loss of bone in the supporting hemisphere of the acetabulum. Cavitary deficiencies (type II) are defined as a volumetric loss in bone substance of the acetabular cavity with retention of an intact rim. These are further subclassified by their location. Type III deficiencies are designated when both type I and type II features coexist. Type IV is added if there is a pelvic discontinuity, and type V is designated for a hip arthrodesis.

AAOS classification for femoral bone loss is similar to that of acetabular loss. Segmental femoral deficiency is defined as loss of bone in the supporting cortex with subcategories based on location of the defect. Cavitary deficiency is divided into cancellous, cortical, and ectasia. Most femoral revisions will have cancellous deficiency. In cortical deficiencies, the endosteum of the

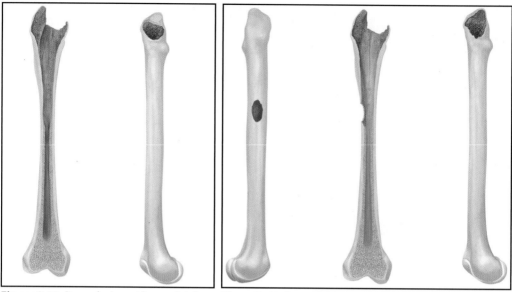

Figure 3-10. Paprosky type I femoral defect.   **Figure 3-11.** Paprosky type II femoral defect.

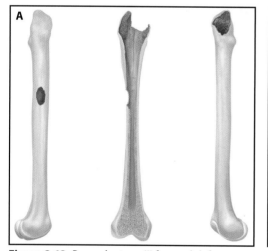

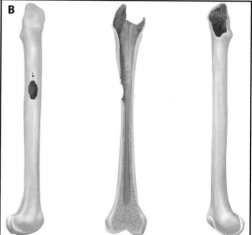

Figure 3-12. Paprosky type III femoral defect.

surrounding cortex is eroded. Ectasia occurs when the femur suffers a complete loss of cancellous bone over time and expands the femur commonly seen in chronic implant failure. Type III is once again a combined segmental and cavitary deficiency. Type IV is alteration of the medullary canal due to femoral malalignment; type V refers to cases of femoral stenosis, and type VI is reserved for frank femoral fractures.

Paprosky et al classify femoral defects as types I through IV. A type I defect involves minimal cancellous bone loss with an intact diaphysis (Figure 3-10). Type II defects involve more extensive cancellous bone loss in metaphysis with an intact diaphysis (Figure 3-11). Type III is divided into 2 subgroups: A and B (Figure 3-12). Type IIIA involves extensive loss of the metaphyseal bone to the point where it cannot support an implant (Figure 3-13). There remains, however, greater than 4 cm of diaphyseal bone that can support a scratch-fit. Type IIIB lacks a supportive metaphysis and less than 4 cm bone remains in the diaphysis for a scratch fit (Figure 3-14). In type IV defects, there is no appreciable isthmus for an uncemented stem to obtain a press-fit (Figure 3-15).

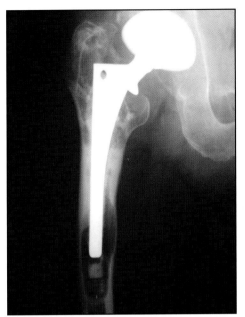

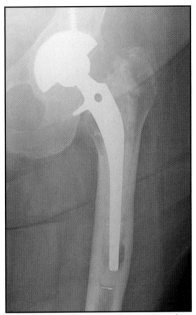

Figure 3-13. Radiograph of Paprosky type IIIA femoral defect.

Figure 3-14. AP radiograph of a Paprosky type II femur with osteolysis and bone loss. Note delamination of the lateral shoulder of the implant consistent with loosening as well.

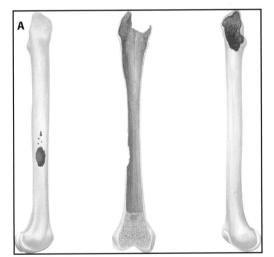

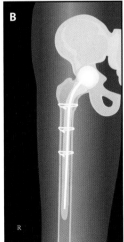

Figure 3-15. (A) Paprosky type IV femoral defect. (B) Radiograph of Paprosky type IV femoral defect. Note there is no appreciable isthmus for an uncemented stem to obtain a press fit.

Using the radiographic techniques described to diagnose bone loss in the arthroplasty patient, the surgeon can have the required augments, bone graft, and any additional tools needed to reconstruct these complicated cases. In the case of Paprosky types I, IIA, and IIB acetabular defects, there is enough bone stock remaining to support a hemispherical shell. Cancellous bone graft can be used when necessary to fill cavitary defects. Paprosky type IIC will usually require cancellous allograft medially in addition to a hemispherical cup impacted onto the remaining intact rim. Type IIIA defects will usually require a hemispherical cup with either a superior distal femoral structural graft (number 7 graft), a bi-lobed acetabular component, or a modular superior augment to provide additional initial support to the acetabular cup. Type IIIB defects without a pelvic discontinuity can be treated with a cage construct, a hemispherical shell with augments, or a custom prosthesis such as a triflange implant. If a pelvic discontinuity is diagnosed, it can be treated in compression with internal plates in addition to a cage construct or porous metal acetabular shell.[40-43] A pelvic discontinuity can also be treated with a novel distraction technique using an oversized trabecular metal shell with or without augments.[44] Whole acetabular transplants as well as custom triflange prostheses have also been employed in the treatment of pelvic discontinuity.[45,46] Implant choices for managing femoral bone loss are covered extensively elsewhere in this text.

PREOPERATIVE TEMPLATING

Acetabular Templating

At this point the history, physical, and radiographic examinations are complete and have led to a clear diagnosis that necessitates revision surgery. The next step is preoperative templating of the patient's hip, which will allow the surgeon to plan out which prostheses best fit the patient's individual anatomy (Figure 3-16). It also allows anticipation of difficulties that may arise intraoperatively so that the surgeon can have the proper tools and components to deal with them. As in primary THAs, the templating process begins with the acetabular component. Using the AP hip radiograph, place the acetabular template to maximize bony contact at the acetabulum. The inferomedial edge should be adjacent to the teardrop. Often in a revision patient, there is acetabular bone loss or lysis and the cup must be placed more proximally to maximize this contact. This is usually offset by using a larger shell to restore the hip center in as close to the anatomical position as possible while still maintaining maximal bony contact with the acetabulum. Once the acetabular component is placed in the appropriate orientation, the amount of lateral "uncoverage" should be noted. If over 20% of the shell is not covered laterally, as in a Paprosky IIIA defect, the surgeon should be prepared intraoperatively to use either a superior augments or a structural bone graft. Sporer et al showed a high success rate using either distal femoral allograft or superior augments in the setting of Paprosky IIIA type defects.[47,48] The optimum angle of cup placement on an AP radiograph is at 45 degrees of verticality. On the lateral radiograph, approximately 20 degrees of cup anteversion is desirable. Vertical cups are at increased risk of polyethylene wear and osteolysis, and incorrect version can increase dislocation risks postoperatively. For type II defects, good long-term results have been reported using a trabecular metal shell since there is adequate host bone available for biologic fixation.[49] If the defect is medial, such as in protrusio acetabuli, or a Paprosky IIC defect, the implant should be templated to be medialized to Kohler's line, however, care must be taken to retain the hip center as excessive medialization can result in failure to restore offset with associated laxity of the hip abductors causing weakness and difficulty ambulating. Likewise, excess lateralization can increase joint reactive forces and muscle tension causing postoperative pain and bursitis. Very large diameter revision cups, or jumbo cups, have been used with good results in an effort to try and maintain maximal bony contact with the acetabulum while maintaining the anatomic hip center.

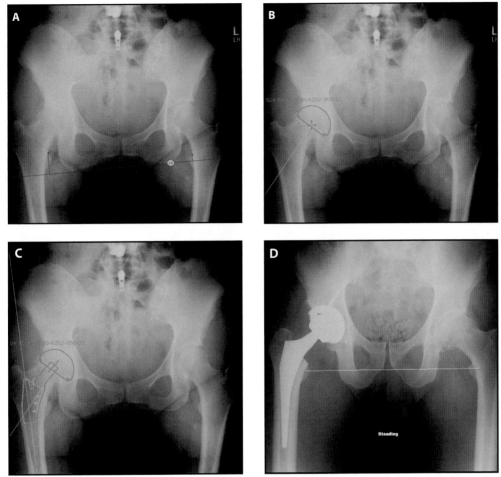

Figure 3-16. Templating. (A) Measurement of the transischial line to determine leg length inequality. (B) Placing the acetabulum to determine the center of rotation. (C) Restoring leg length equality by templating the femoral component. (D) Postoperative radiograph showing restored leg length equality.

Femur Templating

Templating of the femoral component is based off of the center of rotation assigned from templating the acetabulum. Particular goals of femoral templating are determining the type and size of implant that provides axial stability while restoring adequate offset and leg length. To accomplish this, the AP and lateral radiographs must be of good quality as described in the radiographic examination section. Externally rotated radiographs can underestimate the amount of offset and can result in intraoperative instability secondary to bone-bone impingement. If for any reason the leg cannot be placed in the proper 15 degrees of internal rotation, femoral templating should be done using the contralateral hip. In cases where the leg lengths are equal preoperatively, the femoral component can be templated to the center of rotation already established. However, if lengthening is needed, then the femoral template should be placed above the center of rotation by the amount needed to be lengthened. Once the level of the femoral head center is determined, the stem should be templated to allow a good intramedullary fit in the femoral canal. Templating guides for uncemented stems should be measured to allow close ongrowth and ingrowth to the stem. Templating guides for cemented stems have markers showing how much of the canal should be cement and how much should be the stem itself. Once this is measured, the level of the neck cut can be assessed. Stem lengths should be chosen to bypass femoral defects by 2 canal diameters.[50] Cases that require long stems should be carefully templated to the tip of the prosthesis and often require a curve to match the femoral bow. Failing to template the entire long stem prosthesis can result in anterior cortex perforation. Likewise in cases where the anatomy is altered, such as with varus remodeling, long stems should be carefully templated to avoid breaching the cortex intraoperatively. If the latter appears likely, this usually requires an extended trochanteric osteotomy for safe and proper placement of a long-stem femoral prosthesis.[51] Appropriate femoral templating should provide intraoperative options to either lengthen or shorten the construct depending upon the final seating of the femoral component. Consequently, it is advised to template with a +0 neck length in order to offer the surgeon the option of intraoperative adjustment. Extended offset stems are available in many revision systems if extra offset is required.

If a cemented stem is being used, it is desirable to have a 2-mm cement mantle circumferentially around the stem. If an uncemented extensively coated stem is being used, there should be 4 to 6 cm of press-fit bony contact with the diaphyseal bone for adequate fixation. Proximally coated stems are rarely used in revision cases due to proximal bone loss and a subsequent high rate of subsidence. Modular stems can be employed when obtaining adequate axial and rotation stability is difficult to obtain with a monoblock stem. Modular options include a modular proximal sleeve, which can obtain a press-fit in the metaphysis while the stem obtains diaphyseal contact. In cases of more severe bone loss, a modular distally based tapered design can allow distal fixation while proximal body segments can be used to restore leg length, offset, and independently adjust the amount of anteversion. In cases of severe proximal femur bone loss, proximal femoral allograft or proximal femoral replacements can also be considered. Proximal femoral replacements suffer from high complication rates, such as dislocation from poor attachment of the abductors, and proximal femoral allograft carries the risk of disease transmission, infection, and limited healing capacity, though it offers better biologic attachment of the abductor muscle group. These options for management of femoral bone loss are covered extensively elsewhere in this textbook.

Removal of Well-Fixed Components

Once the indication for the revision is made and the new prostheses are templated, the surgeon must be prepared to remove the current acetabular and/or femoral implants. Failure to be prepared for a difficult prosthesis removal can lead to increased operative time, bone loss, iatrogenic fracture, bleeding, and surgeon frustration. The major goal whenever removing any existing hardware is to remove it in its entirety while disrupting as little host bone as possible. In a cemented all-polyethylene liner, the removal should start by disrupting the cement-component interface with a thin curved osteotome.[52] If needed, the acetabular rim can be expanded using a rongeurs or a pencil-tip burr. If the component remains difficult to remove, a high-speed burr can section the implant for piece-by-piece removal. If the component and cement construct are loose, it can be removed by drilling a hole into the cup and using a threaded acetabular extractor in the hole to remove the implant.[52]

When attempting to remove a cementless acetabular shell, first the rim must be exposed. All bony and soft tissue layers covering the rim should be removed. The liner should then be removed. It is important to know what manufacturer makes the cup and liner preoperatively, because some hip systems require special tools to remove them. If these tools are not readily available, an osteotome can be inserted between the metal shell and the liner in order to disrupt to the locking mechanism. Sectioning the liner using a high-speed burr may be necessary in acetabular components with very secure locking mechanisms. Once the liner is out, the screws should be removed if present. If the screw heads are worn and cannot be removed, the screw heads can be burred down, and a screw removal kit can be used to retrieve them. Once the screws are removed, either a trial liner can be used or the previously removed liner can be reinserted. Explant osteotome systems can then be used of varying diameters to remove the well-fixed shell with minimal bone loss.

Alternatively, sequentially longer curved osteotomes can be used to disrupt the bone-prosthesis interface. Other options include using a reciprocating saw that is pre-bent to the shell radius or a high-speed burr can once again be employed to remove the shell in pieces.

Removing a well-fixed cemented stem is achieved by disrupting the stem-cement interface. This can be done using a high-speed pencil-tip burr or an osteotome. Care must be taken to make sure the shoulder and collar of the prosthesis is clear of any bone overgrowth and trochanteric bone before attempting removal. If the cement-prosthesis interface is adequately disrupted, a tamp or extraction device can be used to remove the stem. An extended trochanteric osteotomy or a cortical window may need to be performed to safely remove a cemented stem, especially in cases where there is good distal cement prosthesis bonding. Textured cemented stems are often more difficult to remove than smooth stems and often require an extended trochanteric osteotomy (ETO) as well. When performing an ETO the hip should be placed in internal rotation and extension with the knee flexed to minimize traction on the sciatic nerve. After mobilizing the vastus lateralis anteriorly, the desired osteotomy length should be marked with electrocautery and the cut should be made in a posterolateral to anterolateral orientation, starting anterior to the linea aspera. Using an oscillating saw, angle it medially when making the longitudinal cut to maximize the width of the osteotomy and ensure the entire greater trochanter is released with the osteotomy. When making the distal transverse cut, using a pencil-tip burr and rounding the corners will prevent stress risers and fracture. Wide osteotomes can be used to lever the greater trochanter anteriorly with the vastus lateralis and the abductors. A pencil-tip burr can be used to break up the remaining implant-bone interface distally, and a Gigli saw can be used to free the stem proximally. If necessary, the stem can be transected with a metal cutting burr and the distal stem can be trephined. After the component is removed, the surgeon must diligently remove the remaining cement without removing bone from the femoral canal. Metaphyseal cement is often in large segments and can be broken apart with high-speed burrs and osteotomes and removed. After the metaphyseal cement is removed, the proximal diaphyseal bone can be removed using hooks and osteotomes in a circumferential manner. Distal cement can be removed once the more proximal cement is removed. This can be done with hooks and specialized osteotomes, as well as drills to break the distal cement plug. Care should be taken when drilling to not perforate the cortex. An ultrasonic device can also be employed to extract well-fixed cement, bypass the distal cement plug as well as remove the cement restrictor. If an extended trochanteric osteotomy is done, the cement can simply be removed under direct visualization. Once the cement is removed, the femoral canal should be thoroughly curetted to remove fibrous tissue and expose the endosteal surface for placement of the revision prosthesis.

Removal of a well-fixed cementless stem should begin by identifying whether it is fully coated or proximally coated. Cementless stem fixation can be categorized as stable with bony ingrowth, stable with fibrous ingrowth, and unstable.[52] Unstable stems should have any bony overgrowth and bone superior to the implant shoulder removed prior to attempts at removal. Although a cementless stem may appear unstable, extraction may remain difficult even with appropriate extraction tools. In a stem with bony and fibrous ingrowth, the bone-prosthesis interface should be disrupted using an osteotome. With proximally coated stems, this can be done circumferentially around the femoral neck; however, an extended trochanteric osteotomy may need to be used even in proximally fitted stems.[52] For fully coated stems, osteotomes should be used sequentially distally, breaking the stem-bone interface. If this proves difficult, an extended trochanteric osteotomy will be required. If the stem is still not able to be removed under direct visualization after an extended trochanteric osteotomy, then the stem can be transected with a metal cutting burr and the distal portion can be removed with a trephine.

Well-fixed modular stems can be extremely difficult to remove. Whenever possible, the explants system for the particular modular stem should be used. These systems will allow the proximal body segment to be disengaged from the more distal segment. Often the distal portion of the stem will remain well fixed and a long extended trochanteric osteotomy to the level of the stem tip needs to be performed. This method will allow direct visualization of the prosthesis-bone interface to minimize bone loss.

SUMMARY

Preoperative planning serves multiple purposes in the revision patient. A proper history and physical examination, radiographic interpretation, and selective laboratory test will establish the correct diagnosis and the need for revision surgery in most cases. Careful examination of the preoperative radiographs along with preoperative templating can minimize operative time and surgeon frustration by preparing him or her for potential complications. Having the proper surgical tools, knowledge of component extraction techniques, and appropriate revision prostheses available will decrease operative time, minimize complications, and maximize patient outcomes.

REFERENCES

1. Zhan C, Kaczmarek R, Loyo-Berrios N, Sangl J, Bright RA. Incidence and short-term outcomes of primary and revision hip replacement in the United States. *J Bone Joint Surg Am.* 2007;89(3):526-533.
2. Bozic KJ, Kurtz SM, Lau E, Ong K, Vail TP, Berry DJ. The epidemiology of revision total hip arthroplasty in the United States. *J Bone Joint Surg Am.* 2009;91(1):128-133.
3. Pritchett JW. Lumbar decompression to treat foot drop after hip arthroplasty. *Clin Orthop Relat Res.* 1994(303):173-177.
4. Harris WH. Wear and periprosthetic osteolysis: the problem. *Clin Orthop Relat Res.* 2001(393):66-70.
5. McCollum DE, Gray WJ. Dislocation after total hip arthroplasty. Causes and prevention. *Clin Orthop Relat Res.* 1990;(261):159-170.
6. Turner RS. Postoperative total hip prosthetic femoral head dislocations. Incidence, etiologic factors, and management. *Clin Orthop Relat Res.* 1994;(301):196-204.
7. Bhattacharyya T, Iorio R, Healy WL. Rate of and risk factors for acute inpatient mortality after orthopaedic surgery. *J Bone Joint Surg Am.* 2002;84-A(4):562-572.
8. Jasty M, Schutzer S, Tepper J, Willett C, Stracher MA, Harris WH. Radiation-blocking shields to localize periarticular radiation precisely for prevention of heterotopic bone formation around uncemented total hip arthroplasties. *Clin Orthop Relat Res.* 1990;(257):138-145.
9. Jacobs JJ, Kull LR, Frey GA, et al. Early failure of acetabular components inserted without cement after previous pelvic irradiation. *J Bone Joint Surg Am.* 1995;77(12):1829-1835.
10. Cameron HU. Hip surgery in aortofemoral bypass patients. *Orthop Rev.* 1988;17(2):195-197.
11. Eggli S, Hankemayer S, Muller ME. Nerve palsy after leg lengthening in total replacement arthroplasty for developmental dysplasia of the hip. *J Bone Joint Surg Br.* 1999;81(5):843-845.
12. Engh CA, Massin P, Suthers KE. Roentgenographic assessment of the biologic fixation of porous-surfaced femoral components. *Clin Orthop Relat Res.* 1990;(257):107-128.
13. Harris WH, McCarthy JC, Jr., O'Neill DA. Femoral component loosening using contemporary techniques of femoral cement fixation. *J Bone Joint Surg Am.* 1982;64(7):1063-1067.
14. Moore MS, McAuley JP, Young AM, Engh CA Sr. Radiographic signs of osseointegration in porous-coated acetabular components. *Clin Orthop Relat Res.* 2006;444:176-183.
15. Hodgkinson JP, Shelley P, Wroblewski BM. The correlation between the roentgenographic appearance and operative findings at the bone-cement junction of the socket in Charnley low friction arthroplasties. *Clin Orthop Relat Res.* 1988;(228):105-109.
16. Devane PA, Robinson EJ, Bourne RB, Rorabeck CH, Nayak NN, Horne JG. Measurement of polyethylene wear in acetabular components inserted with and without cement. A randomized trial. *J Bone Joint Surg Am.* 1997;79(5):682-689.
17. Zicat B, Engh CA, Gokcen E. Patterns of osteolysis around total hip components inserted with and without cement. *J Bone Joint Surg Am.* 1995;77(3):432-439.
18. Emerson RH Jr, Sanders SB, Head WC, Higgins L. Effect of circumferential plasma-spray porous coating on the rate of femoral osteolysis after total hip arthroplasty. *J Bone Joint Surg Am.* 1999;81(9):1291-1298.
19. Fransen M, Neal B. Non-steroidal anti-inflammatory drugs for preventing heterotopic bone formation after hip arthroplasty. *Cochrane Database Syst Rev.* 2004(3):CD001160.
20. Pakos EE, Ioannidis JP. Radiotherapy vs. nonsteroidal anti-inflammatory drugs for the prevention of heterotopic ossification after major hip procedures: a meta-analysis of randomized trials. *Int J Radiat Oncol Biol Phys.* 2004;60(3):888-895.
21. Brooker AF, Bowerman JW, Robinson RA, Riley LH Jr. Ectopic ossification following total hip replacement. Incidence and a method of classification. *J Bone Joint Surg Am.* 1973;55(8):1629-1632.

22. Schneider DJ, Moulton MJ, Singapuri K, et al. The Frank Stinchfield Award. Inhibition of heterotopic ossification with radiation therapy in an animal model. *Clin Orthop Relat Res.* 1998;(355):35-46.

23. Pellegrini VD Jr, Gregoritch SJ. Preoperative irradiation for prevention of heterotopic ossification following total hip arthroplasty. *J Bone Joint Surg Am.* 1996;78(6):870-881.

24. Ghelman B, Kepler CK, Lyman S, Della Valle AG. CT outperforms radiography for determination of acetabular cup version after THA. *Clin Orthop Relat Res.* 2009;467(9):2362-2370.

25. Berger R, Fletcher F, Donaldson T, Wasielewski R, Peterson M, Rubash H. Dynamic test to diagnose loose uncemented femoral total hip components. *Clin Orthop Relat Res.* 1996;(330):115-123.

26. Cyteval C, Hamm V, Sarrabere MP, Lopez FM, Maury P, Taourel P. Painful infection at the site of hip prosthesis: CT imaging. *Radiology.* 2002;224(2):477-483.

27. Palestro CJ, Kim CK, Swyer AJ, Capozzi JD, Solomon RW, Goldsmith SJ. Total-hip arthroplasty: periprosthetic Indium[111]-labeled leukocyte activity and complementary technetium-99m-sulfur colloid imaging in suspected infection. *J Nucl Med.* 1990;31(12):1950-1955.

28. Deirmengian C, Hallab N, Tarabishy A, et al. Synovial fluid biomarkers for periprosthetic infection. *Clin Orthop Relat Res.* 2010;468(8):2017-2023.

29. Patterson BM, Cornell CN, Carbone B, Levine B, Chapman D. Protein depletion and metabolic stress in elderly patients who have a fracture of the hip. *J Bone Joint Surg Am.* 1992;74(2):251-260.

30. Marin LA, Salido JA, Lopez A, Silva A. Preoperative nutritional evaluation as a prognostic tool for wound healing. *Acta Orthop Scand.* 2002;73(1):2-5.

31. Lavernia CJ, Sierra RJ, Baerga L. Nutritional parameters and short term outcome in arthroplasty. *J Am Coll Nutr.* 1999;18(3):274-278.

32. Greene KA, Wilde AH, Stulberg BN. Preoperative nutritional status of total joint patients. Relationship to postoperative wound complications. *J Arthroplasty.* 1991;6(4):321-325.

33. Gherini S, Vaughn BK, Lombardi AV Jr, Mallory TH. Delayed wound healing and nutritional deficiencies after total hip arthroplasty. *Clin Orthop Relat Res.* 1993;(293):188-195.

34. Del Savio GC, Zelicof SB, Wexler LM, et al. Preoperative nutritional status and outcome of elective total hip replacement. *Clin Orthop Relat Res.* 1996;(326):153-161.

35. Canner GC, Steinberg ME, Heppenstall RB, Balderston R. The infected hip after total hip arthroplasty. *J Bone Joint Surg Am.* 1984;66(9):1393-1399.

36. Spangehl MJ, Masri BA, O'Connell JX, Duncan CP. Prospective analysis of preoperative and intraoperative investigations for the diagnosis of infection at the sites of two hundred and two revision total hip arthroplasties. *J Bone Joint Surg Am.* 1999;81(5):672-683.

37. Schinsky MF, Della Valle CJ, Sporer SM, Paprosky WG. Perioperative testing for joint infection in patients undergoing revision total hip arthroplasty. *J Bone Joint Surg Am.* 2008;90(9):1869-1875.

38. Valle CJ, Paprosky WG. Classification and an algorithmic approach to the reconstruction of femoral deficiency in revision total hip arthroplasty. *J Bone Joint Surg Am.* 2003;85-A(Suppl 4):1-6.

39. D'Antonio JA, Capello WN, Borden LS, et al. Classification and management of acetabular abnormalities in total hip arthroplasty. *Clin Orthop Relat Res.* 1989;(243):126-137.

40. Berry DJ, Lewallen DG, Hanssen AD, Cabanela ME. Pelvic discontinuity in revision total hip arthroplasty. *J Bone Joint Surg Am.* 1999;81(12):1692-1702.

41. Berry DJ. Identification and management of pelvic discontinuity. *Orthopedics.* 2001;24(9):881-882.

42. Della Valle CJ, Berger RA, Rosenberg AG, Galante JO. Cementless acetabular reconstruction in revision total hip arthroplasty. *Clin Orthop Relat Res.* 2004;(420):96-100.

43. Paprosky W, Sporer S, O'Rourke MR. The treatment of pelvic discontinuity with acetabular cages. *Clin Orthop Relat Res.* 2006;453:183-187.

44. Sporer SM, Paprosky WG. Acetabular revision using a trabecular metal acetabular component for severe acetabular bone loss associated with a pelvic discontinuity. *J Arthroplasty.* 2006;21(6 Suppl 2):87-90.

45. DeBoer DK, Christie MJ, Brinson MF, Morrison JC. Revision total hip arthroplasty for pelvic discontinuity. *J Bone Joint Surg Am.* 2007;89(4):835-840.

46. Holt GE, Dennis DA. Use of custom triflanged acetabular components in revision total hip arthroplasty. *Clin Orthop Relat Res.* 2004;(429):209-214.

47. Sporer SM, Paprosky WG. The use of a trabecular metal acetabular component and trabecular metal augment for severe acetabular defects. *J Arthroplasty.* 2006;21(6 Suppl 2):83-86.

48. Sporer SM, O'Rourke M, Chong P, Paprosky WG. The use of structural distal femoral allografts for acetabular reconstruction. Average ten-year follow-up. *J Bone Joint Surg Am.* 2005;87(4):760-765.

49. Park DK, Della Valle CJ, Quigley L, Moric M, Rosenberg AG, Galante JO. Revision of the acetabular component without cement. A concise follow-up, at twenty to twenty-four years, of a previous report. *J Bone Joint Surg Am.* 2009;91(2):350-355.

50. Maurer SG, Baitner AC, Di Cesare PE. Reconstruction of the failed femoral component and proximal femoral bone loss in revision hip surgery. *J Am Acad Orthop Surg.* 2000;8(6):354-363.

51. Della Valle CJ, Paprosky WG. The femur in revision total hip arthroplasty evaluation and classification. *Clin Orthop Relat Res.* 2004;(420):55-62.

52. Paprosky WG, Martin EL. Removal of well-fixed femoral and acetabular components. *Am J Orthop (Belle Mead NJ).* 2002;31(8):476-478.

4

Surgical Exposure in Revision Total Hip Arthroplasty

Robert M. Cercek, MD

One of the most important components of the preoperative surgical plan for revision total hip arthroplasty (THA) is selection of the most appropriate surgical approach. The ideal approach should provide sufficient exposure of all surgical components, surrounding bone stock, and any bone defects that may be present. It must also account for and protect the important surrounding neurovascular structures. In addition, it should not result in uncontrolled bone or soft tissue damage during implant removal. Adequately planned incisions and extensile techniques that can be properly repaired are always preferable over unpredictable, iatrogenic injury. The exposure should also avoid unnecessary devascularization of bone, particularly in the face of infection, as devascularized bone will serve as a nidus for harboring ongoing infection.

For simple revision procedures, one of the standard approaches commonly utilized in primary THA generally will provide adequate surgical exposure. More complex revision cases may necessitate a more extensive technique developed specifically for revision THA. No single surgical approach is indicated for all revision procedures; therefore, the revision surgeon should be comfortable with all possible surgical approaches. Before embarking on revision THA, several key factors must be considered. These factors include the following:

- The presence of previous surgical incisions
- The indication for the revision procedure
- The type of implant currently in place and the type of implant to be used for the revision procedure
- The presence of acetabular or femoral bone loss

The first consideration is the location of previous skin incision(s). The approach should utilize as much of the prior incision as possible without unduly compromising the surgical exposure in order to minimize additional soft tissue scarring. Multiple skin incisions also increase the risk of wound edge necrosis. There is a tendency for a laterally based hip incision to migrate posteriorly over time. However, there is generally sufficient skin and soft tissue laxity surrounding the hip to allow use of a less than ideally placed prior incision. Care must be taken to then make the correct fascial incision. In this regard, the deep dissection is also ideally best performed along the route of the previous surgical exposure. This decision may depend upon the proper execution and subsequent healing of the prior incision. An effort should be made to maintain remaining

Jacofsky DJ, Hedley AK.
Fundamentals of Revision Hip Arthroplasty:
Diagnosis, Evaluation, and Treatment (pp 51-66).
© 2013 SLACK Incorporated.

normal tissue planes whenever possible. For instance, a poorly healed anterolateral approach may be the most appropriate route for the revision procedure, as a proper repair may be performed at the completion of the procedure, and the remaining intact posterior tissues will not be compromised in addition to the already compromised anterior tissues. Similarly, a nonunited greater trochanter may provide an obvious route of access to the hip.

The next consideration is the indication for the revision procedure. Common indications include aseptic loosening of one or both components, extensive osteolysis, recurrent dislocation, and periprosthetic infection. In all cases other than aseptic loosening, the surgical implants may be solidly fixed at the time of revision. This must be taken into account when selecting the surgical approach. In the case of an acute postoperative infection, the prior surgical approach should be reused. In the case of a chronically infected prosthesis, the surgical approach should take into account the need to remove all foreign material and infected or necrotic tissue, while avoiding devascularization of viable, healthy tissue. This may necessitate advanced techniques to remove material from areas not readily accessible via ordinary exposure, such as inside the pelvis or femoral shaft. This may also be the case in revision being performed for débridement of osteolysis, and the approach chosen will depend upon whether the components are cemented or press-fit and whether or not they are solidly fixed.

Special consideration should be given to the surgical approach when planning a revision for the unstable, recurrently dislocating hip. The soft tissue structures that lend stability to the hip joint must be respected, especially the abductors. The direction of instability should be clearly delineated from the history and physical examination and from examination under anesthesia during closed reduction(s) of the unstable hip. The instability may be anterior, posterior, or multidirectional. This will aid in determining whether preservation of the anterior or the posterior soft tissue envelope is more important during the surgical exposure.

The next consideration will be the type and stability of the implant to be removed. The design of the acetabular component will not usually influence the surgical approach, as circumferential visualization is required for removal of all acetabular components, regardless of design. More extensive exposure of the outer table of the ilium may be required if a reconstruction cage is to be inserted or removed or if reconstruction of a superolateral or posterior column deficiency will be necessary. The main factor to consider will be the design type and stability of the retained femoral component. When a loose, cemented femoral stem is being revised, solidly bonded cement will often remain in the femoral canal after the prosthesis has been removed. There may be a long column of cement extending distally from the tip of the original implant if an intramedullary cement restrictor was not used during the previous procedure. The need to remove this cement should be determined during preoperative planning depending upon the possible presence of infection and the type of revision femoral stem to be inserted. If the removal of solidly fixed distal cement is deemed necessary, consideration should be given to more extensive exposure to improve visualization of the bone-cement interface, as the risk of damage and perforation of the femoral shaft is considerable when an attempt is made to remove solidly fixed distal cement from above.

The removal of osseointegrated cementless femoral stems requires a familiarity with the particular stem design. The preoperative x-rays should be scrutinized for the location and extent of the ingrowth/ongrowth surface, the modularity of the prosthesis, the presence or absence of a collar, and the level at which the metaphyseal flare of the prosthesis joins the more tubular distal end. An extended trochanteric osteotomy is often necessary when removing a solidly fixed cementless stem. The osteotomy should be extended past the distal extent of the porous coating in order to minimize the risk of damage to femoral bone stock. Even in cases where the stem does not appear to be solidly osseointegrated on preoperative radiographs, dense fibrous ingrowth may still be present,[1] and the extended trochanteric osteotomy may be necessary for the removal of this stem. Cemented stems which have been precoated with methyl methacrylate also can cause difficulty during revision, and this design should be identified during preoperative planning if possible. These stems are designed to achieve a very rigid bond within the cement mantle. When this stem is solidly fixed, it can be extremely difficult to remove from above, as it will not debond from the cement. Removal of a solidly fixed precoated stem usually will require extensive visualization of the cement mantle, which is most readily achieved via the extended trochanteric osteotomy.

The next factor in consideration of the surgical exposure is the amount of bone loss in the proximal femur and acetabulum. A failed THA may be associated with significant bone loss as a result of osteolysis, infection, component migration, prior surgeries, or stress shielding of the proximal femur. The surgical exposure must allow for adequate access for these deficiencies to be properly addressed. Multiple classification systems for the assessment of acetabular bone loss have been described. These systems have shown poor intra- and interobserver agreement,[2] and their ability to provide statistically reliable information for preoperative assessment has been questioned. However, regardless of classification of the acetabular defect, the widest exposure of the acetabulum is provided by the standard trochanteric osteotomy with proximal retraction of the trochanteric fragment and the attached abductor muscles. While this technique has in large part given way to the extended trochanteric osteotomy, it may still be indicated in the case of significant medial migration of the femur and acetabular component into the pelvis. The sciatic nerve can become very superficial secondary to medial femoral migration, and great care must be taken to avoid it. The trochanteric osteotomy, regardless of type, will provide the widest exposure of the superolateral rim of the acetabulum when required for the placement of a reconstruction cage or bulk allograft.[3]

The femur may also be affected by a range of bony defects, including ectasia, stenosis, malalignment from loosening, fracture, or osteotomy, and cavitary, segmental, or combined defects.[4] The surgeon should have a low threshold for more comprehensive exposure of the femur in revision THA. In a matter of minutes, the femoral shaft can be readily visualized through anterior mobilization of the vastus lateralis and an extended trochanteric osteotomy, and potentially serious unnecessary damage to the femoral shaft can be avoided.

The final factor to consider in planning the surgical approach in revision THA is the previous training, familiarity, and preferences of the individual operating surgeon. Most surgeons will be most familiar and confident with a single surgical approach, which will generally be the technique to which the surgeon was most widely exposed to during residency and/or fellowship training. This will most likely be the approach that the surgeon will choose to utilize in the revision setting. However, it cannot be overemphasized that no singular surgical approach is the most appropriate approach for all revision THAs. The sound revision THA surgeon must be well trained and familiar with the full range of surgical approaches to the hip so that the most appropriate one can be used in each individual revision case.

Common Surgical Approaches to the Hip

All approaches used for primary THA can be used for revision surgery. The requirement for a more extensive exposure becomes much more important, however, in the revision setting. We will review each of the standard approaches below, and discuss the advantages and disadvantages to their use, as well as the ease with which each can be converted into a more extensive surgical approach.

Anterolateral Approach to the Hip

The anterolateral approach to the hip is derived from the Watson-Jones approach that was described for the treatment of hip fractures in 1935,[5] and was popularized for use in arthroplasty in the 1970s by Charnley, Harris, and Müller.[6] The approach exploits the intermuscular plane between the tensor fascia lata and the gluteus medius. For the anterolateral approach (and revision THA in general), the patient is placed in the lateral decubitus position, with the operative leg draped free. The leg is then flexed approximately 30 degrees, which will bring the tensor fascia lata anteriorly. The skin incision is centered over the tip of the greater trochanter, and is gently curved posteriorly as it passes superior to the tip of the trochanter. The subcutaneous fat is incised in line with the skin incision to reach the deep fascia of the thigh. A lap sponge can be used to gently tease the fat from the fascia lata for better visualization. Once visualization and orientation is achieved, starting at the tip of the trochanter, the fascia lata is incised in line with the shaft of femur heading distally, and the gluteus maximus muscle fibers are bluntly separated in line with the skin incision proximally. Blunt dissection is used to develop the interval between the tensor fascia lata and the underlying gluteus medius, and then a Charnley retractor is placed deep to retract the tensor fascia lata anteriorly.

The anterior and posterior borders of the gluteus medius are then identified, and the anterior 40% to 50% of the tendinous attachment to the trochanter is elevated with the use of a curving periosteal incision. A split is made proximally in the line of the gluteus medius muscle fibers for 3 to 4 cm. Further proximal dissection should be avoided in order to avoid injury to the superior gluteal nerve. Placing the limb in a position of flexion, adduction, and external rotation will place the anterior capsule on stretch, making the capsule easier to identify and dissect. This position also will move the femoral neurovascular structures anteriorly, lessening the risk that they will be injured during the approach. The anterior hip capsule is then incised with a longitudinal incision in line with the femoral neck. This is then converted into a T- or H-shaped capsulotomy for later capsular repair, or alternatively, the capsule may be excised. The hip is then dislocated anteriorly by further flexing and externally rotating the adducted limb. The limb is brought over the edge of the operating table and placed in the sterile pocket of the drape.

Further exposure will be dictated by the nature of the revision procedure being performed. Acetabular exposure will be readily available with the placement of Homan-type retractors anteriorly, posteriorly, and superiorly. Care must be taken during placement of the anterior retractor to stay directly on bone and not pierce the iliopsoas muscle belly, as the femoral neurovascular bundle lies on this muscle's superficial surface. The acetabular exposure that is obtained facilitates accurate placement of the prosthetic acetabular component, which likely contributes in part to the historically reported lower dislocation rate associated with this approach as compared to the posterior approach.[7-9] However, the anterolateral approach provides relatively poor access to the posterior column of the acetabulum and is therefore not recommended if complex reconstruction of the posterior column will be required. Other advantages of the anterolateral approach include avoidance of direct exposure of the sciatic nerve, possibly reducing the risk of iatrogenic nerve damage, and preservation of the posterior soft tissue structures.

Disadvantages of the anterolateral approach include the potential risk of injury to the superior gluteal nerve and a slower recovery of abductor strength and function. The issues of abductor dysfunction and gait abnormalities are largely theoretical, however, and have not been substantiated in randomized controlled trials. The incidence of limp is 0% to 16% for the posterior approach and 4% to 20% for the anterolateral approach.[7,8] Ritter et al[10] directly compared the postoperative gait between the anterolateral and posterolateral approach and could not demonstrate a statistically significant difference between the 2 groups. However, Madsen et al[11] examined the gait pattern of THA patients 6 months after surgery compared to control patients without hip pathology. Their study demonstrated that 30% of patients who underwent THA via the posterior approach had a normal gait pattern, whereas none of the patients who underwent THA via the anterolateral approach had a normal gait pattern.

Another disadvantage of the anterolateral approach is its nonextensive nature. Proximal dissection is limited by the risk of damage to the superior gluteal nerve, which restricts extended exposure of the acetabulum. The proximal femoral shaft can be accessed only through extensive muscle stripping and devascularization, which limits the usefulness of the exposure in the removal of well-fixed femoral stems or débridement of osteolysis or infection. In addition, adequate access to the femoral canal can result in iatrogenic damage to the substance of the gluteus medius muscle fibers that are still attached to the posterior aspect of the greater trochanter. For all the reasons listed above, the anterolateral approach is largely reserved for simple revisions or revisions in which the femoral component will be retained. For more complex reconstructions, strong consideration should be given to one of the approaches listed below.

MODIFIED LATERAL APPROACH TO THE HIP

Multiple modifications of the anterolateral approach have been described which involve detaching a portion of the gluteus medius in continuity with the vastus lateralis. McFarland and Osborne[12] first described this modification in 1954. Their technique involved detaching the gluteus medius in its entirety, but maintaining the periosteal sleeve overlying the greater trochanter in continuity with the vastus lateralis, thus providing the potential for better postoperative abductor function. This approach was later modified by Hardinge,[13] who stressed the advantage of preserving the attachment of the thick posterior portion of the gluteus medius tendon to the greater trochanter.

The superficial exposure for the Hardinge approach is performed in a similar fashion to the anterolateral approach as described above. The gluteus medius is then split in line with its muscle fibers, taking care to detach no more than the anterior 50% of the muscle belly. Once again, the split should not be extended more than 3 to 4 cm proximal to the tip of the greater trochanter to avoid injury to the superior gluteal nerve. This split is then extended distally over the greater trochanter into the vastus lateralis, encompassing the anterior 40% to 50% of the vastus lateralis. This musculotendinous sleeve is then elevated in a subperiosteal fashion off the bone and is reflected anteriorly, providing excellent exposure of the joint. The insertion of the gluteus minimus will then need to be detached from the anterior aspect of the greater trochanter. The exposure can be extended distally as necessary by extending the vastus lateralis split down the lateral femoral shaft.

Multiple variations of this technique have been described that vary on the location of the longitudinal split in the musculotendinous sleeve overlying the greater trochanter. Distal extension of the vastus split reduces the risk of inadvertent proximal extension, thus reducing the risk of injury to the superior gluteal nerve. Osteotomy of an anterior wafer of greater trochanteric bone can aid in the reattachment of the gluteus medius and vastus lateralis musculotendinous sleeve.[14] At the superior rim of the acetabulum, additional exposure of the outer aspect of the ilium can be safely achieved through elevation of the gluteal musculature off the bone (as compared to additional proximal splitting of the gluteus medius).

The modified lateral approach can provide adequate exposure in revision THA when a reasonable soft tissue envelope exists between the pelvis and the proximal femur. This approach has the advantage, similar to the standard anterolateral approach, of avoiding the potentially higher dislocation rate classically attributed to the posterior approach.[7] Another additional advantage is the ability to extend this approach into an extended trochanteric osteotomy.[15] Potential drawbacks of the Hardinge approach in THA include the following:

- Difficulty in achieving wide exposure of the posterior column of the acetabulum (unless a supplementary subfascial plane is developed behind the femur and posterior border of the abductors)
- Inability to adjust abductor muscle tension
- Difficulty with advancement of the abductors if lengthening of more than 1 cm is accomplished
- Increased incidence of prolonged abductor weakness and limp[16]
- The potential for damage to the superior gluteal nerve
- A higher incidence of heterotopic bone formation[8]

This approach is unsuitable when the need for more than 1 cm of lengthening is anticipated. The risk of prolonged abductor weakness is related partly to damage to the inferior branches of the superior gluteal nerve,[17] and partly to avulsion of the tendon repair.[18] The superior gluteal nerve passes approximately 5 cm above the tip of the greater trochanter; every effort should be made to avoid splitting the gluteus medius muscle fibers above this point.

Posterior Approach to the Hip

The posterior approach to the hip was first described by Langenbeck. His description involved an incision extending from the posterior-superior iliac spine to the posterior border of the greater trochanter. Kocher later described shifting the incision to the anterior aspect of the trochanter and then continuing distally 10 to 12 cm along the axis of the femoral shaft. The Kocher-Langenbeck approach was popularized for use in pelvic fracture surgery. The distal end was subsequently modified by extending it more posterior to improve the exposure. The proximal incision was also moved to the upper border of the gluteus maximus to preserve muscle function. The approach was popularized for use in THA by Moore.[19] Moore termed this the Southern exposure, as he considered the best exposure for an operating room to be facing the south.

The patient is positioned in the lateral decubitus position as described above. A curvilinear incision is then made along the greater trochanter. The proximal portion begins 5 to 6 cm proximal and posterior to the greater trochanter. This will run in line with the fibers of the gluteus maximus. At the tip of the trochanter, the incision is carried distally in line with the posterior half of the femoral shaft. If the hip is flexed to 90 degrees and a straight line is drawn over the posterior aspect of the trochanter, it will curve into the desired incision when the limb is brought straight. The exact length of the incision will vary depending on the nature of the revision being performed.

The fascia lata is then incised over the lateral aspect of the femur, uncovering the underlying vastus lateralis. The fascial split is extended proximally in line with the skin incision, and the fibers of the gluteus maximus are separated by blunt dissection. The fascial covering of the gluteus maximus can be quite thin, especially in the elderly patient. The gluteus maximus receives its blood supply from the superior and inferior gluteal arteries, which enter from the deep surface of the muscle, and then splay out in a radial pattern; hence, splitting the muscle inevitably causes some arterial and venous bleeding. This split does not denervate the muscle, however, as the nerve supply enters well medial to this split. The fascial layers are then held with deep Charnley retractors, and the hip is internally rotated by the surgeon's assistant, exposing the posterolateral aspect of the hip joint. Internal rotation will put the short external rotators on stretch, and will also pull the operative field away from the posteriorly based sciatic nerve.

There may be fat overlying the short external rotators; this should bluntly be retracted posteromedially to expose their tendinous insertion into the greater trochanter. The sciatic nerve will lie within the substance of the fatty tissue; it can be palpated, but should not be dissected out unless necessary. Stay sutures can be inserted into the piriformis and obturator internus tendons if desired, and then the tendons are peeled directly off the trochanteric insertion. The short rotators are then reflected backward over the sciatic nerve, protecting it during the remainder of the procedure. The quadratus femoris lies distal to the short rotators, and may also need to be released from its femoral insertion depending on the extent of the revision procedure being performed. This muscle contains ascending branches of the lateral femoral circumflex artery; vigorous bleeding can be encountered when this muscle is released. The posterior capsule of the hip joint is then exposed, if still present, and can be incised or excised according to surgeon preference. The posterior capsulotomy will expose the femoral head and neck; the hip is then dislocated through further internal rotation of the limb.

The posterior approach has the advantage of minimal disturbance to the abductor mechanism, which likely contributes in large part to the excellent functional outcomes and decreased gait disturbance.[11,16] There is a lower rate of heterotopic ossification (HO) when performing the posterior approach when compared to the anterolateral and modified lateral approaches.[20] The posterior approach provides excellent visualization of the posterior wall and column of the acetabulum and the proximal femur. Finally, the posterior approach can be extended distally into a trochanteric slide or extended trochanteric osteotomy whenever necessary.

The main disadvantage of the posterior approach is the historically reported higher rate of postoperative dislocation.[7-10] This is due in part to potential loss of the integrity of the posterior joint capsule and short external rotators, and also due to the tendency to place the acetabular component in insufficient anteversion due to insufficient anterior retraction of the femur. One large meta-analysis which included data from 13,203 primary THAs showed a 3% dislocation rate for the posterior approach compared to a 2% rate for the anterolateral approach and a 0.5% dislocation rate for the direct lateral approach.[21] The authors urged caution when selecting the posterior approach over the direct lateral approach for primary THA. A subsequent review published in the Cochrane Database with more stringent inclusion criteria, however, found no statistically significant difference in the dislocation rates between the posterior and direct lateral surgical approach.[22] The authors concluded that the data were insufficient to recommend any one technique as the optimal surgical approach for primary THA. This conclusion has been substantiated by other studies that have demonstrated no effect of the surgical approach on the postoperative dislocation rate.[23,24]

Furthermore, recent studies have shown that with sufficient posterior soft tissue repair, the incidence of postoperative dislocation with the posterior approach for primary THA has been reduced to 1% to 2% and is comparable with the dislocation rates for the anterolateral and direct lateral surgical approaches.[21,25,26] This has also been studied in the revision THA setting. Suh et al,[27] in a retrospective study, reported a dislocation rate of 10% following revision THA prior to posterior soft tissue repair, and this was reduced to 2% after posterior soft tissue repair was added to their surgical technique.

Several different methods of posterior soft tissue repair have been described, all of which appear to be effective. Generally, the capsule is either sewn together or reattached to bone at the insertion into the greater trochanter. The short external rotators are reattached either in conjunction with the capsule or separately into the posterior aspect of the greater trochanter. The repair should be performed with nonabsorbable suture and through transosseous tunnels if possible. A cadaveric study[28] demonstrated that transosseous repair was superior with regard to torsion strength, and the magnitude of the angle of rotation prior to dislocation increased by 83% compared with that of no repair, and it increased by 46% compared with that of soft tissue repair without transosseous tunnels. Complications reported with this technique include external rotation contractures, failure of the repair, and avulsion of a portion of the trochanter. These complications, however, have relatively low associated morbidity.

TRANSTROCHANTERIC APPROACH TO THE HIP

The term *transtrochanteric* implies that an osteotomy of the greater trochanter is performed. The routine use of a trochanteric osteotomy in primary THA was popularized by Charnley[29] in the 1970s. Its routine use in primary THA has declined for multiple reasons, including symptomatic hardware, increased surgical time, increased blood loss, nonunion, and proximal trochanteric migration. However, the trochanteric osteotomy is an extensive approach that remains a valuable tool for difficult primary and revision THAs. Attempts to remove a solidly ingrown femoral stem, extensive cement, or a broken femoral stem can result in serious damage to the remaining bone stock and can jeopardize the revision procedure. A trochanteric osteotomy can facilitate hip dislocation, acetabular exposure, femoral component extraction, and access to the proximal femur. It also affords the ability to adjust the tension and offset of the abductors and allows increased exposure of the hip without excessive torque applied to the femur, which is at risk for fracture in patients with extensive osteolysis or osteoporosis.

Figure 4-1. The paths of the standard trochanteric osteotomy (A), the trochanteric slide (B), and the extended trochanteric osteotomy (C). Note that the trochanteric slide and the extended trochanteric osteotomy incorporate the origin of the vastus lateralis muscle, but the standard osteotomy does not. (© 2003 American Academy of Orthopaedic Surgeons. Reprinted with permission from the *Journal of the American Academy of Orthopaedic Surgeons*, Volume 11[3], p. 164.)

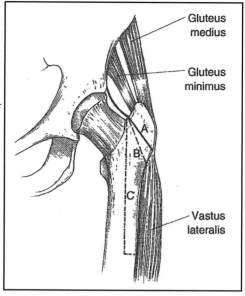

The level of the trochanteric osteotomy can be categorized into 3 basic types:

1. The standard single-plane osteotomy and its modifications (ie, chevron, partial, horizontal, vertical)[30]
2. The trochanteric slide
3. The extended trochanteric osteotomy (Figure 4-1)

Fixation options include wires or cables, with or without claws, trochanteric bolts, and cable plates with a proximal claw. Each type of trochanteric osteotomy has relatively unique indications, contraindications, and complications. Individual variations of each technique and multiple fixation methods have been developed, providing options to enhance the effectiveness of trochanteric osteotomy during revision THA.

Standard Trochanteric Osteotomy

Indications for the standard trochanteric osteotomy are now relatively rare. One indication is the case of lax abductor musculature after THA or revision THA with resulting global instability. This can generally be avoided with appropriate restoration of the anatomic hip center, leg length, and offset. Occasionally, however, despite these measures, a lax abductor mechanism may still be present. If adjustments in modular implants such as offset and lipped acetabular liners, offset femoral stems, and longer neck lengths do not provide sufficient stability without excessive lengthening, a standard trochanteric osteotomy with distal advancement can be performed (a trochanteric slide may still be preferable, however). A second indication for the standard trochanteric osteotomy is the need for extensive acetabular exposure, such as during implantation of an antiprotrusio cage with a large flange on the ilium. The trochanteric osteotomy, along with superior retraction of the abductor muscles, provides excellent acetabular and pelvic exposure, allows avoidance of excessive torque on the proximal femur, and avoids excessive tension on the superior gluteal neurovascular bundle. However, this can generally be performed with the trochanteric slide or extended trochanteric osteotomy, which both maintain the continuity of the abductor mechanism. A relative contraindication to the standard trochanteric osteotomy is its use with the anterolateral or modified lateral approach, because a portion of the abductor mechanism has already been released from the greater trochanter prior to the osteotomy being performed. This makes subsequent abductor

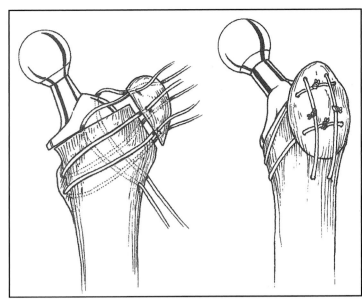

Figure 4-2. The 4-wire technique of fixation of the trochanteric osteotomy. (© 1996 American Academy of Orthopaedic Surgeons. Reprinted with permission from the *Journal of the American Academy of Orthopaedic Surgeons*, Volume 4[5], p. 260.)

muscle repair difficult and tenuous. Therefore, if a trochanteric osteotomy is anticipated, the posterior approach is preferred.

Exposure for the standard trochanteric osteotomy is done by releasing the proximal portion of the vastus lateralis muscle origin, exposing the underlying vastus tubercle. A blunt instrument is inserted over the superior femoral neck in the interval between the joint capsule and the gluteus medius. The osteotomy is begun distally on the lateral femur with an oscillating saw or osteotome, and is extended in a proximal-medial direction at an angle of 45 degrees to the femoral shaft. Once the osteotomy is complete, any attached short external rotators are released from the trochanteric fragment, allowing it to be retracted proximally. Capsular resection then provides excellent exposure of the hip. Elevation of the abductor musculature off the outer table of the iliac wing will provide more extensive acetabular exposure; as always, care must be taken to avoid injury to the superior gluteal neurovascular bundle.

Fixation of the osteotomy site at the conclusion of the case continues to be a source of discussion and investigation.[31-34] Successful fixation must provide compression at the osteotomy site and also resist both vertical displacement and rotatory forces placed on the hip by the abductors. Charnley initially described fixation with a monofilament wire. Variations of wire constructs have since been described utilizing 2, 3, or 4 wires. Published nonunion rates with wire fixation have ranged from 1% to 25%[31-34]; a 99% union rate has been reported with a 4-wire technique, which involves 2 vertical wires and 2 transverse wires.[31] The vertical wires are placed through drill holes in the lateral femoral cortex, exiting 1 to 2 cm distal to the cut surface. The holes are drilled further distally if advancement of the trochanteric fragment is desired. The horizontal wires are placed around the proximal femur through drill holes in the lesser trochanter (Figure 4-2). A total of 6 holes are drilled in the trochanteric fragment from the cut surface for passage of the wires; 2 are placed proximally for the vertical wires, and 4 are placed distally for the transverse wires. The vertical wires are tensioned first, followed by the transverse wires. Although this technique provides secure fixation, it is technically difficult. It also can severely damage an osteoporotic trochanteric fragment. Additionally, the presence of intramedullary wires can interfere with femoral component insertion and fixation. It is also difficult to perform the repair after the femoral component has been implanted, such as the case of unexpected abductor laxity and resultant instability.

Nonunion is the most common complication of the standard trochanteric osteotomy; this can result in hip pain, abductor muscle insufficiency, and hip instability. Symptomatic nonunion generally requires revision of fixation in conjunction with bone grafting. Other complications include trochanteric bursitis and HO. Lateral hip pain after trochanteric osteotomy is often attributed to prominent trochanteric hardware; pain relief after hardware removal is unpredictable, however, with less than 50% of patients obtaining pain relief.[35] A trial injection of local anesthetic should be performed prior to surgical intervention, and the patient must be thoroughly educated regarding the possibility that the procedure may not alleviate his or her pain. The relationship between trochanteric osteotomy and HO is unclear. While some studies have found an increase in the incidence and severity of clinically significant HO when the osteotomy is performed, other studies have failed to substantiate this finding.[36,37] Because the evidence is inconclusive, performance of the trochanteric osteotomy should not be influenced by the concern for HO; high-risk patients should be treated prophylactically, regardless of approach.

Trochanteric Slide Osteotomy

The trochanteric slide technique was described for use in revision THA by Glassman[38] in 1987. This approach has the advantage of preserving the origin of the vastus lateralis muscle, thus lessening the risk of proximal migration of the trochanteric fragment. The attachment of the vastus lateralis muscle on the trochanteric fragment has a tethering effect on the osteotomy fragment; in addition, a compressive effect is applied to the fragment because the gluteus medius and vastus lateralis muscles provide a medially directed force couple. The trochanteric slide also has the advantage of better preserving the blood supply to the trochanteric fragment. Indications for this approach include acetabular revisions, protrusio acetabuli, and femoral revisions involving extensive cement removal.

The skin incision should not be curved as far posteriorly when a trochanteric slide is anticipated, in order to provide optimal access to the anterior aspect of the trochanter. Once the superficial exposure is complete, the posterior border of the gluteus medius muscle is identified, and the interval between the gluteus minimus muscle and the capsule is developed bluntly in a posterior-to-anterior direction. The vastus lateralis muscle is incised along its posterior aspect for a length of 10 cm distal to the vastus ridge, leaving a cuff of fascia intact posteriorly. The osteotomy is then performed with an oscillating saw in a posterior to anterior direction with the leg in internal rotation. The proximal extent of the osteotomy is just medial to the piriformis fossa, and the distal extent is just distal to the vastus ridge. The attachment of the gluteus minimus muscle to the trochanter should be preserved whenever possible to maintain maximum abductor strength after repair. Once the osteotomy is complete, the trochanteric fragment and its attached proximal and distal musculature are retracted anteriorly.

At the conclusion of the case, the osteotomy is repaired with 2 monofilament wires or cables, with or without a claw construct. Drill holes through the trochanteric fragment are generally not necessary. The cables are passed medially around the proximal femur and laterally around the trochanteric fragment, passing them deep to any muscle tissue whenever possible. If the osteotomy fragment will not seat neatly on the medial femoral bone due to a prominent revision femoral component, the fragment should be contoured with a high-speed burr to achieve good bony apposition. Once provisional fixation is achieved, the hip is taken through a range of motion to check for any impingement caused by malpositioning of the trochanteric fragment. The cables are then tightened once proper placement has been confirmed. In the case of tenuous fixation or poor bone stock, a cable grip system can be used. Various fixation techniques exist, including cables, claws, or cable plates. The cable grip system developed by Dall and Miles[39] has been used extensively for this purpose. The cable grip system provides greater resistance to displacement compared to an isolated wire or cable construct.[34] The cables should be placed at least 2 cm apart medially, and the distal cable should be placed distal to the lesser trochanter to prevent proximal migration. Clinical results of the cable grip system are variable, however, with reported rates of nonunion ranging from 2% to 38%, and cable fraying or breakage occurring in up to 47% of cases.[40,41] Fraying of the cable can generate metallic debris that may be a source of third-body wear; some surgeons prefer wires over cables due to this concern.

Outcome studies for the trochanteric slide osteotomy during revision THA report a nonunion rate of 2% to 10%.[38,42,43] The proximal migration of the nonunited fragment averaged 7 mm in one study.[38] Only one patient in this study demonstrated clinically significant abductor muscle insufficiency, although 28% of the patients demonstrated a Trendelenburg sign or abductor lurch. While there are many confounding variables which make direct comparison across clinical series difficult, the trochanteric slide seems to improve the resistance to proximal migration of the trochanteric fragment and also has a higher reported rate of union than the standard trochanteric osteotomy. Therefore, the trochanteric slide osteotomy is generally preferred in the revision setting when a limited trochanteric osteotomy is necessary.

Extended Trochanteric Osteotomy

The extended trochanteric osteotomy was pioneered by Wagner,[44] who described an extended anterior trochanteric osteotomy in which the anterior portion of the gluteus medius was reflected in continuity with the anterior third of the proximal femur. This technique was later modified by Younger et al[45] into an osteotomy in which the abductors are reflected anteriorly in their entirety with the lateral third of the proximal femur. Indications for the extended femoral osteotomy in the revision THA setting include removal of a well-fixed cemented or cementless femoral component, femoral revision with difficult cement removal, varus remodeling of the proximal femur, and the need for more extensive acetabular exposure. The extended trochanteric osteotomy greatly enhances the ability to remove cement through direct visualization; in the case of revision for infection, the osteotomy will help ensure that the entire extent of the cement mantle, including the distal plug, is removed. The presence of varus remodeling of the proximal femur makes eccentric reaming and cortical perforation difficult to avoid in the absence of an osteotomy, as the reamers can pass through the lateral cortex at the apex of the deformity. With the extended trochanteric osteotomy, direct access to the diaphysis is provided, which allows straight reaming of the diaphysis for revision femoral stem insertion. The extended trochanteric osteotomy requires use of a femoral component designed to obtain diaphyseal fixation in the femur distal to the osteotomy site. Relative contraindications to the extended trochanteric osteotomy include impaction grafting or femoral revisions in which the prosthesis will be fixed with cement. There is a higher reported rate of osteotomy nonunion when performed in association with impaction grafting,[46] and it is difficult to avoid cement extrusion into the osteotomy site, which can also contribute to nonunion.

The length of the osteotomy to be performed should be determined during preoperative planning to ensure that the full extent of the porous coating of the component or the retained cement can be readily accessed. The osteotomy is generally 12 to 15 cm in length measured from the tip of the greater trochanter; it is critical to maintain at least 5 cm of isthmic diaphyseal cortex for revision component fixation. While the osteotomy is generally performed in conjunction with the posterior approach, it has been described in conjunction with the modified lateral approach as well.[15] It may be performed at any time during the revision procedure—before or after dislocation and stem removal. It is easier to perform the osteotomy after the stem has been removed; however, this is often not possible. Therefore, the osteotomy is usually performed after dislocation, but before stem removal. When dislocation proves difficult, the extended trochanteric osteotomy provides excellent exposure and is extremely helpful in assisting dislocation of the stiff hip.

To obtain adequate exposure for the osteotomy, the posterior approach to the hip is extended distally over the posterior aspect of the greater trochanter and along the posterior fascia overlying the vastus lateralis. The vastus lateralis is reflected anteriorly from the intermuscular septum, and perforating vessels are ligated or cauterized. The insertion of the gluteus maximus muscle is released subperiosteally from the posterolateral femur, or alternatively, the dissection is curved anteriorly to maintain the gluteus maximus insertion. The osteotomy is then initiated along

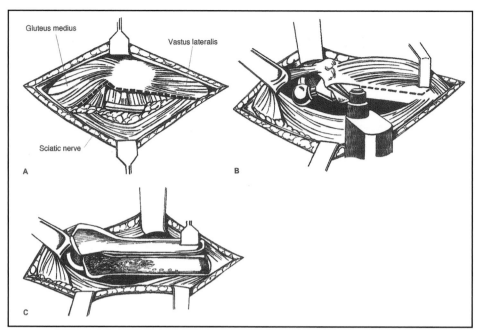

Figure 4-3. The extended trochanteric osteotomy. (A) Initial exposure is provided by identifying the posterior border of the gluteus medius proximally and the posterior border of the vstus muscles distally. (B) Detachment of the posterior capsule, external rotators, and gluteus maximus, coupled with posterior dislocation and removal of the stem, will facilitate the osteotomy. Retention of the stem will be necessary in some cases (as illustrated in this diagram). With use of an oscillating saw or high-speed burr, the proximal lateral femur is detached as far distally as necessary, as determined during preoperative planning. (C) The proximal lateral fragment is hinged forward, with the gluteus and vastus muscles attached, to expose the femoral medullary canal, after which the stem and cement are removed. (© 1998 American Academy of Orthopaedic Surgeons. Reprinted with permission from the *Journal of the American Academy of Orthopaedic Surgeons*, Volume 6[2], p. 89.)

the posterior aspect of the greater trochanter with an oscillating saw (Figure 4-3). The saw is positioned in a posterior to anterior direction and is carefully advanced distally along the posterior femur to the preoperatively determined distance (12 to 15 cm). A high-speed burr is then used to make rounded corners at the distal aspect of the osteotomy in order to lessen the stress risers associated with sharp corners. The transverse portion is then cut to include approximately one-third of the femoral diaphyseal circumference. The distal anterior portion of the osteotomy is advanced 2 cm proximal to the transverse osteotomy. The proximal extent of the anterior limb is then made by passing the saw from posterior to anterior between the prosthetic femoral neck and the medial trochanter, cutting at least 2 cm if possible. An osteotome can be used to score the anterior extension of the osteotomy in a distal to proximal direction. A prophylactic cable can be passed 2 to 3 cm distal to the transverse osteotomy site prior to completion of the osteotomy. The osteotomy is then carefully hinged open anteriorly with the sequential insertion of broad osteotomes into the posterior limb of the osteotomy. This procedure creates an intact muscle-osseous sleeve composed of the gluteus medius, greater trochanter, anterolateral femoral diaphysis, and vastus lateralis. It is important to release the anterior proximal soft tissue and capsule from the osteotomy fragment prior to elevation of the osteotomy fragment. This will prevent anterior tethering of the proximal fragment that can lead to fracture; it will also allow the fragment to retract posteriorly for reattachment at the conclusion of the case.

The proximal femoral shaft is generally retracted anteriorly for acetabular exposure; the anterior Charnley retractor can be placed on the undersurface of the osteotomy fragment. After addressing the acetabulum, the femoral diaphysis is prepared for the revision stem prior to reduction of the osteotomy. A cementless revision stem with at least 5 cm of distal fixation is generally used. Hip stability is then assessed with the osteotomy still open. The osteotomy can be advanced if necessary to obtain proper abductor tension. After stability is ensured and the acetabular and femoral components are in place, the extended trochanteric osteotomy is closed. The medial surface of the trochanteric fragment often requires sculpting with a high-speed burr to accommodate the lateral profile of the revision femoral component.

Fixation of the extended trochanteric osteotomy is often less troublesome than that of the standard trochanteric osteotomy or the trochanteric slide. The osteotomy fragment is reapproximated back to the lateral femur. Care must be taken to not place the fragment too anterior, as this may result in anterior impingement and possible posterior hip dislocation. It is helpful to abduct the leg and internally rotate the femur during osteotomy repair. Contracted anterior capsule and scar tissue can also impair reattachment and limit external rotation; this should be released if necessary. The posterior aspect of the osteotomy should be closely reapproximated, leaving any longitudinal gap anteriorly. In the case of varus remodeling of the proximal femur, the medial aspect of the proximal femur will not be adjacent to the femoral prosthesis. Once the osteotomy is reduced, 2 to 4 wires or cables are passed around the femoral diaphysis and trochanteric fragment. The use of cables offers improved tensile strength and resistance to fatigue. It is important to pass the cables in a submuscular fashion to not strangulate the vascular supply to the osteotomy site or inadvertently entrap neurovascular structures. The cables are generally passed in a posterior to anterior direction to avoid inadvertently incarcerating the sciatic nerve. One cable should be placed just distal to the lesser trochanter, and another cable should be placed 2 to 3 cm proximal to the transverse portion of the osteotomy. Additional cables are then used as necessary depending on the length of the osteotomy. The most tenuous portion of the osteotomy is just distal to the vastus tubercle; therefore, the proximal cables are not secured as tightly as the distal cables to lessen the likelihood of osteotomy fracture. Once fixation is secured, range of motion is again tested to ensure stability without impingement. An allograft strut can be used to span the distal extent of the osteotomy in the case of an attenuated or fractured osteotomy fragment, although this has been found to prolong the time to union.[43] Postoperatively, the osteotomy is protected with touch-down weightbearing and no active abduction for 6 weeks. Although used in the past, abduction orthoses are not currently in routine use except in patients at high risk for dislocation.[47] After 6 weeks, the patient is progressed to weightbearing as tolerated, and active abduction and progressive ambulation are initiated.

Controversy still exists regarding the optimal mode of fixation. A recent cadaveric study[48] demonstrated no statistically significant difference between 2 and 3 cables with regard to stiffness, peak force, or displacement. Combined vertical and horizontal cable fixation, which was employed in the past for fixation of the standard trochanteric osteotomy, has recently been described for fixation of the extended trochanteric osteotomy. The authors reported a 100% union rate,[47] and no incidence of proximal trochanteric migration. Nonunion and proximal migration are the major complications reported with the standard and sliding osteotomes; the reported rates are much lower with the extended osteotomy. The rate of union is very high, ranging from 98% to 100%, and proximal migration rates range from 0% to 10%.[44-49] Other complications include anterior malunion, component subsidence, and intra- or postoperative fracture of the osteotomy fragment. The base of the greater trochanter just distal to the vastus tubercle is the area most susceptible to fracture. Intraoperative measures to avoid fracture include release of the anterior capsular and scar tissues from the proximal trochanteric fragment to increase its mobility, gentle exposure of the acetabulum with broad retractors, and delayed removal of retained cement in the trochanteric fragment. If an intraoperative fracture of the osteotomy fragment occurs, fixation with a trochanteric claw or plate is recommended. In cases of marked cortical attenuation, prophylactic fixation with a claw or plate may be considered.

Transfemoral Osteotomy

Occasionally, it may be necessary to transect the femoral shaft during a revision procedure. The proximal femur may be malaligned as a result of varus remodeling around a loose prosthesis or after remodeling of a periprosthetic fracture; in this case, it may be impossible to reach the distal intramedullary canal. It may also be necessary in order to remove a retained distal cement plug or a broken femoral stem. Glassman et al[50] described a transverse osteotomy in revision THA that was repaired with internal fixation in addition to the use of a revision femoral stem. Wagner's description of the extended trochanteric osteotomy included a complete transverse femoral osteotomy at its distal end.[44] Jansson et al[51] described a transverse femoral osteotomy performed at least 12 cm from the tip of the trochanter without the concomitant use of an extended trochanteric osteotomy. While their technique has the advantage of not splitting the proximal femur, this will only be possible in the case of a loose femoral stem; an extended trochanteric osteotomy will likely be unavoidable otherwise.

An alternative to the transfemoral osteotomy is the creation of a femoral cortical window. With distal extrusion of the cement mantle, visualization of the bone-cement interface is extremely difficult, and the risk of cortical perforation increases the further distal the cement is located. It may be preferable to perform a controlled perforation of the proximal femoral shaft to permit direct visualization of the intramedullary canal and enable the cement to be more effectively removed. Sydney and Mallory[52] described placing one or more 9-mm drill holes in the anterior femur after subperiosteal mobilization of the vastus lateralis. It is important to leave at least 2 femoral diameters between adjacent perforations in order to prevent cumulative stress risers. Masterson et al[53] described the creation of an oval longitudinal window to access a solidly fixed distal cement plug; they termed this the *pencil box osteotomy*. This is performed by elevating the vastus lateralis anteriorly, exposing the posterolateral aspect of the femoral shaft. An oval osteotomy is then produced with the combination of an oscillating saw and high-speed burr. The oval shape will reduce the risk of fracture through an acute angle. The cortical fragment is then hinged forward with soft tissues attached to access the intramedullary canal. It is important to preserve the attachment of the vastus lateralis to the osteotomy fragment, as this preserves the periosteal blood supply. After removal of the retained cement and/or implant, the window is closed with cerclage wires or cables.

Summary

The revision THA surgeon should be comfortable with the entire range of possible surgical approaches to the hip. The most appropriate exposure for each case should be determined through careful preoperative planning based upon the type and stability of the implant to be removed, the extent of bone deficiency present, and the presence or absence of infection. In general, the anterolateral approach should be reserved for acetabular revisions. This approach is nonextensive and cannot be converted to a trochanteric osteotomy without compromising the blood supply to the trochanteric fragment. If a trochanteric osteotomy is necessary for removal of a well-fixed femoral stem or an extended cement mantle, it should be performed in conjunction with the posterior approach. Adequate soft tissue repair with the posterior approach will reduce the risk of postoperative dislocation significantly and should be performed whenever possible.

References

1. Cruz-Pardos A, Garcia-Cimbrelo E. The Harris-Galante total hip arthroplasty: a minimum 8-year follow-up study. *J Arthroplasty*. 2001;16(5):586-597.
2. Campbell DG, Garbuz DS, Masri BA, Duncan CP. Reliability of acetabular bone defect classification systems in revision total hip arthroplasty. *J Arthroplasty*. 2001;16(1):83-86.

3. Jando VT, Greidanus NV, Masri BA, Garbus DS, Duncan CP. Trochanteric osteotomes in revision total hip arthroplasty: contemporary techniques and results. *Instr Course Lect.* 2005;54:143-155.

4. Della Valle CJ, Paprosky WG. Classification and an algorithmic approach to the reconstruction of femoral deficiency in revision total hip arthroplasty. *J Bone Joint Surg Am.* 2003;85-A(Suppl 4):1-6.

5. Watson-Jones R. Fractures of the neck of the femur. *Br J Surg.* 1935;23:787.

6. Müller ME. Total hip prosthesis. *Clin Orthop Relat Res.* 1970;72:46-68.

7. Vicar AJ, Coleman CR. A comparison of the anterolateral, transtrochanteric, and posterior surgical approaches in primary total hip arthroplasty. *Clin Orthop Relat Res.* 1984;188:152-159.

8. Horwitz BR, Rockowitz NL, Goll SR, et al. A prospective randomized comparison of two surgical approaches to total hip arthroplasty. *Clin Orthop Rel Res.* 1993;291:154-163.

9. Mallory TH, Lombardi AV Jr, Fada RA, Herrington SM, Eberle RW. Dislocation after total hip arthroplasty using the anterolateral abductor split approach. *Clin Orthop Relat Res.* 1999;358:166-172.

10. Ritter MA, Harty LD, Keating ME, Faris PM, Meding JB. A clinical comparison of the anterolateral and posterolateral approaches to the hip. *Clin Orthop Relat Res.* 2001;385:95-99.

11. Madsen MS, Ritter MA, Morris HH, et al. The effect of total hip arthroplasty surgical approach on gait. *J Orthop Res.* 2004;22:44-50.

12. McFarland B, Osborne G. Approach to the hip: a suggested improvement on Kocher's method. *J Bone Joint Surg Br.* 1954;36:364-367.

13. Hardinge K. The direct lateral approach to the hip. *J Bone Joint Surg Br.* 1982;64:17-19.

14. Dall D. Exposure of the hip by anterior osteotomy of the greater trochanter: a modified anterolateral approach. *J Bone Joint Surg Br.* 1986;68:382-386.

15. MacDonald SJ, Cole C, Guerin J, Rorabeck CH, Bourne RB, McCalden RW. Extended trochanteric osteotomy via the direct lateral approach in revision hip arthoplasty. *Clin Orthop Relat Res.* 2003;417:210-216.

16. Masonis JL, Bourne RB. Surgical approach, abductor function, and total hip arthroplasty dislocation. *Clin Orthop Relat Res.* 2002;405:46-53.

17. Ramesh M, O'Byrne JM, McCarthy N, Jarvis A, Mahalingham K, Cashman WF. Damage to the superior gluteal nerve after the Hardinge approach to the hip. *J Bone Joint Surg Br.* 1996;78:903-906.

18. Baker AS, Bitounis VC. Abductor function after total hip replacement: an electromyographic and clinical review. *J Bone Joint Surg Br.* 1989;71:47-50.

19. Moore AT. The Moore self-locking Vitallium prosthesis in fresh femoral neck fractures: a new low posterior approach (the southern exposure). *Instr Course Lect.* 1959;16:309-321.

20. Bischoff R, Dunlap J, Carpenter L, DeMouy E, Barrack R. Heterotopic ossification following uncemented total hip arthroplasty. Effect of the operative approach. *J Arthroplasty.* 1994;9(6):641-644.

21. Masonis JL, Bourne RB. Surgical approach, abductor function, and total hip arthroplasty dislocation. *Clin Orthop Relat Res.* 2002;405:46-53.

22. Jolles BM, Bogoch ER. Posterior versus lateral surgical approach for total hip arthroplasty in adults with osteoarthritis. *Cochrane Database Syst Rev.* 2006;19(3):CD003828.

23. Khatod M, Barber T, Paxton E, Namba R, Fithian D. An analysis of the risk of hip dislocation with a contemporary total joint registry. *Clin Orthop Relat Res.* 2006;447:19-23.

24. Gulati A, Dwyer AJ, Shardlow DL. The impact of posterior approach for total hip arthroplasty on early complications. *Acta Orthop Belg.* 2008;74(2):200-205.

25. Weeden SH, Paprosky WG, Bowling JW. The early dislocation rate in primary total hip arthroplasty following the posterior approach with posterior soft-tissue repair. *J Arthroplasty.* 2003;18(6):709-713.

26. Kwon MS, Kuskowski M, Mulhall KJ, Macaulay W, Brown TE, Saleh KJ. Does surgical approach affect total hip arthroplasty dislocation rates? *Clin Orthop Relat Res.* 2006;447:34-38.

27. Suh KT, Roh HL, Moon KP, Shin JK, Lee JS. Posterior approach with posterior soft tissue repair in revision total hip arthroplasty. *J Arthroplasty.* 2008;23(8):1197-1203.

28. Sioen W, Simon JP, Labey L, Van Audekercke R. Posterior transosseous capsulotendinous repair in total hip arthroplasty: a cadaver study. *J Bone Joint Surg Am.* 2002;84-A(10):1793-1798.

29. Charnley J. The long-term results of low-friction arthroplasty of the hip performed as a primary prevention. *J Bone Joint Surg Br.* 1972;54:61-76.

30. McGrory BJ, Bal BS, Harris WH. Trochanteric osteotomy for total hip arthroplasty: six variations and indications for their use. *J Am Acad Orthop Surg.* 1996;4(5):258-267.

31. Jensen NF, Harris WH. A system for trochanteric osteotomy and reattachment for total hip arthroplasty with a ninety-nine percent union rate. *Clin Orthop Relat Res.* 1986;208:174-181.

32. Hodgkinson JP, Shelley P, Wroblewski BM. Reattachment of the ununited trochanter in Charnley low friction arthroplasty. *J Bone Joint Surg Br.* 1989;71:523-525.

33. Nercessian OA, Newton PM, Joshi RP, Sheikh B, Eftekhar NS. Trochanteric osteotomy and wire fixation: a comparison of 2 techniques. *Clin Orthop Relat Res.* 1996;333:208-216.

34. Hersh CK, Williams RP, Trick LW, Lanctot D, Athanasiou K. Comparison of the mechanical performance of trochanteric fixation devices. *Clin Orthop Relat Res.* 1996;329:317-325.

35. Bernard AA, Brooks S. The role of trochanteric wire revision after total hip replacement. *J Bone Joint Surg Br.* 1987;69:352-354.

36. Errico TJ, Fetto JF, Waugh TR. Heterotopic ossification: incidence and relation to trochanteric osteotomy in 100 total hip arthroplasties. *Clin Orthop Relat Res.* 1984;190:138-141.

37. Morrey BF, Adams RA, Cabanela ME. Comparison of heterotopic bone after anterolateral, transtrochanteric, and posterior approaches for total hip arthroplasty. *Clin Orthop Relat Res.* 1984;188:160-167.

38. Glassman AH, Engh CA, Bobyn JD. A technique of extensive exposure for total hip arthroplasty. *J Arthroplasty.* 1987;2(1):11-21.

39. Dall DM, Miles AW. Reattachment of the greater trochanter: the use of the trochanter cable-grip system. *J Bone Joint Surg Br.* 1983;65:55-59.

40. McCarthy JC, Bone JV, Turner RH, Kremchek T, Lee J. The outcome of trochanteric reattachment in revision total hip arthroplasty with a Cable Grip System: mean 6-year followup. *J Arthroplasty.* 1999;14(7): 810-814.

41. Silverton CD, Jacobs JJ, Rosenberg AG, Kull L, Conley A, Galante JO. Complications of a cable grip system. *J Arthroplasty.* 1996;11(4):400-404.

42. English TA. The trochanteric approach to the hip for prosthetic replacement. *J Bone Joint Surg Am.* 1975;57:1128-1133.

43. Chen WM, McAuley JP, Engh CA Jr, Hopper RH Jr, Engh CA. Extended slide trochanteric osteotomy for revision total hip arthroplasty. *J Bone Joint Surg Am.* 2000;82:1215-1219.

44. Wagner H. Revisionsprothese für das Hüftgelenk. *Orthopäde.* 1989;18:438-453.

45. Younger TI, Bradford MS, Magnus RE, Paprosky WG. Extended proximal femoral osteotomy: a new technique for femoral revision arthroplasty. *J Arthroplasty.* 1995;10(3):329-338.

46. Hellman EJ, Capello WN, Feinberg JR. Nonunion of extended trochanteric osteotomes in impaction grafting femoral revisions. *J Arthoplasty.* 1998;13(8):945-949.

47. Huffman GR, Ries MD. Combined vertical and horizontal cable fixation of an extended trochanteric osteotomy site. *J Bone Joint Surg Am.* 2003;85A:273-277.

48. Schwab JH, Camacho J, Kaufman K, Chen Q, Berry DJ, Trousdale RT. Optimal fixation for the extended trochanteric osteotomy: a pilot study comparing 3 cables vs 2 cables. *J Arthroplasty.* 2008;23(4):534-538.

49. Mardones R, Gonzalez C, Cabanela ME, Trousdale RT, Berry DJ. Extended femoral osteotomy for revision of hip arthroplasty: results and complications. *J Arthroplasty.* 2005;20(1):79-83.

50. Glassman AH, Engh CA, Bobyn JD. Proximal femoral osteotomy as an adjunct in cementless revision total hip arthoplasty. *J Arthroplasty.* 1987;2(1):47-63.

51. Jansson V, Müller PE, Pellengahr C. Transverse femoral osteotomy for revision surgery—an alternative to the transfemoral approach. *Orthop Traumatol.* 2002;10:83-91.

52. Sydney SV, Mallory TH. Controlled perforation: a safe method of cement removal from the femoral canal. *Clin Orthop Relat Res.* 1990:253:168-172.

53. Masterson EL, Masri BA, Duncan CP. Surgical approaches in revision hip replacement. *J Am Acad Orthop Surg.* 1998;6(2):84-92.

Component Removal in
Revision Total Hip Arthroplasty

Viktor E. Krebs, MD; Ian M. Gradisar, MD; Creighton C. Tubb, MD;
and Kenneth A. Greene, MD

Component removal in revision total hip arthroplasty (THA) can be a time-consuming and arduous task. Through good preoperative planning, this stress can be minimized. The primary goal of implant removal is the preservation of host bone through a safe and efficient approach. Host bone loss can be minimized with the use of special tools and thorough knowledge of a variety of removal techniques. Proper selection of the most appropriate surgical approach can enable better reconstruction and therefore an enhanced patient outcome.

Preoperative planning for revision total hip surgery is imperative. It ensures that the appropriate equipment is available for both the extraction and reimplantation. Planning begins with an evaluation of the patient including a proper history and physical exam as well as obtaining previous operative reports. Examination of the operative site may give clues as to the previous approach used.

Selecting the surgical approach for a revision hip procedure is based on surgeon preference, the previously used approach, and the approach that provides the best access to a particular known defect. Most total hip revision surgeries in the United States are performed through either the posterior or direct lateral approaches. Although it is possible to use any previous incisions, each approach has its advantages. The posterior approach can be used after any previous approach and can be easily extended to improve femoral exposure. However, anterior pelvic or anterior column defects are not easily managed through this approach. The posterior approach is particularly useful after a previous anterior approach has been attempted and there is a history of posterior instability where posterior capsular repair is desired. A previous direct lateral or anterolateral approach requiring a débridement, liner exchange, or whole acetabular revision can be done through a direct lateral or anterolateral incision. Indeed, some surgeons prefer a direct lateral approach for all their revisions except for those cases with a total absence of posterior soft tissue.[1]

For very complex revisions, an extended trochanteric osteotomy (ETO) may be necessary and has been described from both a posterior and direct lateral approach.[2,3] It should be reserved for cases when the femoral component cannot be removed by other means. This approach can reduce the risk of a fracture of the greater trochanter and can protect weakened proximal bone. While preserving muscular abductor attachments, ETO can also aid in abductor tensioning with a trochanteric slide.[4] It allows for excellent exposure of the femur and, in turn, enhances

Jacofsky DJ, Hedley AK.
Fundamentals of Revision Hip Arthroplasty:
Diagnosis, Evaluation, and Treatment (pp 67-78).
© 2013 SLACK Incorporated.

Figure 5-1. U-shaped osteotomes can be useful for interrupting component-bone and cement-bone interfaces.

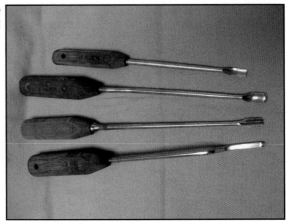

Figure 5-2. A bipolar tissue sealer can help keep the wound dry by aiding in tissue cautery.

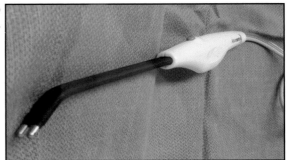

acetabular exposure. Indications include the removal of the femoral cement mantle and removal of well-fixed or extensively coated or tapered cementless stems. There are some disadvantages that may include increased bone trauma, increased potential for blood loss, the need for cerclage wires, and possible nonunion.

The minimum preoperative radiograph requirements include an anteroposterior (AP) pelvis film with AP and lateral views of the hip including the proximal femur. Full-length femur films are preferable and may alert the surgeon to distal bone quality and geometry or the presence of any distal hardware or cement. Preoperative x-rays can help classify any osteolysis and help determine component positioning and loosening. Serial films can show progressive characteristics, such as osteolysis or heterotopic bone. Stress shielding or spot welding can be identified on plain films and can indicate the quality of bone ongrowth or bone ingrowth. Other imaging, such as computed tomography scans, can be used to evaluate for adequate bone stock and help define component relationships to other pelvic structures.

All efforts should be made to obtain the original operative report to discern the exact manufacturer and type and size of total hip implants in place. Special equipment needs can also be identified from the postoperative radiographs. This will streamline the revision process and can be used to ensure that the correct components, extractors, liners, screwdrivers, and other special tools are available for component removal. Implant-specific extractors can aid in removal. Universal extractors, modular component separators, vice-grips, and slap hammers are all noncomponent-specific tools that should be available. More simple tools, such as bone tamps and a wide range of osteotomes including curved acetabular and U-shaped osteotomes, can be useful to disrupt the fixation interface (Figure 5-1). A broken screw removal set should also be readily available. In addition, a bipolar tissue sealer can be useful to aid in rapid tissue cautery and maintenance of interface visibility (Figure 5-2).

TABLE 5-1. COMPONENT REMOVAL TOOLS FOR REVISION TOTAL HIP ARTHROPLASTY

Hand tools	Power tools
■ Mallet	■ Saw
■ Bone tamp	□ Sagital
■ Bone hook	□ Reciprocating
■ Vice-grips	■ High-speed burr
■ Graspers	■ Midas Rex (Fort Worth, TX)
□ Pituitary	■ Drill
□ Cartilage-clamp	■ Ultrasonic cement remover
■ Currettes	Acetabular component-specific tools
□ Straight	■ Component-specific extractor
□ Curved	■ Acetabular gouges
□ Uterine	■ Threaded extractor
□ McElroy	■ Explant acetabular cup removal system (Zimmer, Inc, Warsaw, IN)
■ Osteotomes	Femoral component-specific tools
□ Straight	■ Component-specific extractor
□ Curved	■ Universal femoral component extractor
□ Flexible	■ Modular component separators
□ U-shaped	■ Head-lamp/light on a stick
■ Gouges	■ Cable cutters
■ Cement hooks	■ Trephines
■ Cement splitter	□ Straight
■ Slap hammer	□ Flexible
■ Bipolar sealer	
■ Broken screw removal set	

Power tools, such as a high-speed burr, a sagittal saw, as well as reciprocating saws, can be useful for breaking up component interfaces. Metal cutting burrs like the Midas-Rex (Medtronic, Fort Worth, TX) are sometimes needed to cut metal or polyethylene components into pieces for access and removal. Ultrasound devices have been shown to be effective for cement removal.[5] A checklist of tools likely required for component removal can be useful (Table 5-1).

FEMORAL COMPONENT

Indications for femoral component removal include chronic infection, aseptic loosening, hip instability due to component malposition, prosthesis impingement, periprosthetic fracture, and component failure. The most common indication for revision of the femoral component is mechanical loosening as noted by Bozic et al in a recent study.[6] In this study, the investigators found that only 13.2% of total hip revisions in the United States over a 15-month interval were for isolated femoral component revisions. It is important to note that with an osteointegrated stem, it is rare to have late loosening. As with all surgeries, medical illness preventing safe surgery is a contraindication.

Cementless Stem Removal

Engh and Bobyn classified fixation status of cementless stems into 3 classes:
1. Stable with bony ingrowth
2. Stable with fibrous ingrowth
3. Unstable[7]

The stem may be visually loose on radiographs or found to be grossly loose at the time of surgery. On the contrary, although the stem may appear loose on x-ray, it may have significant fibrous ingrowth and bony overgrowth preventing easy extraction. For unstable or loose stems, after clearing the femoral shoulder of any overlying bone or soft tissue, the extraction device is used. This may be a component-specific extractor, such as a slap hammer that screws into the shoulder of the component, a universal slap hammer, or a modular stem extractor made to attach to the trunnion of multiple manufacturers.[8] If there is no visible movement of the stem after repeated attempts with an extractor device, then stop and do not risk fracture with repeated disimpaction. In these situations there is either a bone or fibrous interface present that must be approached directly.

Stable Proximally Coated Stems

Stems that are stable proximally require patience to clear the stable interface to prevent a femoral fracture. Clearing of the shoulder along the medial aspect of the greater trochanter cannot be overemphasized. Using a burr or a combination of straight and flexible osteotomes, any medial overhanging of the greater trochanter needs to be removed to prevent a trochanter fracture when extracting the stem straight out of the canal. Care must be taken to preserve the lateral pillar of the greater trochanter and its soft tissue attachments. Do not lever an osteotome against the greater trochanter as this could easily create a greater trochanter fracture, especially in osteoporotic and osteopenic bone.

Additionally, removing bone proximal to the lesser trochanter in the calcar region can facilitate direct access to the bone-implant interface. This maneuver can make it easier to pass a burr or osteotome down along the anteromedial and posteromedial aspect of the prosthesis without risking structural compromise. This does, however, require a calcar replacing reconstruction. For stems with collars, the collar may need to be removed with a metal cutting burr to allow for medial access. The collar can also be used as a disimpacting surface.

Once the shoulder region and calcar areas are cleared, it is important to free up the implant in a proximal-to-distal fashion. For proximally coated stems, rigid and flexible osteotomes can be used around proximally ingrowth segment. The goal is to free up the implant without splitting the femur. Exercise particular care when using osteotomes because their wedge shape could cause cortical fracture. Flexible osteotomes with thinner blades and less wedge effect can be more forgiving, but can also be deflected by rigid spot-welds and penetrate the cortex above the point of stem fixation. Thin U-shaped osteotomes are available and may be a better option because they are less likely to deflect and also follow the contour of the implant. When thick areas of ongrowth are present a pencil-tip high-speed burr can be useful in breaking up the implant-bone interface, but can quickly violate cortical bone if misdirected (Figure 5-3). Alternatively, small oscillating and reciprocating saw blades can be used to initiate bone implant separation.

Once the bone-component interface is loose, extraction can then be attempted with a slap hammer. If the procedures are performed in a meticulous fashion, extraction should be possible. If the surgeon is unable to substantially loosen the interface, then a trochanteric slide or extended trochanteric osteotomy may be necessary. A posterior longitudinal split osteotomy has also been described with some success.[9]

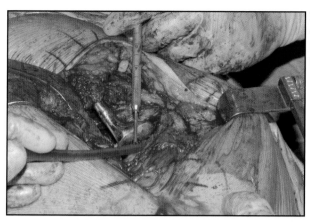

Figure 5-3. A high-speed pencil-tip burr can be useful in breaking up the proximal implant-bone interface of the femoral component.

Fully Porous Coated Stems

Extracting a fully porous coated stem can be challenging and exhausting. The firmly ingrown distal portion of the femoral stem may require the use of a cortical window. The corners of the window are drilled to prevent stress concentration and fracture propagation along the femur. The drill holes are then connected with a saw or high-speed burr. A cortical window can be used to tap on the distal part of the stem with a bone tamp or can aid in cutting the implant in cross section with a metal cutting burr to allow for distal stem removal with trephines. The cortical window is then replaced to maintain cortical integrity.

Paprosky et al described a technique that minimizes bone loss and the risk of femoral fracture. An ETO is made to the level of the cylindrical portion of the stem. A Gigli saw is then used to free the medial proximal bone-stem interface. A trial of extraction is then attempted. If unsuccessful after 3 to 5 blows, then the stem is transected with a metal cutting burr. Multiple burrs should be readily available. Trephines are then used to remove the distal cylindrical portion of the cut stem.[10] It is important to use the smallest trephine that fits over the stem. A trephine that is too large may leave excessive bone attached to the ingrown stem or perforate the cortex.

Extended trochanteric osteotomes are becoming more common. Avoid making the ETO too distal. The reconstruction stem will require about 4 to 6 cm of diaphysis for fixation. It is best to determine the osteotomy length preoperatively.

Cemented Stem Removal

A loose or smooth cemented stem should be extracted easily from the cement mantle. A well-fixed or precoated stem may be more difficult to remove. In this instance, attention should be turned to disrupting the cement-implant interface. Again, care should be taken to clear the shoulder area of the prosthesis to prevent a greater trochanter fracture. In cemented components, there may be proximal cement in this area preventing its extraction. A combination of osteotomes and burrs can be used to disrupt the proximal cement-implant junction.

A well-fixed cemented stem may require an ETO, especially if the cement extends distal to the isthmus. An ETO allows direct access to the cement-bone interface. A pencil-tip burr and osteotomes can then be used to remove any remaining cement mantle. Distal cement can also be accessed through a cortical window, which permits tool access to the femoral diaphysis.[11]

Retained cement removal from the femoral canal can be tedious. If, however, the femoral cement mantle is intact, it is possible to recement into that mantle with excellent fixation shown to be biomechanically stronger than recementing into a smooth cortical tube.[12] Cross and Bostrom described 3 common indications for the cement-in-cement technique:

1. When the original stem is broken, but the cement mantle is intact

Figure 5-4. Hand tools such as a grasper, chisel, cement splitter, and crochet hook are useful for cement removal.

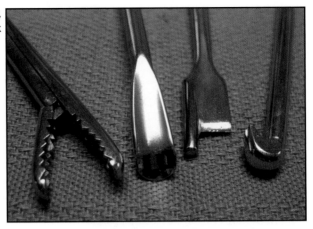

Figure 5-5. Radiograph of a large retained distal cement mantle.

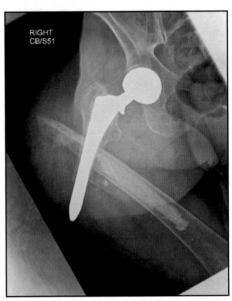

2. When removing and replacing a well-fixed, cemented stem

3. When removing a debonded femoral component[13]

One study showed this cement-in-cement technique done successfully with no revisions for aseptic loosening in 136 hips for a mean 8-year follow-up period.[14] It is therefore not necessary to remove a well-fixed cement mantle in cases of aseptic loosening if the new stem is to be cemented into place.

For a broken cement mantle or when the new stem requires biointegration, then complete cement removal is necessary. There are multiple techniques described in the literature to ease and expedite femoral cement removal. Lombardi described a technique using specialized hand tools for proximal cement removal followed by controlled perforations and a high-speed burr to remove the remaining canal cement.[15] A loose cement mantle can sometimes be removed with hand tools, however, osteotomes risk fracture in a circumferentially intact proximal femoral cement mantle, and a pencil-tip burr may be less destructive (Figure 5-4). Remember to clear proximally first, then advance distally (Figure 5-5). Retained canal cement can also be removed by inserting new cement and a threaded rod then allowing the bonded pieces to extract the cement in segments.[16] It can be difficult to prevent femoral canal perforation with any of the previously described

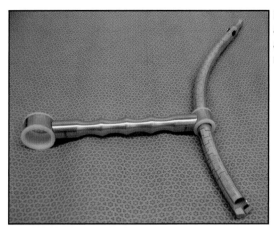

Figure 5-6. A flexible trephine can be passed over a drill bit and be useful for cement plug extraction as well as coring out modular stems in the intramedullary canal.

methods. If there is suspicion at any point of a cortical breach, then an intraoperative x-ray should be obtained. Radiographs can also be used to assess for any retained cement, especially prior to any reaming. Retained hard cement will deflect a reamer into the softer cortical bone resulting in cortical thinning and perforation.

One technique for removing the distal cement plug uses a drill with a centralizer to drill down the center of the plug. Once the plug is drilled, a tap can be used to extract it. A new tool that can be used for cement plug removal uses flexible trephines (Shukla Medical, Piscataway, NJ; Figure 5-6). With the flexible trephine, a drill is passed through the cement plug and a trephine of the appropriate size is passed over the drill, capturing the cement plug in the trephine. Intraoperative fluoroscopy can help guide the drill safely. Distal cement plug removal is also a good indication for use of ultrasound devices.

Ultrasonic devices have been shown to be a safe and efficient means of removing cement in revision surgery.[5] Proponents of ultrasound state it facilitates selective cement removal, preserves bone, decreases cortical perforation risk, and eliminates the need for osteotomy.[17] One pitfall to ultrasonic devices is the heat build-up that can cause thermal necrosis, and in one case a radial nerve palsy.[18] Users must be aware of this possibility and familiar with proper techniques in its use.

Often an extended trochanteric osteotomy can expedite cement removal and protect the surgeon and patient from inadvertent, uncontrolled femoral fracture or cortical perforation in patients with poor bone quality. Other cement removal techniques include robot-assisted 3-dimensional cement removal and the use of a flexible endoscope for femoral canal visualization.[19,20]

Fractured Femoral Stem

Metal fatigue from cantilever bending in cemented and noncemented stems can result in femoral stem fracture. Usually, the proximal piece is loose and easily extracted. Trephines can be used to extract the usually well-fixed distal piece of the stem. In some cases, curved or tapered stem geometry is not amenable to trephines. For these stems, a cortical window placed just distal to the stem tip can allow space for a high-impact carbon punch to drive the component proximally with a mallet.[21] In the most stubborn cases, an ETO can gain access to the entire stem. Be sure to carry the ETO just distal to the stem.

ACETABULUM

Once the decision has been made to save or remove the femoral component, attention can then be turned to the acetabulum. Obviously, removal of the femoral component will greatly enhance the exposure of the acetabulum. Complete visualization may require an enhanced exposure technique, such as a trochanteric osteotomy. Another technique to aid in visualization is the removal and reinsertion technique of a cemented femoral stem as described by Nabors et al.[22] This allows for cemented femoral component removal for acetabular exposure followed by reinsertion into a stable cement mantle. The goal of acetabular component removal is to protect the posterior column and superior dome of the pelvis, as these are important for revision cup fixation.

Indications for removal of the acetabular component include mechanical loosening, chronic infection, polyethylene wear in a nonmodular cup, and component malposition resulting in instability, impingement, or wear. Periacetabular osteolysis can be an indication especially in a nonmodular cup incapable of easy bearing exchange. A recent study by Bozic et al found the most common reason for isolated acetabular revision in the United States over a 15-month period was instability and dislocation involving 33% of all acetabular revisions.[6] Component malposition is the primary cause for dislocation. In this same study, mechanical loosening was the second major cause for isolated acetabular revisions at 24.2%. Although an asymptomatic or mildly symptomatic acetabular loosening with nonprogressive osteolysis can be observed with close follow-up, any symptomatic or progressive osteolysis requires acetabular revision. Stable osteolysis itself is not an indication for cup removal, any more than it is for stem removal. An acetabular component can be retained if the cup is well fixed without supplemental fixation, positioning is appropriate with no instability or impingement, and there are no signs of significant wear. Only when these criteria are satisfied can the acetabulum remain. Conversely, any loose acetabular component as observed intraoperatively must be revised. Components with a historically high failure rate are also a relative indication for acetabular component removal.

Isolated Liner Exchange

Acetabular liner exchange for poly wear can be considered when the acetabular component is well fixed. Moderate wear of the polyethylene liner can eventually lead to osteolysis and instability. Replacing a worn liner can help prevent loosening of the component by osteolysis and prevent later catastrophic failure from bearing wear-through.[23] Polyethylene liner exchanges are appropriate even in moderate osteolysis.[24,25] Bone grafting of osteolytic acetabular lesions behind a well-fixed cup at the time of a liner exchange has shown good results with no progression of the osteolytic defect and, in most cases, an increase in radiographic density is seen on follow-up x-rays.[26]

It is important preoperatively to be familiar with the different polyethylene locking mechanisms and to know which type of locking mechanism is present. Some mechanisms require special instruments for a locking ring. Others have a wire that inevitably will be damaged with poly removal. If the locking ring is damaged, it must be replaced with a new ring.

Some manufacturers supply special instruments for extraction of existing liners. For a polyethylene liner, if liner locking mechanism tools are not needed or are unavailable, there are several techniques that can be used to remove the poly. One technique involves using a narrow-bladed osteotome that can be used to spear the outer rim of the polyethylene and drive the osteotome inferiorly into the opposite rim of the liner. The poly can then be gently levered out by pulling the osteotome in an inferior direction. Another well-described method for liner extraction is the screw technique. A 3.2-mm drill hole is made in the poly, and a 6.5-mm screw is advanced into the poly. The bottomed-out screw will elevate the poly from the metal acetabular shell. Beware of possible drill or screw penetration through any open screw holes or apical holes in the acetabular shell. If necessary, more than one screw can be used. If poly removal is still unsuccessful, a burr can be used to section the poly into quadrants for removal.

If the type of implanted system is unknown at the time of surgery and the correct poly is not readily available or the locking mechanism becomes damaged, then cementing a new polyethylene into a well-fixed acetabular shell is an acceptable alternative.[27]

Once the polyethylene liner is removed, the fixation of the acetabular shell should be tested. It is recommended that all acetabular screws be removed at the time of revision for accurate assessment of component fixation.[28] Supplemental fixation screws can give a false sense of fixation. Any motion of the component indicates it is loose and requires a complete acetabular revision.

Removal of Loose Acetabular Component

Removal of a loose acetabular component rarely requires much more than good exposure of the entire rim and a firm grasp of the component. Care must be taken to ensure all screws are removed prior to extraction to avoid additional bone loss. Components that appear loose on radiographs but do not show any motion intraoperatively due to fibrous ingrowth should be removed in a way similar to removing a well-fixed noncemented component. Loose cemented components can be removed by drilling a centering hole into the polyethylene and screwing in a threaded acetabular extractor.[10] The surgeon should note that a loose modern acetabular component today is rare and should raise suspicion for infection.

Removal of Well-Fixed Acetabular Component

Revision of a stable cementless acetabular component on the basis of its duration alone is not necessary.[28] However, the acetabulum must be removed in cases of chronic infection, gross malposition, or a damaged cup that can no longer support weightbearing.

If the acetabulum has supplemental screw fixation, the polyethylene liner and screws must be removed prior to extraction of the cup. Once the screws are removed, the liner can be replaced if not destroyed or a trial liner can be inserted. The previous operative report can provide component manufacturer, type, and size. This is important for not only the component-specific retractors but also knowing the specific liner locking mechanism, trial liners, or screwdriver type needed. The polyethylene liner is removed using either the osteotome levering technique or screw technique, as described previously. For metal and ceramic liners, one technique for liner removal is a forceful blow using a mallet and a bone tamp at the rim of the acetabular shell. This is usually enough to dislodge the metal-metal or ceramic-metal interface.

Once the liner is removed, any remaining screws must be removed before extraction of the cup to avoid periacetabular bone loss. If an appropriate screwdriver is not available, a high-speed metal cutting burr can be used to cut-off the screw heads. After cup extraction remaining broken screws can be removed using a broken screw removal set, small trephines, or even vice grips. Broken screws can also be left in place if they do not interfere with acetabular reaming and are not infected.

Removal of a noncemented well-fixed acetabulum requires excellent visualization of the entire rim and careful dissection of the bone-component interface to preserve acetabular bone stock. A high-speed burr or osteotomes can be used to expose the bone-prosthesis interface. Curved acetabular Aufranc or Moreland osteotomes have historically been used to separate the interface. Their space-occupying thickness can lead to bone loss and pelvic fracture even if used carefully.[29] When using these osteotomes, particular care should be taken to preserve the medial and posterior rim of bone for revision fixation.

The recent introduction of the Explant Acetabular Cup Removal System (Zimmer, Inc, Warsaw, IN) allows for cup removal with minimal bone loss (Figure 5-7). The Explant system centers itself with 22-, 26-, 28-, or 32-mm heads in the liner and uses short- and long-curved radius osteotomes that circumferentially disrupt the bone-component interface. The curved osteotomes are thin and match the exact radius of the cup, allowing for minimal bone damage. In a study of 31 procedures using the Explant system, the median difference between the diameter of the implant removed and the final reamer used was 4 mm. This small difference indicated that there was no more bone loss than the thickness of the blades, and the time for the removal of the shell did not exceed 5 minutes.[30] For large metal-on-metal liners, the Explant system can be used with modifications because there are no head sizes currently larger than 32 mm. One solution is to cement a smaller diameter poly into the metal liner for use with the Explant system.[31] Another technique for metal-on-metal shell removal is to place an appropriately sized trial Trilogy (Zimmer, Inc) liner into the shell and use the Explant system.[32]

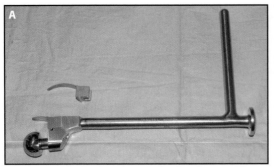
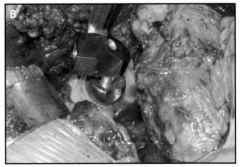

Figure 5-7. The Explant Acetabular Cup Removal System (Zimmer, Inc, Warsaw, IN) contains cutting blades that match the radius of the implant (A), allowing for bone-implant interface disruption with minimal bone loss (B).

Figure 5-8. Radiograph of a spiked acetabular component. The area behind the spikes can have significant bone ingrowth.

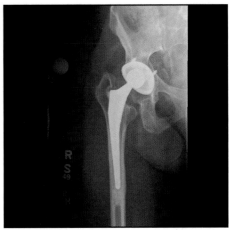

For medialized cups that approach Kohler's line, use caution to prevent bone destruction. A loss of the columns will create a pelvic dissociation requiring a cage construct for revision. Some investigators recommend the use of a high-speed burr to section the cup prior to removal.[10] This method may leave metal filings in the hip joint, and if not entirely removed, may cause future bearing wear. Severe protrusion of the cup, defined as migration of the component medial to the iliopectineal line, may require a retroperitoneal approach or a manipulation maneuver to dislodge the migrated cup as described by Ahmad et al.[33]

Cups that contain spikes for additional fixation can be troublesome to remove with traditional cup extraction techniques (Figure 5-8). The area behind these spikes has been found to have significant bone ingrowth, which can lead to large defects if forcefully removed. One technique uses an overlay template to identify the spike positions, and then a carbide-tipped burr is used to remove the portion of the metal shell that contains the spikes.[34]

Cemented Acetabular Component

Revision of a well-fixed cemented acetabular component solely on the basis of the duration it was in place is not warranted.[35] However, revision of well-fixed cemented acetabular components with Ranawat grade E or F osteolysis or any cup that is malpositioned or has unacceptable wear is supported.[35]

The key to cemented cup removal is to disrupt the poly-cement interface first, as this will prevent bone damage. Curved osteotomes or gouges, such as the Moreland cemented revision set, can be used to create this separation. The poly can also be removed in piecemeal fashion by sectioning it with a burr and osteotomes. Another technique involves making several drill holes in the poly to place multiple 4.5-mm screws to separate the poly-cement interface.[36] Alternatively, acetabular reamers can be used to ream away the polyethylene down to the level of the cement.[37] Once the cement is exposed, a combination of hand tools and high-speed burrs can then be used to remove the residual cement.[15]

Component removal in revision THA is an important step in the reimplantation process. Removal of components in a controlled and timely manner requires thorough preoperative planning with an adequate array of instruments and the ability to execute multiple removal techniques. Successful component removal with minimal damage to host bone and tissue is the key to a successful outcome for the patient.

REFERENCES

1. Lombardi AV Jr, Berend KR. Surgical approach to the hip: direct lateral. In: Hozack W, Parvizi J, Bender B, eds. *Surgical Treatment of Hip Arthritis: Reconstruction, Replacement and Revision*. Philadelphia, PA: Saunders; 2009:272-277.
2. MacDonald SJ, Cole C, Guerin J, Rorabeck CH, Bourne RB, McCalden RW. Extended trochanteric osteotomy via the direct lateral approach in revision hip arthroplasty. *Clin Orthop Relat Res*. 2003;(417):210-216.
3. Meek RM, Greidanus NV, Garbuz DS, Masri BA, Duncan CP. Extended trochanteric osteotomy: planning, surgical technique, and pitfalls. *Instr Course Lect*. 2004;53:119-130.
4. Chen WM, McAuley JP, Engh CA Jr, Hopper RH Jr, Engh CA. Extended slide trochanteric osteotomy for revision total hip arthroplasty. *J Bone Joint Surg Am*. 2000;82(9):1215-1219.
5. Klapper RC, Caillouette JT, Callaghan JJ, Hozack WJ. Ultrasonic technology in revision joint arthroplasty. *Clin Orthop Relat Res*. 1992;(285):147-154.
6. Bozic KJ, Kurtz SM, Lau E, Ong K, Vail TP, Berry DJ. The epidemiology of revision total hip arthroplasty in the United States. *J Bone Joint Surg Am*. 2009;91(1):128-133.
7. Engh CA, Bobyn JD. *Biological Fixation in Total Hip Arthroplasty*. Thorofare, NJ: SLACK Incorporated; 1985:89-107.
8. Bohn WW. Modular femoral stem removal during total hip arthroplasty using a universal modular stem extractor. *Clin Orthop Relat Res*. 1992;(285):155-157.
9. Bauze AJ, Charity J, Tsiridis E, Timperley AJ, Gie GA. Posterior longitudinal split osteotomy for femoral component extraction in revision total hip arthroplasty. *J Arthroplasty*. 2008;23(1):86-89.
10. Paprosky WG, Weeden SH, Bowling JW Jr. Component removal in revision total hip arthroplasty. *Clin Orthop Relat Res*. 2001;(393):181-193.
11. Klein AH, Rubash HE. Femoral windows in revision total hip arthroplasty. *Clin Orthop Relat Res*. 1993;(291):164-170.
12. Quinlan JF, O'Shea K, Doyle F, Brady OH. In-cement technique for revision hip arthroplasty. *J Bone Joint Surg Br*. 2006;88(6):730-733.
13. Cross M, Bostrom M. Cement mantle retention: filling the hole. *Orthopedics*. 2009;32(9):pii
14. Duncan WW, Hubble MJ, Howell JR, Whitehouse SL, Timperley AJ, Gie GA. Revision of the cemented femoral stem using a cement-in-cement technique: a five- to 15-year review. *J Bone Joint Surg Br*. 2009;91(5):577-582.
15. Lombardi AV Jr. Cement removal in revision total hip arthroplasty. *Semin Arthroplasty*. 1992;3(4):264-272.
16. Schurman DJ, Maloney WJ. Segmental cement extraction at revision total hip arthroplasty. *Clin Orthop Relat Res*. 1992;(285):158-163.
17. Goldberg SH, Studders EM, Cohen MS. Ultrasonic cement removal in revision arthroplasty. *Orthopedics*. 2007;30(8):632-635.
18. Goldberg SH, Cohen MS, Young M, Bradnock B. Thermal tissue damage caused by ultrasonic cement removal from the humerus. *J Bone Joint Surg Am*. 2005;87(3):583-591.
19. de la Fuente M, Ohnsorge JA, Schkommodau E, Jetzki S, Wirtz DC, Radermacher K. Fluoroscopy-based 3-D reconstruction of femoral bone cement: a new approach for revision total hip replacement. *IEEE Trans Biomed Eng*. 2005;52(4):664-675.
20. Takagi M, Tamaki Y, Kobayashi S, Sasaki K, Takakubo Y, Ishii M. Cement removal and bone bed preparation of the femoral medullary canal assisted by flexible endoscope in total hip revision arthroplasty. *J Orthop Sci*. 2009;14(6):719-726.

21. Moreland JR, Marder R, Anspach WE Jr. The window technique for the removal of broken femoral stems in total hip replacement. *Clin Orthop Relat Res.* 1986;(212):245-249.

22. Nabors ED, Liebelt R, Mattingly DA, Bierbaum BE. Removal and reinsertion of cemented femoral components during acetabular revision. *J Arthroplasty.* 1996;11(2):146-152.

23. Lombardi AV Jr, Berend KR. Isolated acetabular liner exchange. *J Am Acad Orthop Surg.* 2008;16(5):243-248.

24. Maloney WJ, Paprosky W, Engh CA, Rubash H. Surgical treatment of pelvic osteolysis. *Clin Orthop Relat Res.* 2001;(393):78-84.

25. O'Brien JJ, Burnett RS, McCalden RW, MacDonald SJ, Bourne RB, Rorabeck CH. Isolated liner exchange in revision total hip arthroplasty: clinical results using the direct lateral surgical approach. *J Arthroplasty.* 2004;19(4):414-423.

26. Schmalzried TP, Fowble VA, Amstutz HC. The fate of pelvic osteolysis after reoperation. No recurrence with lesional treatment. *Clin Orthop Relat Res.* 1998;(350):128-137.

27. Bonner KF, Delanois RE, Harbach G, Bushelow M, Mont MA. Cementation of a polyethylene liner into a metal shell. Factors related to mechanical stability. *J Bone Joint Surg Am.* 2002;84-A(9):1587-1593.

28. Beaule PE, LeDuff MJ, Dorey FJ, Amstutz HC. Fate of cementless acetabular components retained during revision total hip arthroplasty. *J Bone Joint Surg Am.* 2003;85-A(12):2288-2293.

29. Maloney WJ, Wadey VM. Removal of well-fixed cementless components. *Instr Course Lect.* 2006;55:257-261.

30. Mitchell PA, Masri BA, Garbuz DS, Greidanus NV, Wilson D, Duncan CP. Removal of well-fixed, cementless, acetabular components in revision hip arthroplasty. *J Bone Joint Surg Br.* 2003;85(7):949-952.

31. Olyslaegers C, Wainwright T, Middleton RG. A novel technique for the removal of well-fixed cementless, large-diameter metal-on-metal acetabular components. *J Arthroplasty.* 2008;23(7):1071-1073.

32. Taylor PR, Stoffel KK, Dunlop DG, Yates PJ. Removal of the well-fixed hip resurfacing acetabular component: a simple, bone preserving technique. *J Arthroplasty.* 2009;24(3):484-486.

33. Ahmad MA, Biant LC, Tayar R, Thomas PR, Field RE. A manoeuvre to facilitate acetabular component retrieval following intra-pelvic migration. *Hip Int.* 2009;19(2):157-159.

34. Della Valle CJ, Stuchin SA. A novel technique for the removal of well-fixed, porous-coated acetabular components with spike fixation. *J Arthroplasty.* 2001;16(8):1081-1083.

35. Berger RA, Quigley LR, Jacobs JJ, Sheinkop MB, Rosenberg AG, Galante JO. The fate of stable cemented acetabular components retained during revision of a femoral component of a total hip arthroplasty. *J Bone Joint Surg Am.* 1999;81(12):1682-1691.

36. Sabboubeh A, Al Khatib M. A technique for removing a well-fixed cemented acetabular component in revision total hip arthroplasty. *J Arthroplasty.* 2005;20(6):800-801.

37. de Thomasson E, Mazel C, Gagna G, Guingand O. A simple technique to remove well-fixed, all-polyethylene cemented acetabular component in revision hip arthroplasty. *J Arthroplasty.* 2001;16(4):538-540.

The opinions and assertions contained herein are the private views of the authors and are not to be construed as official or reflecting the views of the Department of the Army or Department of Defense.

Reconstruction and Management Options for Femoral Bone Loss in Revision Total Hip Arthroplasty

Jared R. H. Foran, MD and Craig J. Della Valle, MD

Total hip arthroplasty is one of the most successful procedures in all of medicine and results in reliable improvements in pain and function. Despite this great success, the need for revision in some cases remains inevitable. Revising femoral components in the setting of femoral bone loss can be challenging. An understanding of the treatment options for femoral bone loss in revision arthroplasty is essential for the surgeon taking on these potentially challenging cases.

Modes of failure necessitating total hip revision are varied and include aseptic loosening, infection, instability, polyethylene wear, osteolysis, periprosthetic fracture, and catastrophic implant failure secondary to implant fracture. Loss of femoral bone stock may occur with each of these failure modes and may be exacerbated by iatrogenic bone loss during implant removal.[1] Recognizing femoral bone loss, and having a framework with which to classify it, is crucial in guiding management decisions.

Management strategies are based on the pattern and extent of femoral bone loss as well as the quality of the remaining bone. Options for reconstruction include cemented or noncemented fixation, proximally coated stems (modular or nonmodular), extensively coated stems that obtain fixation distally (modular or nonmodular), impaction grafting, allograft prosthetic composites, and proximal femoral replacing prostheses (megaprostheses). Although there is a dearth of high quality, randomized, prospective studies comparing femoral revision techniques,[2] there are several studies that detail the results of specific fixation strategies, and these are helpful in guiding decision making. Regardless of the type of reconstruction that is undertaken, the ultimate goal of revision surgery is to provide a stable construct that decreases pain, improves function, preserves native bone and soft tissue, and provides options for potential future revisions.

PREOPERATIVE RADIOGRAPHIC EVALUATION

A thorough review of plain radiographs is an essential part of preoperative planning for femoral revision. Although not the focus of this chapter, it is essential to perform a thorough evaluation of the acetabulum because the acetabular status may influence management options on the femoral side. Several acetabular classifications have been proposed.[3-6] We find the Paprosky classification[4] to be of particular utility in guiding treatment. The acetabular component should be

Jacofsky DJ, Hedley AK.
*Fundamentals of Revision Hip Arthroplasty:
Diagnosis, Evaluation, and Treatment (pp 79-90).*
© 2013 SLACK Incorporated.

Figure 6-1. Loose cemented femoral component. A fractured cemented femoral component is a sign of definite loosening.

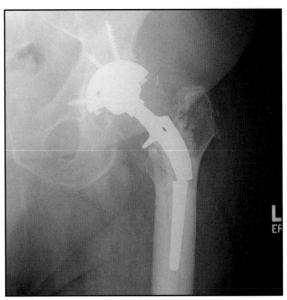

evaluated for implant model, position, type, and size so that appropriate trials and replacement liners, including offset, elevated rim, and constrained will be available. Additionally, signs of loosening, polyethylene wear, osteolysis, component migration, fracture, and/or pelvic discontinuity should be noted. The acetabular component may be retained if the cup is adequately positioned and well fixed.

When planning for femoral revision, high quality, anteroposterior (AP) pelvis as well as AP, lateral, and shoot-through radiographs of the hip should be closely scrutinized. Radiographs should be of adequate length to evaluate the entire prosthesis as well as the quality, quantity, and location of remaining bone stock. Particular attention should be paid to visualizing the femoral isthmus where fixation is often times obtained for the revision component. Additionally, the radiographs should be of sufficient clarity to allow visualization of subtle interface changes that may suggest loosening. Radiographs should be inspected for evidence of loosening, osteolysis, stress shielding, varus remodeling, fracture, heterotopic ossification, trochanteric overgrowth, and periosteal reaction (which may indicate infection). Serial radiographs can be helpful in identifying subtle changes.

Signs of definite loosening of cemented stems include component migration, fracture of the cement mantle, or fracture of the femoral component. A continuous radiolucent line at the bone-cement interface indicates probable loosening. Possible loosening is suggested by a radiolucent line of 50% to 90% of the bone-cement interface (Figure 6-1).[7]

Signs of loosening of cementless femoral components may be more subtle. Cementless femoral components can be categorized as ingrown, stable fibrous, or unstable. In general, well-ingrown femoral components lack reactive lines in the area of porous coating and have "spot welds" of endosteal bone at the bone-porous surface interface. Stable fibrous components may show nonprogressive reactive lines between the porous surface and host endosteum. Additionally, there may be a small pedestal, but component migration or subsidence is absent. Unstable components reveal progressive, nonlinear radiolucencies between the bone-porous surface interface, component migration or subsidence, and depending on the design of the stem, may have a distal pedestal. Bead shedding may also occur (Figure 6-2).[8]

In the setting of a loose femoral component, the femur often remodels into varus and retroversion (so-called "proximal femoral remodeling") (Figure 6-3). It is important to recognize such remodeling during preoperative templating because, when present, there is a heightened

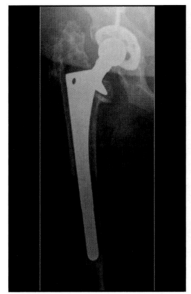

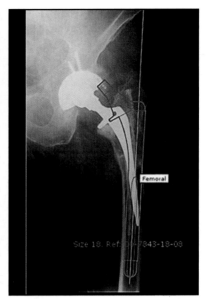

Figure 6-2. Loose cementless femoral component. There is a complete radiolucent line at the bone-prosethesis interface, an absence of "spot-welds," component subsidence, and a large distal bony pedestal.

Figure 6-3. Varus femoral remodeling. The distal portion of a clear overlay template fits in the center of the medullary canal, but the proximal portion lies outside of the femur indicating varus femoral remodeling. An extended trochanteric osteotomy is required for reconstruction.

risk of cortical perforation while reaming, fracture during implant insertion, and undersizing the implant. An extended trochanteric osteotomy is usually required in the presence of such remodeling to correct it.[9]

PREOPERATIVE PLANNING

Every attempt should be made to obtain preoperative records—particularly if the patient's previous procedures were performed at an outside institution. Operative reports should be reviewed to identify the size, make, and model of the implanted components as well as the indication for the previous arthroplasty, other previous procedures about the hip, intraoperative or postoperative complications, and previous surgical approaches. Additionally, any history of infection should be recognized. In our practice patients undergoing revision for any reason undergo an infection workup, which includes a C-reactive protein (CRP) and erythrocyte sedimentation rate (ESR) prior to the first visit to the office. If these inflammatory markers are elevated, or if there is clinical suspicion for infection, then a preoperative aspiration will be performed.

Templating is an essential part of planning for reconstruction of the deficient femur. It is important to take into account preoperative bone loss as described above, and also to anticipate bone loss that may occur secondary to exposure and implant removal. Clear overlays are used to plan for the appropriate length and diameter of the revision component to obtain adequate fixation. For example, if an extensively coated, diaphyseal-fitting stem is planned, then there should be a minimum of 4 cm of intact cortical bone present at the isthmus (Figure 6-4). If there is less than 4 cm of intact cortical bone, then consideration should be given to alternative techniques such as the use of modular tapered stems. Additionally, a mismatch in fit between the clear overlay and the

Figure 6-4. Type IIIA femur. There is a minimum of 4 cm of isthmus available for scratch-fit. An extensively coated femoral component achieves reliable fixation in this setting.

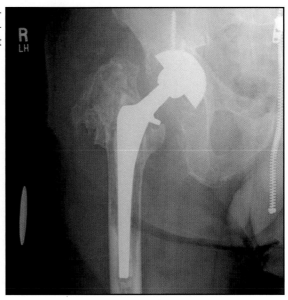

femoral canal may be an indication that significant bony remodeling has occurred and may alert the surgeon regarding the need for an extended trochanteric osteotomy to correct the deformity.

Preoperative radiographs may underestimate the actual amount of bone loss, and host bone can be significantly damaged or lost during difficult extractions of the femoral component. As such, the preoperative plan may need to be modified based on the intraoperative findings at the time of revision. It follows that orthopedic surgeons taking on revision hip arthroplasty should be comfortable with a range of fixation techniques. When preoperative planning, the surgeon should anticipate alternative scenarios and have the appropriate instruments and implants available should they be necessary.

Manufacturer-specific explantation devices should be available whenever possible. Additionally, universal explantation devices, flexible osteotomes, high speed burrs, trephines, and ultrasonic cement removal instrumentation are invaluable tools for disrupting the implant-bone or bone-cement interfaces. The goal is to efficiently extract implants while minimally disrupting host bone.

CLASSIFICATION OF FEMORAL BONE LOSS

Multiple classification systems have been developed to characterize femoral bone loss.[6,10-13] We find that the Paprosky classification (Table 6-1), which describes the relative amounts of residual metaphyseal and diaphyseal bone, provides a straightforward algorithm for defining bone loss and directing the appropriate choices for femoral revision techniques.

Type I Defects

A type I defect is characterized by minimal loss of metaphyseal cancellous bone and an intact diaphysis (Figure 6-5). This pattern is rare and is typically associated with undersized, nonporous coated cementless femoral components (such as an Austin-Moore type of prostheses) or a failed hip resurfacing. Type I defects can be reconstructed with techniques similar to those used in primary total hip arthroplasty. A proximally coated stem can be used if rotational and axial stability can be obtained intraoperatively. If a cemented implant is chosen then a meticulous cement technique should be employed to remove the "neocortex" to allow for adequate cement interdigitation.[14]

TABLE 6-1. THE PAPROSKY CLASSIFICATION

TYPE	METAPHYSIS	DIAPHYSIS	RECONSTRUCTION TECHNIQUE/IMPLANT TYPE	NOTES
I	Minimal bone loss	Completely intact	1. Extensively coated, noncemented; OR 2. Proximally coated, noncemented; OR 3. Cemented implant	Similar to primary THA
II	Moderate bone loss	Completely intact	1. Extensively coated, noncemented implant; OR 2. Proximally coated, noncemented implant with diaphyseal stabilization	Watch for varus femoral remodeling: may need ETO
IIIA	Severe bone loss	4 cm or greater of intact cortical bone at femoral isthmus	1. Extensively coated, noncemented; OR 2. Modular tapered cementless implant; OR 3. Impaction grafting	1. Watch for varus femoral remodeling 2. Ensure prosthesis long enough for 4 cm scratch fit
IIIB	Severe bone loss	Less than 4 cm of intact cortical bone at isthmus	1. Modular tapered cementless implant; OR 2. Impaction grafting	
IV	Severe bone loss	Severe bone loss: isthmus nonsupportive	1. Modular tapered cementless implant 2. Impaction grafting (if proximal femoral cortex intact); OR 3. APC (if proximal femoral cortex deficient); OR 4. Megaprosthesis (if proximal femoral cortex deficient)	In low demand or elderly patients a megaprosthesis or long cemented femoral prosthesis may be used

THA indicates total hip arthroplasty; ETO, extended trochanteric osteotomy; APC, allograft-prosthesis composite.

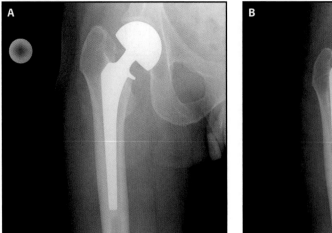
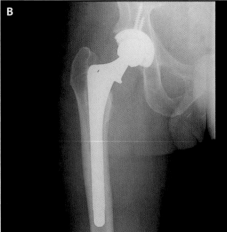

Figure 6-5. Pre- and postoperative radiographs (A, B) of a type I defect. There is minimal metaphyseal or diaphyseal bone loss. Type I defects can be reconstructed with techniques similar to those used in primary total hip arthroplasty.

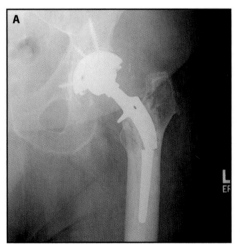
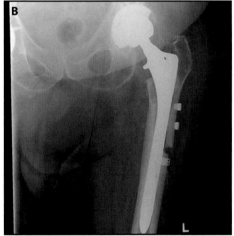

Figure 6-6. Pre- and postoperative radiographs (A, B) of a type II defect. There is moderate metaphyseal bone loss with a completely intact diaphysis. Extensively coated implants achieve reliable diaphyseal fixation in this setting.

Type II Defects

In a type II defect, there is moderate metaphyseal bone loss, however, the metaphysis can still be relied upon for primary fixation of the revision stem; the diaphysis is intact (Figure 6-6). Type II defects are relatively common in the revision setting and are often encountered when a cementless or cemented component is revised in the early stages of loosening. Given the loss of metaphyseal cancellous bone, there is typically inadequate cancellous bone for sufficient cement interdigitation, and therefore cemented femoral fixation is not recommended.[14] Because the metaphysis is supportive, a proximally coated, noncemented implant with diaphyseal stabilization (typified by the S-ROM stem [Depuy, Warsaw, IN]) may be used. As the diaphysis is intact, an extensively porous-coated cylindrical 6-inch implant reliably achieves stable fixation and is our preference for reconstruction given the ease of surgical technique and the excellent long-term results.[15] A

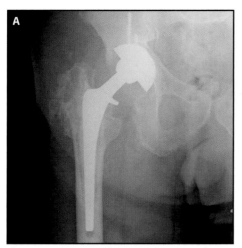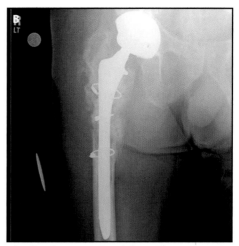

Figure 6-7. Pre- and postoperative radiographs (A, B) of a type IIIA defect. There is severe metaphyseal bone loss and moderate diaphyseal bone loss. Because there is 4 cm or more of isthmic bone available for scratch-fit, an extensively coated implant achieves reliable fixation.

minimum of 4 cm of scratch-fit is required to obtain initial component stability and to allow for subsequent ingrowth. When using an extensively coated implant, the canal is sequentially reamed until the endosteal cortex is engaged. Underreaming by 0.5 mm allows for the appropriate press-fit of the component.

Type IIIA Defects

Type IIIA defects are characterized by severe metaphyseal bone loss (the metaphysis is not supportive) with a minimum of 4 cm of intact cortical bone at the femoral isthmus (Figure 6-7). In our experience an extensively coated, diaphyseal-fitting implant achieves excellent fixation in type IIIA defects. It is essential to use an implant of adequate length to ensure that there is at least 4 cm of scratch-fit between the implant and cortical bone to allow initial mechanical stability and eventual biologic fixation to the porous surface. However, it is equally important to recognize that the use of a fully porous-coated implant that is longer than necessary greatly complicates the surgical technique, and we therefore recommend the use of the shortest stem that will achieve between 4 and 6 cm of diaphyseal engagement. Other options for reconstruction include the use of modular[16] or nonmodular tapered[17-19] stems, or impaction grafting.[20-22] However, an extensively coated, diaphyseal-fitting stem is technically easier, the implant is less expensive, and is associated with a lower complication rate than the latter options.[15,23,24] The one caveat would be large femoral canals in which the diameter of the revision implant is found to be greater than 18 mm in diameter; in this scenario we have found a higher rate of failed ingrowth with a fully porous-coated stem and thus we presently use a modular taper in this setting. Cemented revision in this setting has historically been associated with a high rate of failure and is not recommended.[25-31]

Type IIIA femurs are also frequently associated with proximal femoral remodeling into varus and retroversion (seen in approximately one-third of cases) and may require an extended trochanteric osteotomy to correct the deformity. With remodeling there is a significant risk of anterior femoral perforation during reaming and component insertion. The use of an extended trochanteric osteotomy and hand reaming helps mitigate this risk. Intraoperative radiographs with a reamer or a trial stem in place are useful to verify that femoral perforation has not occurred and that the diameter and length of the proposed revision implant are appropriate.

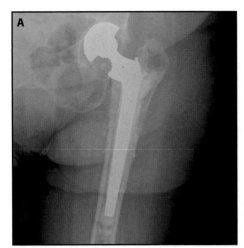
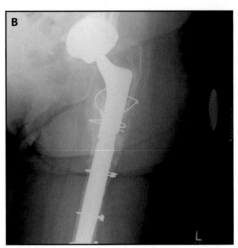

Figure 6-8. Pre- and postoperative radiographs (A, B) of a type IIIB defect. There is severe metaphyseal bone loss and moderate diaphyseal bone loss. Because there is less than 4 cm of isthmic bone available for scratch-fit, a modular tapered implant achieves bony ingrowth more reliably than an extensively coated implant.

Type IIIB Defects

Type IIIB defects are characterized by severe metaphyseal bone loss (the metaphysis is not supportive) with some (less than 4 cm) intact bone at the femoral isthmus (Figure 6-8). These defects are often associated with loosening of longer cementless implants or loosening of longer cemented implants inserted with second-generation techniques. It is important to differentiate type IIIB from type IIIA femurs. While extensively coated stems reliably achieve bony fixation in type IIIA femurs, placement of an extensively porous-coated stems in femurs with less than 4 cm of cortical bone available for scratch-fit at the femoral isthmus (type IIIB) results in higher rates of fibrous stable fixation as opposed to bony ingrowth.[32] For this reason, we currently use a modular, tapered cementless implant for the reconstruction of type IIIB defects, as these implants have the ability to gain adequate stability and subsequent ingrowth in situations with less than 4 cm of femoral isthmus.

Impaction grafting may also be used to reconstruct IIIB defects but may require mesh, plates, or strut grafts to create an intact tube to contain the graft if sufficient cortical bone is not present. Impaction grafting is technically demanding and associated with risk of iatrogenic fracture both intraoperatively and in the early postoperative period.[33] Advocates of this technique cite the ability to restore bone stock in younger, higher demand patients. Again, type IIIB femurs may be associated with femoral remodeling and may require the use of an extended trochanteric osteotomy for safe component extraction and insertion.

Type IV Defects

In a type IV defect there is severe metaphyseal and diaphyseal bone loss without a structurally competent isthmus for distal fixation (Figure 6-9). As such, femoral fixation cannot be achieved proximally and is very difficult to achieve distally. Modular tapered stems have been used with success in selected cases with type IV defects.[34,35] Impaction grafting can also be used successfully, particularly if the proximal femoral "tube" is intact.[20-22] Alternatively, if the cortical bone is insufficient, then a proximal femoral allograft-prosthesis composite (APC) may be used.[36,37] The revision component must be cemented into the allograft, and achieving stable fixation at the host-allograft junction is critical for success. It is imperative to keep the junction between

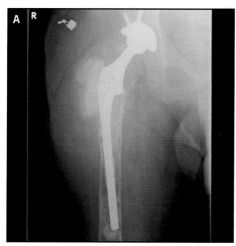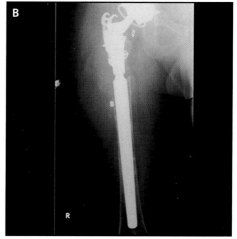

Figure 6-9. Pre- and postoperative radiographs (A, B) of a type IV defect. There is severe metaphyseal and diaphyseal bone loss. This femur was revised with a modular tapered component.

the APC and host bone free of cement to allow for bony healing at the interface. Other salvage options in elderly or low demand patients include cementing a long femoral component or the use of a proximal femoral replacement (megaprosthesis).[38] If an APC or proximal femoral replacement is utilized, abductor attachment is usually difficult or absent and strong consideration should be given to the use of a constrained liner to avoid instability.[39] Poor quality tissue may lead to poor abductor integrity, even if repaired to the cadaveric tendon of an APC. In these settings, postoperative abduction bracing may be beneficial to minimize the tension placed on the repair until 6 to 8 weeks postoperatively.

Summary

Revising femoral components can be challenging, especially when there is significant femoral bone loss. The surgeon taking on revision arthroplasty should anticipate alternative scenarios and be comfortable with a range of fixation techniques. Thoughtful preoperative planning is important. Recognizing femoral bone loss, and having a framework with which to classify it, is crucial in guiding management decisions. The Paprosky classification provides a straightforward algorithm for defining bone loss and directing the appropriate method of fixation for that loss. An extensively coated femoral component reliably provides adequate fixation for Paprosky type I, II, and IIIA defects. Type IIIB and IV defects may require a modular component, impaction grafting, proximal femoral allograft, or in salvage cases, a proximal femoral replacing prosthesis. Outcomes continue to improve with refinements in understanding, instrumentation, and technique.

References

1. Maurer SG, Baitner AC, Di Cesare PE. Reconstruction of the failed femoral component and proximal femoral bone loss in revision hip surgery. *J Am Acad Orthop Surg.* 2000;8(6):354.
2. Iorio R, Healy WL, Presutti AH. A prospective outcomes analysis of femoral component fixation in revision total hip arthroplasty. *J Arthroplasty.* 2008;23(5):662.
3. D'Antonio JA. Periprosthetic bone loss of the acetabulum. Classification and management. *Orthop Clin North Am.* 1992;23(2):279.
4. Paprosky WG, Perona PG, Lawrence JM. Acetabular defect classification and surgical reconstruction in revision arthroplasty. A 6-year follow-up evaluation. *J Arthroplasty.* 1994;9(1):33.

5. Garbuz D, Morsi E, Mohamed N, Gross AE. Classification and reconstruction in revision acetabular arthroplasty with bone stock deficiency. *Clin Orthop Relat Res.* 1996;(324):98.

6. Johnston RC, Fitzgerald RH Jr, Harris WH, Poss R, Muller ME, Sledge CB. Clinical and radiographic evaluation of total hip replacement. A standard system of terminology for reporting results. *J Bone Joint Surg Am.* 1990;72(2):161.

7. Harris WH, McCarthy JC Jr, O'Neill DA. Femoral component loosening using contemporary techniques of femoral cement fixation. *J Bone Joint Surg Am.* 1982;64(7):1063.

8. Engh CA, Bobyn JD, Glassman AH. Porous-coated hip replacement. The factors governing bone ingrowth, stress shielding, and clinical results. *J Bone Joint Surg Br.* 1987;69(1):45.

9. Della Valle CJ, Paprosky WG. The femur in revision total hip arthroplasty evaluation and classification. *Clin Orthop Relat Res.* 2004;(420):55.

10. D'Antonio J, McCarthy JC, Bargar WL, et al. Classification of femoral abnormalities in total hip arthroplasty. *Clin Orthop Relat Res.* 1993;(296):133.

11. Mallory TH. Preparation of the proximal femur in cementless total hip revision. *Clin Orthop Relat Res.* 1988;(235):47.

12. Saleh KJ, Holtzman J, Gafni AL, et al. Development, test reliability and validation of a classification for revision hip arthroplasty. *J Orthop Res.* 2001;19(1):50.

13. Longjohn DL. *Bone Stock Loss and Allografting: Femur.* New York, NY: Springer; 1999.

14. Dohmae Y, Bechtold JE, Sherman RE, Puno RM, Gustilo RB. Reduction in cement-bone interface shear strength between primary and revision arthroplasty. *Clin Orthop Relat Res.* 1988;(236):214.

15. Weeden SH, Paprosky WG. Minimal 11-year follow-up of extensively porous-coated stems in femoral revision total hip arthroplasty. *J Arthroplasty.* 2002;17(4 Suppl 1):134.

16. Kwong LM, Miller AJ, Lubinus P. A modular distal fixation option for proximal bone loss in revision total hip arthroplasty: a 2- to 6-year follow-up study. *J Arthroplasty.* 2003;18(3 Suppl 1):94.

17. Bohm P, Bischel O. The use of tapered stems for femoral revision surgery. *Clin Orthop Relat Res.* 2004;(420):148.

18. Isacson J, Stark A, Wallensten R. The Wagner revision prosthesis consistently restores femoral bone structure. *Int Orthop.* 2000;24(3):139.

19. Grunig R, Morscher E, Ochsner PE. Three-to 7-year results with the uncemented SL femoral revision prosthesis. *Arch Orthop Trauma Surg.* 1997;116(4):187.

20. Leopold SS, Berger RA, Rosenberg AG, Jacobs JJ, Quigley LR, Galante JO. Impaction allografting with cement for revision of the femoral component. A minimum four-year follow-up study with use of a precoated femoral stem. *J Bone Joint Surg Am.* 1999;81(8):1080.

21. Elting JJ, Mikhail WE, Zicat BA, Hubbell JC, Lane LE, House B. Preliminary report of impaction grafting for exchange femoral arthroplasty. *Clin Orthop Relat Res.* 1995;(319):159.

22. Gie GA, Linder L, Ling RS, Simon JP, Slooff TJ, Timperley AJ. Impacted cancellous allografts and cement for revision total hip arthroplasty. *J Bone Joint Surg Br.* 1993;75(1):14.

23. Krishnamurthy AB, MacDonald SJ, Paprosky WG. 5- to 13-year follow-up study on cementless femoral components in revision surgery. *J Arthroplasty.* 1997;12(8):839.

24. Moreland JR, Bernstein ML. Femoral revision hip arthroplasty with uncemented, porous-coated stems. *Clin Orthop Relat Res.* 1995;(319):141.

25. Callaghan JJ, Salvati EA, Pellicci PM, Wilson PD Jr, Ranawat CS. Results of revision for mechanical failure after cemented total hip replacement, 1979 to 1982. A two to five-year follow-up. *J Bone Joint Surg Am.* 1985;67(7):1074.

26. Kavanagh BF, Fitzgerald RH Jr. Multiple revisions for failed total hip arthroplasty not associated with infection. *J Bone Joint Surg Am.* 1987;69(8):1144.

27. Kavanagh BF, Ilstrup DM, Fitzgerald RH Jr. Revision total hip arthroplasty. *J Bone Joint Surg Am.* 1985;67(4):517.

28. Pellicci PM, Wilson PD Jr, Sledge CB, et al. Long-term results of revision total hip replacement. A follow-up report. *J Bone Joint Surg Am.* 1985;67(4):513.

29. Katz RP, Callaghan JJ, Sullivan PM, Johnston RC. Results of cemented femoral revision total hip arthroplasty using improved cementing techniques. *Clin Orthop Relat Res.* 1995;(319):178.

30. McLaughlin JR, Harris WH. Revision of the femoral component of a total hip arthroplasty with the calcar-replacement femoral component. Results after a mean of 10.8 years postoperatively. *J Bone Joint Surg Am.* 1996;78(3):331.

31. Mulroy WF, Harris WH. Revision total hip arthroplasty with use of so-called second-generation cementing techniques for aseptic loosening of the femoral component. A fifteen-year-average follow-up study. *J Bone Joint Surg Am.* 1996;78(3):325.

32. Paprosky WG, Aribindi R. Hip replacement: treatment of femoral bone loss using distal bypass fixation. *Instr Course Lect.* 2000;49:119-130.

33. Ornstein E, Atroshi I, Franzen H, Johnsson R, Sandquist P, Sundberg M. Early complications after one hundred and forty-four consecutive hip revisions with impacted morselized allograft bone and cement. *J Bone Joint Surg Am.* 2002;84-A(8):1323.

34. Sporer SM, Paprosky WG. Revision total hip arthroplasty: the limits of fully coated stems. *Clin Orthop Relat Res.* 2003;(417):203.

35. Patel PD, Klika AK, Murray TG, Elsharkawy KA, Krebs VE, Barsoum WK. Influence of technique with distally fixed modular stems in revision total hip arthroplasty. *J Arthroplasty.* 2010;25(6):926-931.

36. Blackley HR, Davis AM, Hutchison CR, Gross AE. Proximal femoral allografts for reconstruction of bone stock in revision arthroplasty of the hip. A nine to fifteen-year follow-up. *J Bone Joint Surg Am.* 2001; 83-A(3):346.

37. Safir O, Kellett CF, Flint M, Backstein D, Gross AE. Revision of the deficient proximal femur with a proximal femoral allograft. *Clin Orthop Relat Res.* 2009;467(1):206.

38. Malkani AL, Settecerri JJ, Sim FH, Chao EY, Wallrichs SL. Long-term results of proximal femoral replacement for non-neoplastic disorders. *J Bone Joint Surg Br.* 1995;77(3):351.

39. Kung PL, Ries MD. Effect of femoral head size and abductors on dislocation after revision THA. *Clin Orthop Relat Res.* 2007;465:170.

Reconstruction and Management Options for Acetabular Bone Loss

Michael D. Ries, MD

Bone loss after total hip arthroplasty (THA) typically results from wear, debris-induced osteolysis, component loosening and migration, infection, implant removal, and surgical preparation of the acetabulum. Acetabular defects can be classified using several systems to describe the location and severity of bone loss and results of reconstruction techniques. Generally, acetabular defects are separated into those that are relatively small and contained or cavitary and larger segmental defects in which a structural segment of the acetabular rim is deficient. Contained defects can be effectively treated with morselized bone graft and a cementless hemispherical cup fixed with screws if the acetabular rim is relatively intact. For segmental defects in which structural support of the acetabular rim is needed to support a revision component, structural augmentation of the defect with either allograft or modular metal augments or a jumbo, bi-lobed or oblong cup is necessary. Structural allografts for segmental defects have been associated with favorable early results, but a relatively high failure rate has been reported in long-term studies. Metal augmentation provides more reliable structural support of segmental defects. Discontinuity represents a separation between the ilium and ischium due to bone loss and has a relatively poor prognosis, particularly if segmental bone loss is present. Results of structural allograft and cage reconstruction for discontinuity have not been favorable. Better results appear to be achieved with custom triflange implants or a cup-cage technique. However, long-term follow-up is needed to determine the durability of these methods in maintaining pelvic stability for treatment of discontinuity.

CLASSIFICATION OF BONE LOSS

Various acetabular defect classification systems have been developed and used during the past 25 years to describe acetabular defects in revision THA.[1-6] The Paprosky system is based on the presence or absence of an intact acetabular rim and its ability to support a revision acetabular component.[1,6] The American Academy of Orthopaedic Surgeons (AAOS) and Engh systems distinguish mainly between cavitary and segmental defects.[2,3,6] The Gross classification was based on an intraoperative assessment of bone loss and need for structural bone graft.[4,6] The Saleh system was developed by a consensus of a panel of 21 experts, followed by an interobserver variability study.[5,6] However, none of the current classification systems include bone quality or relative osteopenia, which may also influence the success of the reconstruction.

Jacofsky DJ, Hedley AK.
Fundamentals of Revision Hip Arthroplasty:
Diagnosis, Evaluation, and Treatment (pp 91-102).
© 2013 SLACK Incorporated.

Johansen et al recently reviewed 6 acetabular defect classification systems.[6] The classification systems were separated into those that aim to describe detailed information about defects for preoperative planning (Paprosky, AAOS, Saleh, and Gustillo) and those that simplify the classification in order to improve reproducibility and communication (Engh, Gross).[1-5,7] However, only the Saleh system demonstrated the reliability and validity required for a standard grading system.[6]

The Saleh system separates acetabular defects into 5 types. Type I defects have little or no notable bone loss. A type II defect is a cavitary lesion with a relatively intact peripheral rim. Type III and IV defects are those with loss of a segment of the acetabular rim. Type III has a deficiency of less than 50% of the rim, and type IV has a deficiency of more than 50% of the rim. Type V defects are acetabular discontinuity. These represent a fracture or nonunion with separation of the ilium from the ischium and pubis.

Management Strategies

Type I: Little or No Notable Bone Loss

Type I defects have little or no notable bone loss. This typically occurs during conversion of a bipolar to total hip replacement or revision of a cementless acetabular cup that has been malpositioned or fails as a result of liner dissociation or wear without significant osteolysis. However, bone loss may occur during removal of a well-fixed component, resulting in a larger defect. Instruments with sharp curved osteotome blades have been developed to remove well-fixed implants without significant loss of bone.[8] Revision is then achieved with a slightly larger cementless acetabular cup.

Osteolysis may also develop around a well-fixed cup, permitting curettage and bone grafting the osteolytic lesion while retaining the acetabular metal shell.[9] Access to the osteolytic lesion is obtained by curettage through the acetabular implant screw holes or through cortical defects or an osteotomized bone window around the periphery of the cup. The head and liner are exchanged while retaining the acetabular metal shell. If an acetabular liner is unavailable to fit the previously implanted shell, a new liner can be cemented into the metal shell.[10] Requirements for this technique include a well-fixed metal shell in good position and a satisfactory revision liner that fits the shell. However, a shell can appear well fixed radiographically, while intraoperative findings demonstrate cup loosening so implants, bone graft, and instrumentation for revision of the shell should also be available during surgery.

Type II: Cavitary Defects

Implant Selection

The treatment and prognosis for smaller cavitary defects is considerably different than that of segmental defects. If small areas of bone loss are present in the acetabular cavity and rim, but the rim is largely intact, reconstruction can be performed with a cementless porous-coated hemispherical cup fixed with screws and morselized bone graft to fill the cavitary lesions. The cup is supported on intact host bone, and bone grafts are not load bearing (Figure 7-1).

The acetabular rim provides the primary mechanical support for a hemispherical revision component. Medial defects can be effectively treated with morselized bone. However, if the bone is osteoporotic, the peripheral rim may not provide adequate structural support for a cementless cup. In a series of 19 revisions performed with an oversized rim fit cup and medial morselized bone grafts for large medial (protrusio) defects involving more than 50% of the acetabulum, satisfactory results were achieved in all cases and none of the acetabular cups required revision at 3-year follow-up.[11] However, 2 cups migrated more than 3 mm, both in female patients aged 85 and 87 years, suggesting that a cage may be necessary for protrusio defects with osteopenia (Figure 7-2).

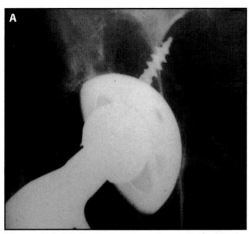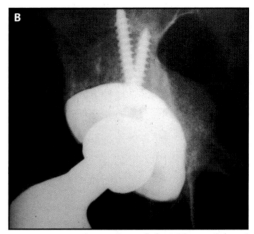

Figure 7-1. (A) An anteroposterior radiograph demonstrates a superior cavitary defect. The peripheral rim appears intact. (B) Revision was achieved with a cementless cup fixed with screws and morselized allograft. Bone graft has extended through a defect in the medial wall, and the peripheral bony rim provides mechanical support for the revision component.

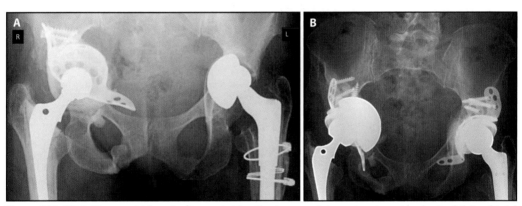

Figure 7-2. (A) A 62-year-old female rheumatoid patient on prednisone treatment had prior bilateral total hip replacements and subsequent revision total hip arthroplasty. Loosening with a protrusio (type II) acetabular defect developed on the left side, and loosening of a previously implanted cage with a large segmental defect (type IV) developed on the right side. (B) Although the acetabular rim was relatively intact on the right side, the bone was osteoporotic and would not provide adequate mechanical support for a rim fit cementless cup. The hip was revised with a cemented cage and morselized allograft. The right hip was revised using a cup-cage technique in which a trabecular metal cup is implanted as a large augment in a medialized position and fixed with screws. A cage is then implanted with fixation to the ilium and ischium, which is intended to protect the cup from weightbearing stresses.

Bone Graft

Type II defects consist of areas of cavitary bone loss with a relatively intact peripheral rim. These can be treated with use of a larger cementless hemispherical cup fixed with screws and morselized bone graft to fill the cavitary lesions. The morselized bone graft is not load bearing and can heal and become replaced by vascularized host bone over time.[12] Bone graft sources include frozen or freeze dried allograft, autograft, and a variety of synthetic bone graft substitutes. Allograft is readily available and avoids donor site morbidity. However, the potential risk of disease transmission may be a concern and immune reactions can occur. The healing rate is less predictable than with autograft. However, autograft availability is limited. Iliac crest graft is associated with donor site morbidity. Autograft can also be obtained from acetabular reamings. However, in revision THA, the acetabular reamings may be contaminated with metallic, or ultrahigh-molecular-weight polyethylene debris, which could limit its utility as a bone void filler. A large number of synthetic bone graft substitutes are commercially available. It is not clear if the results of treatment with synthetic grafts will be more favorable than allograft. Synthetic grafts are usually are more expensive than allograft and may be more appropriate for smaller defects while morselized allograft can be used for large defects in which the cost associated with a large amount of synthetic graft would be a concern.

Reaming

In many primary THAs the femoral head is subluxed laterally and the arthritic acetabulum is shallow so that relative medialization of the acetabulum is necessary to provide adequate bone coverage of the acetabular component and restoration of the normal biomechanical center of the hip. A series of reamers are used that increase concentrically in size until the final reamer engages the acetabular rim. However, in revision THA with type II defects, the peripheral acetabular rim should be enlarged to provide rim support of a slightly larger diameter implant than the previously implanted cup. Minimal medial reaming may be required. Reaming with a relatively large diameter reamer that is held laterally allows concentric reaming of the rim.[13]

Type III: Segmental Defect Less Than 50% of the Rim

Type III defects involve loss of less than 50% of the acetabular rim. These can be treated with several strategies including a high hip center, jumbo hemispherical acetabular cup, bi-lobed or oblong cup, or metal or allograft structural augmentation of the segmental defect. However, many type III defects can be treated with a large hemispherical cup while structural augmentation is usually needed for type IV defects.

High Hip Center

If segmental bone loss is located superiorly, the defect can be reamed into a hemispherical shape and a cementless cup used with direct contact onto host bone. Hendricks and Harris reported on 36 hips (34 patients) treated with a high hip center (at least 35 mm above the inter teardrop line).[14] At average 16.8 years follow-up, 2 shells were revised for loosening and 3 for infection. Since the pelvis is narrower proximal to the acetabulum, this method requires use of a relatively small cup and does not restore the biomechanical center of the normal acetabulum. A very long modular femoral head or proximally placed calcar replacement prosthesis is frequently needed to maintain adequate leg length. However, elevating the position of the acetabulum 1 to 2 cm from its anatomic position does not appear to substantially compromise the cup size or require excessive femoral lengthening.

Jumbo Cup

Large cementless acetabular components are available in diameters up to 80 mm, which is considerably larger than the anatomic acetabulum of most patients. Use of a jumbo acetabular cup permits acetabular preparation with conventional reamers, direct contact between the implant porous coating and host bone over a large surface area, and multiple screw fixation. Clinical results of revision THA with use of oversized (jumbo) cups have been favorable. Whaley et al reported results of jumbo cups used in a series of 89 revision THAs[15]; 79 had segmental or combined segmental and cavitary bone loss. The average cup size was 66 mm for males and 62 mm for females, and at 8 years survivorship for aseptic loosening was 98%. Hendricks and Harris similarly reported no revisions for loosening at 13.9 years follow-up in a series of jumbo (greater than 65 mm) cup revisions.[16]

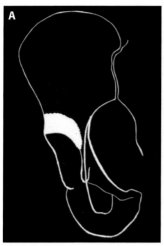
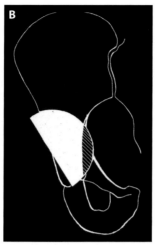
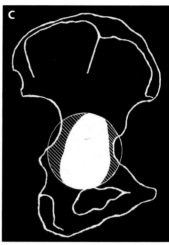

Figure 7-3. (A) A diagram of the pelvis illustrates a superior segmental defect. (B) The defect can be incorporated into a hemispherical shape to accommodate a jumbo cementless cup with large diameter reamers. The reamers and cup may penetrate through the medial wall. (C) A lateral diagram of the pelvis illustrates that circumferential centralized reaming for a jumbo cup can remove the anterior and posterior walls of the acetabulum. Eccentric reaming of the anterior wall should be done to preserve the posterior wall of the acetabulum.

Reaming

Treatment of type III defects with a cementless hemispherical acetabular component requires that the irregular shape of the acetabular cavity be reamed to a larger diameter hemispherical shape. The rim of the acetabulum is expanded to the depth of any posterior and superior segmental bone defects. Weightbearing forces in the hip are directed posteriorly and superiorly. With an oversized (jumbo) cup technique, the posterior wall and superior dome should be preserved to provide mechanical support for the revision cup. When the acetabulum is expanded with hemispherical reamers, bone is removed circumferentially (Figure 7-3). In order to preserve the posterior wall, more bone is reamed anteriorly than posteriorly. Eccentric reaming in this manner is important to provide stable fixation of the revision component since reaming through the posterior acetabular wall can severely compromise the mechanical integrity of the reconstruction. Reaming through the anterior wall with loss of anterior wall support still permits stable fixation of an oversized acetabular component. However, reaming through the anterior wall also means that the anterior rim of the acetabular component can protrude into to the anterior soft tissues and potentially be a source of pain after surgery.

Iliopsoas Tendinitis

A prominent anterior edge of an oversized acetabular cup can impinge on the iliopsoas tendon and cause groin pain.[17-19] This is more apparent if the cup is inadequately anteverted (Figure 7-4). Iliopsoas tendinitis is usually associated with hip flexion activity such as ascending stairs, getting up from a seated position, or bicycle riding. The diagnosis is supported if active hip flexion against resistance causes pain while passive hip flexion is less symptomatic. There may also be tenderness in the region of the iliopsoas tendon. Other causes of groin pain such as acetabular loosening or infection should be ruled out. Symptoms frequently improve with restriction of flexion activities, physical therapy, and nonsteroidal anti-inflammatory drugs. However, confirmation of iliopsoas tendinitis as an etiology of groin pain and pain relief can also be achieved with a cortisone injection into the iliopsoas tendon sheath.[20] This should be performed with fluoroscopic guidance and use of radiographic dye to demonstrate correct location of the injection in the iliopsoas tendon sheath. Occasionally symptoms persist, and surgical treatment is required either to reposition the cup if it is inadequately anteverted or perform iliopsoas tenotomy.[17]

Figure 7-4. An illustration of the pelvis shows a large acetabular cup implanted with a prominent anterior rim. The iliopsoas muscle is also illustrated, which can impinge on the anterior edge of the acetabular component (arrow). (Reprinted with permission from Innovative Medical Design Solutions, Logan, UT.)

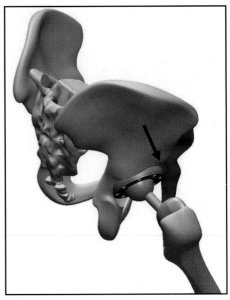

Screw Fixation

Pelvic bone stock available for screw fixation in revisions is often more limited than in primary THA. Screws should not be directed into the anterior or inferior quadrants of the acetabulum, because of the risk of neurovascular injury if the drill bit or screw penetrates into the pelvis. Screws directed superiorly into the intramedullary canal of the ilium usually provide reliable fixation. Large screw fixation of acetabular cups in this region has been used historically with the Ring prosthesis.[21] Typically, a relatively long, 50-mm, screw can be used, which is located within the cancellous bone of the ilium, and does not penetrate through the medial or lateral cortical walls. Shorter, 20- to 30-mm, screws directed posteriorly toward the sciatic notch provide bicortical fixation by penetrating through the posterior column of the pelvis. These should be placed and palpated along the sciatic notch to ensure that screw length is not excessive.

Many large diameter revision acetabular cups permit use of both dome and peripheral screws. Peripheral screws are oriented along the outer face of the cup perpendicular to the cup rim. Since the cup is relatively anteverted, peripheral screws placed through the anterorsuperior area of the rim will be directed posteriorly into the posterior column. This is a safe area of the pelvis in terms of neurovascular anatomy and often permits use of long 50- to 60-mm peripheral screws.

Type IV: Segmental Defect Greater Than 50% of the Rim

Since a large segment of the acetabular rim is deficient in a type IV defect, structural augmentation of the rim is necessary to provide a mechanical buttress to resist displacement of the revision component. Structural augmentation can be achieved with use of a bi-lobed or oblong cup, modular metal augments, or structural allograft.

Structural Allograft

Allograft permits use of bone that can be shaped intraoperatively to fit the defect and potentially restores bone stock. Although early results of allograft reconstruction have been favorable, the outcomes deteriorate considerably over time. Frozen allografts maintained at -80° C are needed to maintain adequate structural integrity, while freeze-dried or femoral head allografts may fail early due to poor mechanical properties of the allograft. The host bone can heal to the allograft surface, but the remaining allograft may remain nonvascularized even after many years in vivo.[22] A distal

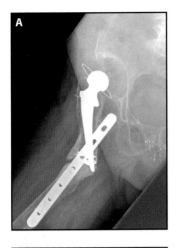

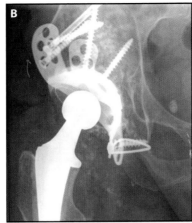

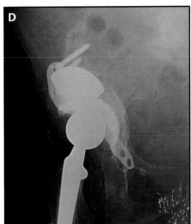

Figure 7-5. (A) An anteroposterior radiograph illustrates a superior segmental acetabular defect in a 72-year-old male patient with osteopenia. (B) The hip was reconstructed with a superior structural allograft and cage. (C) One year after the revision, failure occurred with allograft collapse and nonunion. (D) The acetabulum was revised to a trabecular metal augment and cemented cage. An anteroposterior radiograph 5 years after trabecular metal augmentation and cage reconstruction demonstrates stable position of the implants.

femur, femoral condyle, or proximal tibia allograft provides a large structural augment that can be shaped intraoperatively to fit most segmental defects. If a superior bony buttress is present, then the allograft is fit into the defect and fixed with screws. A "number 7"-shaped allograft can be used to provide a cortical allograft surface along the outer cortex of the ilium, which permits fixation using transversely directed screws across the allograft cortex and lateral ilium.[1] The inferior surface is then reamed to fit the superior dome and rim of the revision component.

Segmental allograft reconstruction with use of a porous-coated cementless cup has been associated with a high failure rate.[23] This is likely related to inability to gain biologic fixation of the cementless cup to allograft. Allograft reconstruction with use of a cage has been associated with more favorable results.[24] A cage is indicated to provide additional fixation to the ilium and ischium and potentially protect the allograft from weightbearing stresses. However, allograft fracture, nonunion, immune rejection, and collapse can all lead to failure of the cage reconstruction[25] (Figure 7-5). Since the cage does not have a porous ingrowth surface, loosening can occur because biologic fixation of the cage to allograft or host bone is not achieved. Cementing the cage directly to the allograft and pelvis by applying cement to the back surface appears to improve the results of structural allograft and cage reconstruction.[26] Although failure can occur after allograft and cage reconstruction, the allograft may also heal to host bone, which improves bone stock for future revisions.[22]

Bi-Lobed and Oblong Cups

Bi-lobed and oblong cups have also been used to treat large superior segmental defects.[27,28] The nonhemispherical shape of the cup permits direct contact of the superior implant surface with host bone in the area of the defect while maintaining the more distal anatomic position of the center of the hip. However, bi-lobed and oblong cups have considerable limitations. A limited number of sizes and shapes are available to fit a large variation in acetabular defects. The orientation of the implant is dependent on the orientation of the superior defect, which may compromise component position and lead to instability. Combined reaming of the superior defect and inferior acetabulum is necessary to accommodate the implant. Although this approach is based on a rational design philosophy, clinical results in revision THA have not been more favorable than allograft techniques. Chen et al reported a 24% failure rate with bi-lobed components in 41 revision THAs, which led the authors abandon the technique.[27]

Modular Metal Augmentation

Metal augments that can be used to fit the defect and then are attached to a revision component with a modular connection or cement permit versatility in positioning the augment and revision component (see Figure 7-5). Trabecular metal augments are available in a variety of shapes and sizes including curved crescent-shaped implants intended to fit into a superior segmental defect and large number 7 augments, which are placed onto the outer cortex of the ilium to provide transversely directed screws through the augment.[29-31] The trabecular metal augment that fits the segmental defect most closely is selected intraoperatively. The bone surface of the defect usually requires additional preparation with a small reamer or burr to accommodate the curved surface of the defect. Fixation of the augment is achieved by placing screws through the augment into the host ilium. However, screw fixation of a crescent-shaped augment can be limited due to poor bone stock in the ilium and limited screw hole positions in the augment. A number 7-shaped augment permits fixation with transversely directed screws through the augment into the ilium similar to a number 7 allograft technique. This technique also requires considerable elevation of the abductors from the outer table of the ilium to permit placement of the augment.

Cavitary defects in the acetabular cavity below the augment are filled with morselized bone graft. The augment can be used with a hemispherical cemented cup, with cement interposed between the augment and cup, or with a reconstructive cage. Superiorly directed screw fixation of the revision acetabular cup or cage is generally obstructed because of the presence of the augment. A cage that is cemented to the augment and pelvis may provide more reliable early fixation of the revision implant than screw fixation.[26]

Trabecular metal augments have a very rough porous metal surface to contact with host bone, which has been associated with reliable bone ingrowth. Early clinical results with trabecular metal augmentation in revision THA have been favorable.[29-31] However, long-term results are not available and bone stock is not improved with this technique.

Type V: Discontinuity

Discontinuity represents a separation of the ilium from the ischium and pubis, due to periacetabular bone loss. The discontinuity may not be apparent on plain x-rays because the metal acetabular shell can obstruct the bone defect seen radiographically. Oblique views or computed tomography (CT) may be helpful to visualize a discontinuity and facilitate preoperative planning.[32] Multiple techniques have been used to treat discontinuity including structural allograft and cage reconstruction, whole acetabular allografts, dual anterior and posterior column plating through combined ilioinguinal and posterior approaches, custom triflange components, and a cup-cage technique.[26,33-37]

Allograft and Cage Reconstruction

The results of revision THA for acetabular discontinuity with allograft and cage reconstruction have generally been poor, particularly if a large amount of bone loss is present.[26,33] For discontinuity with relatively minimal bone loss, healing can be achieved with use of morselized bone allograft and a reconstruction cage. However, for segmental bone loss in association with

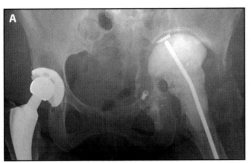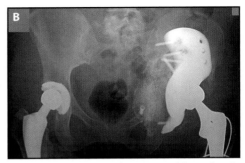

Figure 7-6. (A) An anteroposterior radiograph illustrates a discontinuity with segmental bone loss in a 60-year-old female who developed infection and was treated with removal of the components and insertion of an antibiotic cement spacer. (B) A custom triflange acetabular component was used to span the defect with multiple screw fixation to the iliac wing and use of medial morselized bone graft in the area of the discontinuity.

discontinuity, reliable techniques to achieve a durable reconstruction have not been clearly established. Berry et al reported on 27 patients (31 hips) treated with allograft and cage reconstruction for pelvic discontinuity.[33] The best results occurred in patients who did not have severe bone loss. A satisfactory result was achieved in only 10 of 19 hips with severe segmental or combined segmental and cavitary bone loss and in 3 of 5 hips with prior irradiation.[33]

Custom Triflange

The custom triflange component consists of an iliac wing, and ischial and pubic sections, attached to a conventional acetabular shell (Figure 7-6). DeBoer at al reported on 18 patients (20 hips) treated with a custom triflange acetabular component for pelvic discontinuity.[35] The implant was manufactured from a 3-dimensional model of the pelvis generated using a preoperative CT scan. Morselized bone graft was used to fill cavitary defects and in the area of the discontinuity. Considerable dissection of the posterior column and lateral ilium was required to implant the component. The sciatic nerve was dissected and a portion of the hamstrings released to avoid injury during placement of the ischial portion of the implant. The abductors were elevated from the lateral ilium since the iliac portion of the triflange component is placed along the outer table of the ilium deep to the abductors. The dissection into the sciatic notch was restricted and traction on the superior gluteal nerve minimized by abducting and translating the femur proximally. Healing of the discontinuity occurred in 18 of the 20 hips.[35] Complications included 5 dislocations, 1 sciatic nerve palsy, and broken ischial screws in 1 case. Results with this technique have been more favorable than allograft and cage reconstruction.[35] However, the triflange component is a large implant that requires considerable dissection and elevation of the abductors from the lateral ilium, which may compromise abductor function.

Metal Augmentation

Since healing of a chronic discontinuity with bone loss may not be a realistic goal due to poor vascularity of the periarticular tissues and difficulty in achieving adequate stability of the pelvis with plating or cage reconstruction, use of a cementless metal implant as an intercallary segment between the superior and inferior hemipelvis may permit stabilization of the discontinuity by ligamentotaxis of the soft tissues between the ilium and ischium. Sporer and Paprosky described a technique in which a trabecular metal implant is used to span the discontinuity with the goal of achieving biologic fixation of the acetabular component to the ilium and inferior pelvis.[37] The acetabular component is used with superior augments if necessary to treat segmental bone loss. The authors reported that 12 of 13 patients treated with this technique had radiographically stable hips at 6-year follow-up.[37]

Cup-Cage

A cup-cage technique has been also developed in which a large trabecular metal acetabular component is inserted into the discontinuity defect in an effort to gain biologic fixation of the ilium and inferior pelvis to the cementless implant surface. A cage is then placed along the outer ilium and ischium in order to protect the cementless cup from weightbearing stresses and permit biologic fixation of the ilium and inferior pelvis to the cup (see Figure 7-2). Kosashvili et al reported on 26 hips treated with this technique.[36] In 23 hips (88.5%), there was no clinical or radiographic loosening at an average follow-up of 44 months. The components migrated more than 5 mm in 3 hips (11.5%) at 1 year.[36] Early results with the cup-cage technique appear more favorable than allograft cage reconstruction. However, longer follow-up will be needed to determine the durability of this technique in maintaining pelvic stability.

REFERENCES

1. Paprosky WG, Perona PG, Lawrence JM. Acetabular defect classification and surgical reconstruction in revision arthroplasty. *J Arthroplasty*. 1994;9(1):33-44.
2. D'Antonio JA, Capello WN, Borden LS, et al. Classification and management of acetabular abnormalities in total hip arthroplasty. *Clin Orthop Relat Res*. 1989;243:126-137.
3. Engh CA, Glassman AH. Cementless revision of failed total hip replacement: an update. *Instr Course Lect*. 1991;40:189.
4. Gross AE, Allan DG, Catre M, Garbuz DS, Stockley I. Bone grafts in hip replacement surgery. The pelvic side. *Orthop Clin North Am*. 1993;24(4):679-695.
5. Saleh KJ, Holtzman J, Gafni A, et al. Development, test reliability and validation of a classification for revision hip arthroplasty. *J Orthop Res*. 2001;19(1):50-56.
6. Johanson NA, Driftmier KR, Cerynik DL, Stehman CC. Grading acetabular defects: the need for a universal and valid system. *J Arthroplasty*. 2010;25(3):425-431.
7. Gustilo RB, Pasternak HS. Revision hip arthroplasty with titanium ingrowth prosthesis and bone grafting for failed cemented femoral component loosening. *Clin Orthop Relat Res*. 1988;235:111-119.
8. Taylor PR, Stoffel KK, Dunlop DG, Yates PJ. Removal of the well-fixed hip resurfacing acetabular component. A simple, bone preserving technique. *J Arthroplasty*. 2009;24(3):484-486.
9. Maloney WJ, Herzwurm P, Paprowsky W, Rubash HE, Engh CA. Treatment of pelvic osteolysis associated with a stable acetabular component inserted without cement as part of a total hip replacement. *J Bone Joint Surg*. 1997;79A:1628-1634.
10. Wang JP, Chen WM, Chen CF, Chiang CC, Huang CK, Chen TH. Cementation of cross-linked polyethylene liner into well-fixed acetabular shells: mean 6-year follow-up study. *J Arthroplasty*. 2010;25(3):420-424.
11. Hansen E, Ries MD. Revision total hip arthroplasty for large medial (protrusio) defects with a rim fit cementless acetabular component. *J Arthroplasty*. 2006;21:72-79.
12. Winter E, Piert M, Volkmann R, et al. Allogeneic cancellous bone graft and a Burch-Schneider ring for acetabular reconstruction in revision hip arthroplasty. *J Bone Joint Surg*. 2001;83A:862-867.
13. Ries MD. Total hip arthroplasty in acetabular protrusio. *Orthopaedics*. 2009;32:666.
14. Hendricks KJ, Harris WH. High placement of noncemented acetabular components in revision total hip arthroplasty. A concise follow-up, at a minimum of fifteen years, of a previous report. *J Bone Joint Surg*. 2006;88A:2231-2236.
15. Whaley AL, Berry DJ, Harmsen WS. Extra-large uncemented hemispherical acetabular components for revision total hip arthroplasty. *J Bone Joint Surg*. 2001;83A:1352-1357.
16. Hendricks KJ, Harris WH. Revision of failed acetabular components with use of so-called jumbo noncemented components. A concise follow-up of a previous report. *J Bone Joint Surg*. 2006;88A:559-563.
17. Dora C, Houweling M, Koch P, Sierra RJ. Iliopsoas impingement after total hip replacement: the results of non-operative management, tenotomy, or acetabular revision. *J Bone Joint Surg*. 2007;89B:1031-1035.
18. Abbas AA, Kim YJ, Song EY, Yoon TR. Oversized acetabular socket causing groin pain after total hip arthroplasty. *J Arthroplasty*. 2009;24(7):1144.e5-1144.e8.
19. O'Sullivan M, Tai CC, Richards S, Skyrme AD, Walter WL, Walter WK. Iliopsoas tendonitis: a complication after total hip arthroplasty. *J Arthroplasty*. 2007;22(2):166-170.

20. Nunley R, Wilson J, Gilula LA, Maloney WJ, Barrack R, Clohisy JC. Iliopsoas tendonitis following total hip arthroplasty: how effective are selective steroid injections in treating this uncommon cause of groin pain? *J Arthroplasty.* 2009;24(2):e74.

21. Badhe NP, Howard PW. A stemmed acetabular component in the management of severe acetabular deficiency. *J Bone Joint Surg.* 2005;87B(12):1611-1616.

22. Garbuz D, Morsi E, Gross AE. Revision of the acetabular component of a total hip arthroplasty with a massive structural allograft. Study with a minimum five-year follow-up. *J Bone Joint Surg Am.* 1996;78:693-697.

23. Sporer SM, O'Rourke M, Chong P, Paprosky WG. The use of structural distal femoral allografts for acetabular reconstruction. Average ten-year follow-up. *J Bone Joint Surg.* 2005;87A:760-765.

24. Gill TJ, Sledge JB, Müller ME. The management of severe acetabular bone loss using structural allograft and acetabular reinforcement devices. *J Arthroplasty.* 2000;15(1):1-7.

25. Goodman S, Saastamoinen H, Shasha N, Gross A. Complications of ilioischial reconstruction rings in revision total hip arthroplasty. *J Arthroplasty.* 2004;19(4):436-446.

26. Hansen E, Shearer D, Ries MD. Does a cemented cage improve revision THA for severe acetabular defects? *Clin Orthop Relat Res.* 2011;469(2):494-502.

27. Chen WM, Engh CA, Hopper RH, Mcauley JP, Engh CA. Acetabular revision with use of a bilobed component inserted without cement in patients who have acetabular bone-stock deficiency. *J Bone Joint Surg.* 2000;82A:197-206.

28. Vavrik LP, Jahoda D, Pokorny D, Tawa A, Sosna A. The long oblique revision component in revision arthroplasty of the hip. *J Bone Joint Surg.* 2009;91B:24-30.

29. Van Kleunen JP, Lee, GG, Lementowski PW, Nelson CL, Garino JP. Acetabular revisions using trabecular metal cups and augments. *J Arthroplasty.* 2009;24:64-68.

30. Lingaraj K, Teo YH, Bergman N. The management of severe acetabular bone defects in revision hip arthroplasty using modular porous metal components. *J Bone Joint Surg.* 2009;91B:1555-1560.

31. Flecher X, Sporer S, Paprosky W. Management of severe bone loss in acetabular revision using a trabecular metal shell. *J Arthroplasty.* 2008;23(7):949-955.

32. Giori NJ, Sidky AO. Lateral and high-angle oblique radiographs of the pelvis aid in diagnosing pelvic discontinuity after total hip arthroplasty. *J Arthroplasty.* 2011;26(1):110-112.

33. Berry DJ, Lewallen DG, Hanssen AD, Cabanella ME. Pelvic discontinuity in revision total hip arthroplasty. *J Bone Joint Surg.* 1999;81A:1692-1702.

34. Eggli S, Muller C, Ganz R. Revision surgery in pelvic discontinuity: an analysis of seven patients. *Clin Orthop Rel Res.* 2002;(398):136-145.

35. DeBoer DK, Christie MJ, Brinson MF, Morrison JC. Revision total hip arthroplasty for pelvic discontinuity. *J Bone Joint Surg.* 2007;89A:835-840.

36. Kosashvili Y, Backstein D, Safir O, Lakstein D, Gross AE. Acetabular revision using an anti-protrusion (ilio-ischial) cage and trabecular metal acetabular component for severe acetabular bone loss associated with pelvic discontinuity. *J Bone Joint Surg.* 2009;91B:870-876.

37. Sporer SM, Paprosky WG. Acetabular revision using a trabecular metal acetabular component for severe acetabular bone loss associated with a pelvic discontinuity. *J Arthroplasty.* 2006;21(6 Suppl 1):87-90.

Femoral Component Options in Revision Total Hip Arthroplasty

Michael R. Bloomfield, MD; Carlos A. Higuera, MD; and Wael K. Barsoum, MD

Femoral component revision is a complex procedure that has shown improved outcomes with current technology and the availability of different prosthetic options. In this chapter we will review the indications, techniques, and outcomes for different reconstruction options including one-piece, modular, and cemented stems. We will present an algorithm to assist the surgeon in choosing the optimal reconstructive technique for a given patient. We will also discuss femoral head size in this setting. Some advanced techniques used for massive proximal bone loss, such as allograft-prosthetic composites (APC) and impaction grafting, are addressed in Chapter 7 and will not be discussed in detail here. The authors feel that these uncommon procedures are best done by surgeons experienced in their use to ensure optimal patient outcomes.

The main goals of revision total hip arthroplasty (THA) are to decrease pain and improve function by creating a stable construct that restores hip joint biomechanics. Bone and soft tissue preservation are paramount in providing the foundation for a successful revision procedure and also to facilitate possible future revisions. Recognition of bone loss and its implications on surgical decision making are among the most critical factors in a successful outcome after revision THA.

Multiple different classifications and reporting systems have been described to characterize femoral bone loss.[1-3] The main purpose of all these classification systems is to describe the quantity and location of the remaining bone in a standardized manner. Based on both of these factors, different reconstructive approaches can be used. The quantity and location of bone loss is indicated best on preoperative imaging. Adequate radiographs of the pelvis, including Judet views to evaluate the acetabulum and biplanar views of the hip and femur, are imperative to assess remaining bone stock. Computed tomography (CT) has been shown to be reliable in assessing bone loss,[4] but may be logistically difficult to obtain in every patient undergoing revision THA. The metallic artifact from the previous arthroplasty is also a potential limiting factor. In complex cases where the quantity of bone loss is difficult to assess with radiographs, a CT scan with metallic artifact subtraction may be a helpful adjunct during the preoperative planning.[5]

For standardization purposes, we will use a simplified Paprosky classification,[2] which is one of the most common classification systems cited in the literature to describe femoral bone loss. During the discussion of each reconstructive option, we will review evidence-based indications and outcomes based on these different types of femoral bone loss.

Jacofsky DJ, Hedley AK.
*Fundamentals of Revision Hip Arthroplasty:
Diagnosis, Evaluation, and Treatment (pp 103-118).*
© 2013 SLACK Incorporated.

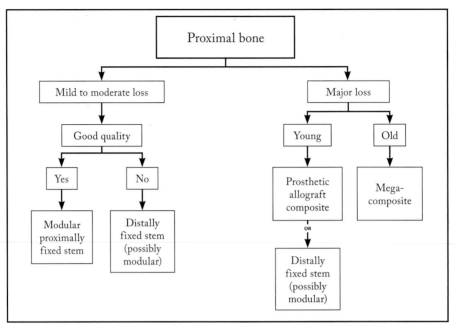

Figure 8-1. An algorithmic approach to femoral component selection in revision THA is summarized. (Adapted from Higuera CA, Capello W, Barsoum WK. Algorithmic approach for reconstruction of proximal femoral bone loss in revision total hip arthroplasty. *Orthopedics.* 2009;32[9]:pii.)

- Type I: There is no significant bone loss. The metaphyseal cancellous bone loss is minimal, and the diaphysis is unaffected. This type of defect is uncommon.
- Type II: There is a significant loss of metaphyseal bone, however, the diaphysis remains intact. The calcar is expanded and may be partially absent, with bone loss anteriorly and posteriorly. This pattern of bone loss is commonly seen.
- Type IIIA: The metaphysis is severely damaged, with bone loss both anteriorly and posteriorly. The available proximal bone may be thin and sclerotic and is incapable of providing mechanical support to a prosthesis. However, the diaphysis is structurally competent, with at least 4 cm of intact cortical bone present in the femoral isthmus. Varus femoral remodeling is common and may rarely require an extended trochanteric osteotomy to correct this deformity during femoral revision. This pattern of bone loss is also commonly seen.
- Type IIIB: As with type IIIA defects, there is complete circumferential bone loss in the metaphysis, however, in these defects less than 4 cm of intact diaphyseal cortical bone is present distal to the isthmus. The anterolateral cortex and supporting subtrochanteric metaphyseal bone are absent and will not offer rotational stability. The stability of the implant is thus dependent on distal diaphyseal fixation. This pattern of bone loss is often seen in cases of multiple previous revisions.
- Type IV: There is extensive circumferential segmental bone loss proximally and extensive cavitary loss and significant ectasia involving the entire diaphysis. Because the isthmus does not confer mechanical stability, a cylindrical, distally fixed implant cannot be used. These defects are rare.

The senior author prefers a simplified algorithm to serve as a guide for surgical planning in revision THA (Figure 8-1),[5] which is based on several classification systems described in the literature.[1,2,6] This approach to address proximal femoral bone loss depends on 2 main factors: the quantity and the quality of the bone available for reconstruction. Quantity is assessed using the radiographs and the above classification system, whereas quality is best assessed intraoperatively.[5] Another important aspect to consider when determining reconstructive options is the expected activity demands of the patient.

NONMODULAR, ONE-PIECE STANDARD STEMS

Many designs for standard cementless femoral stems are available. Standard stems have a monoblock body and neck, with neck length adjustments conferred by the modular femoral head. Many systems have 2 offset options for a given stem size. The location of porous ingrowth surface (either proximal or extensive) and stem geometry determine the location of osteointegration and the loading pattern of host bone.

Despite excellent long-term results in primary THA, the results of proximally porous-coated nonmodular implants for revision THA have been poor. Three studies at midterm follow-up of these implants showed high rates of rerevision, radiographic aseptic loosening, and subsidence.[7-9] These complications occur because significant metaphyseal bone loss is frequently present, and the remaining metaphyseal bone is often sclerotic and of poor quality.[7] These mechanical factors limit initial stability which, compounded by the biologic issues, prevents ingrowth and stable long-term fixation. Use of this implant design in revision THA has largely been abandoned, and thus will not be discussed in detail.

The most durable results of standard femoral stems for revision THA have been seen with extensively porous-coated designs. These stems typically have a cylindrical distal geometry to engage the diaphysis, with a tapered proximal geometry to additionally contact any remaining metaphyseal bone. They are made from cobalt chrome or titanium alloys and are covered over nearly the entire implant with a porous plasma spray and/or hydroxyapatite to promote osteointegration. These designs have the advantage of bypassing deficient metaphyseal bone and securing fixation into the diaphysis. Endosteal scratch-fit fixation provides immediate axial and torsional stability to the implant, which allows for long-term osteointegration.[10] Concerns of proximal stress shielding and thigh pain associated with the modulus mismatch of larger diameter stems in osteopenic bone have been reported,[11,12] but may be of little clinical consequence in the stable, ingrown stem.[13,14]

Multiple series have demonstrated good long-term results in appropriately selected patients using extensively porous-coated standard stems. Moreland and Moreno[13] reported on 137 revision hips at 9.3 years. Five (4%) were removed for fixation problems, with 83% having radiographic evidence of bone ingrowth. Krishnamurthy et al[12] found a 2.4% mechanical failure rate (1.7% revision rate) in 297 hips at mean 8.3 years. Results of rerevision of an extensively porous-coated stem to another stem of the same design were reported by Hamilton et al.[15] Sixteen hips had 100% survivorship (92% with radiographic evidence of ingrowth) at a mean of 9.8 years.

The success of these types of stems appears to be lower in more severe cases of bone loss. Paprosky and Weeden[14] reported on 170 patients undergoing revision using an extensively porous-coated stem. The rate of mechanical failure in their overall series was 4.1% at 14.8 year mean follow-up. However, upon subgroup analysis, 21% of patients with a type IIIB defect at the time of revision went on to failure. They concluded that due to difficulty obtaining stable biologic fixation in this subgroup, alternate reconstruction methods may be used in patients with severe metadiaphyseal bone loss. Similarly, Engh et al[16] found greater than 95% survivorship in 777 patients at 10 and 15 years postoperative. However, in a separate analysis of 26 hips with severe bone loss greater than 10 cm distal to the lesser trochanter, they found 89% survivorship and a 15% aseptic loosening rate at a minimum of 10 years.[17] One series also found a higher incidence of periprosthetic fractures in patients with type III and IV bone loss reconstructed with this stem design.[18]

Indications

Extensively porous-coated cylindrical stems may be used in cases of mild to moderate (type I, II, or IIIA) bone loss. Since immediate stability and long-term bone ingrowth with these stems require a scratch-fit along at least 4 cm of intact diaphysis, there must be adequate intact diaphyseal bone remaining to use this technique. Ideally, bone loss should not extend more than 10 cm below the lesser trochanter for best results. Additionally, it must be recognized that there is no ability to alter femoral neck anteversion in these stems as this version is dictated by the bow of the femur in longer bowed stems.

Fully porous-coated cylindrical stems are relatively contraindicated in major (type IIIB) bone loss. In addition, since patients with bone loss 10 cm or more below the lesser trochanter have a lower likelihood of achieving stable fixation and ingrowth using this technique, other implants (such as modular tapered stems) may be more advisable. Modular implants allow for control of femoral version independent of the femoral bow, and therefore may be an advantageous option when very long stems are needed. Standard stems should not be used in massive (type IV) bone loss. Other options that can be used in these situations include APC, megaprostheses, cemented stems with or without impaction grafting, or occasionally distally fixed modular stems, as discussed below.

Technical Tips

Examples of this stem design include the AML and Solution (Depuy Orthopaedics, Warsaw, IN). Several other manufacturers also offer fully porous-coated stem options within their revision hip systems, including Zimmer, Inc, Biomet, and Smith and Nephew. We recommend selecting a stem supported by good long-term survivorship data.

Preoperative planning and templating are critical in determining the suitability of this type of implant for a given patient. Attention should be paid to recreating leg length and lateral offset; if these cannot be adequately reconstructed using this stem design, a modular component should be utilized. Straight stems are used most commonly for 6- to 10-inch length implants. However, depending on availability in the implant system selected, bowed stems may be useful if a longer length is needed. These stems will maintain anatomic version despite the femoral bow. The stem must be an appropriate length to bypass all defects by 2 cortical diameters and to obtain at least 4 cm of scratch-fit in healthy diaphyseal bone. A calcar-replacing stem should be used when the calcar is damaged to the point that a conventional stem is not supported by the remaining subchondral bone or when having an ability to anchor the greater trochanter into metal with cables or sutures is necessary.

The femur is approached according to the surgeon's preference, and implant removal is accomplished as discussed elsewhere. An extended trochanteric osteotomy (ETO) as detailed in Chapter 5 may be necessary to remove a well-fixed component or retained cement, particularly 10 cm or more distal to the lesser trochanter. In situations where the femur has undergone severe varus remodeling, an ETO is helpful to prevent disruption of the lateral cortex during reaming or stem implantation. In cases of significant varus remodeling requiring a long stem, the use of a modular stem can be a wise choice, as varus remodeling may alter the anatomic femoral version thereby increasing the risk of instability if a monoblock cylindrical stem is chosen.

The femur is next prepared by reaming the canal in a concentric fashion, taking care to avoid varus malpositioning. Reaming depth is chosen based on the preoperative templating of stem length. Sequentially larger diameter straight reamers are used until good endosteal contact is achieved along a 5- to 7-cm segment of the diaphysis. Based on the preoperative templating and the intraoperative findings, the reaming is complete when the diameter is 0.5 mm less than the size of the intended implant. When using a bowed stem, flexible reamers are utilized. In this case, the femur may be reamed line to line or even overreamed by up to 1.5 mm distally to accommodate mismatch of the bow of the prosthesis. The remaining proximal metaphyseal bone is then rasped in the correct version and a clean-up cut is made if necessary on the neck or the calcar, should a calcar-replacing prosthesis be used.

A trial reduction is then performed to check the leg length and stability. The version is rechecked and marked, and the offset for the final stem is determined. The stem is then chosen so that a stable scratch-fit is obtained between the porous coating of the implant and the cortex. The size stem chosen in relation to the size of the final reaming is dependent on the choice of implants as each manufacturer has its own recommendations. This technique will ensure immediate stem stability, lessen the risk of subsidence, and optimize long-term osteointegration.[14] The stem should seat easily until close to the final depth. If the stem is hung up during initial insertion by hand, then additional reaming may be necessary. The final component is impacted and a trial reduction is again performed to determine neck length and check stability. The final head is impacted, and if performed, the ETO is repaired with cables. The final soft tissue repair and the closure technique are paramount in achieving a good final result.

MODULAR STEMS

The variability of options that the concept of modularity imparts can significantly facilitate the management of complex cases. Differing neck lengths, offsets, ingrowth surfaces, and geometries of the proximal and distal components may be chosen. It is therefore feasible to preserve proximal bone and load the femur as physiologically as possible, which helps create a stable construct that optimizes the patient's anatomy and biomechanics. The majority of modular stems currently available are designed to be used with a press-fit technique. Successful outcomes of different types of these modular stem reconstruction techniques have been well documented in the literature.[4,19-23] Additionally, there are some modular stems that can be used as cemented constructs when needed.

Instability has been described as one of the most common complications after revision THA with modular femoral stems.[20-22] Sporer and Paprosky[24] reported mechanical failure and instability with extensively coated modular stems in type IIIB and IV defects due to femoral remodeling in retroversion. However, current modular designs allow the surgeon to independently control femoral version, which may reduce the risk of dislocation.[23] A stable hip center can be established by independently adjusting offset and neck length, correcting tension in the soft tissues and minimizing impingement. The availability of larger femoral heads may also contribute to a lower risk of dislocation, as discussed later in this chapter.

Fretting between the modular components may lead to abnormal third body wear and potentially fracture of the implants.[25,26] Although some fretting does occur, it has been reported as nonclinically significant.[19] While there have been reports of fractures in modular femoral stems, these have been relatively rare.[26] Fracturing of modular stems should become less common with low plasticity burnishing and shot peening and improved rolling techniques. Additionally, ensuring some method to decrease stresses across the distally fixed modular junction have led to decreases in stem fractures. These included ensuring ingrowth proximal to the junction or using strut grafts and cables across the junction when the proximal bone is deficient. Careful attention to surgical technique during milling should minimize the incidence of fractures by providing proper support to the proximal prosthesis by the remaining bone.[23]

With proximally fixed modular stems, it becomes possible to build a "stable base" distally and then work-up from this base proximally. These stems provide a variety of choices to achieve stability in fixation, which has led to their usage in proximal-distal mismatches. Different options to achieve ingrowth can be used, including porous-coated and hydroxyapatite-coated sleeves. Bolognesi et al[27] showed better bone fixation when using hydroxyapatite-coated sleeves in type III defects. Proximal stress shielding can be decreased with the use of proximally coated stems due to more physiologic loading of the remaining metaphyseal bone. Bono et al[28] reported only a 6% incidence of stress shielding in 63 patients who underwent revision using this type of modular stem. Some designs incorporate a metaphyseal sleeve taper fit with a distal body of different length

Figure 8-2. (A) Patient with aseptic loosening and minimal proximal bone loss with good quality. (B) Reconstruction with a proximally fixed modular stem. This particular modular stem (Exactech AccuMatch M-Series, Gainesville, FL) allows for choosing version regardless of the femoral bow. A coronal slot (white arrow) allows this stem to be used without performing an osteotomy to correct the femoral deformity. (Reprinted with permission from Higuera CA, Hanna G, Florjancik K, Allan DG, Robinson R, Barsoum WK. The use of proximal fixed modular stems in revision of total hip arthroplasty. *J Arthroplasty.* 2006;21[4 Suppl 1]:112-116.)

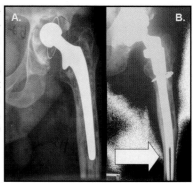

and neck offsets, which provides independent control of version and thus biomechanical optimization.[4,29] Many modular femoral stem systems offer numerous types of distal stems.[29] Fluted stems optimize distal rotational control and offer a lower incidence of thigh pain.[4,19]

Outcomes following proximally fixed modular reconstruction are good when used for the appropriate indications. Our group has reported the results of a proximally fixed modular stem in a cohort of 53 patients who underwent 55 revision procedures.[23] We found significant postoperative improvements in the Harris hip scores and Short Form-12 at an average follow-up of 2.5 years. A small number of complications were reported. Similar results have been described by other authors.[4,19,29]

Distally fixed modular components are used when proximal bone stock is compromised. These extensively porous coated stems offer excellent distal fixation and resistance to varus-valgus, flexion-extension, rotational, and axial forces. Stem options include tapered, fluted, or conical configurations.

Multiple series have shown good results using this design.[24,30-32] However, technical errors have been shown to cause early revisions. Patel et al[33] reported on a series of 43 patients who underwent revision THA using this stem design at our institution. Subsidence from the immediate postoperative films was seen in 25% of patients due to undersizing of the femoral stem, which required rerevision in 9% of the series. Undersizing was found to be the main factor contributing to subsidence. This situation can be avoided by completely filling the canal to achieve a stable distal press-fit with the endosteal bone. As with distally fixed standard stems, higher Paprosky classification has been correlated with higher complication rates after modular reconstruction.[24]

Calcar-replacing stems are used when the calcar is compromised, as is seen with type II and IIIA defects. These types of prostheses were initially used in peritrochanteric hip fractures and pathologic fractures, but are now more commonly used in the revision arthroplasty setting. Good survivorship has been reported in the literature in this patient population.[34]

Indications

Modular stems have multiple indications as described above. They are useful when there is a metaphyseal-diaphyseal mismatch, as independent sizes of both metaphyseal and diaphyseal components improve bone contact in both locations to allow for enhanced stability. They are also indicated when the kinematics of the hip joint are compromised due to laxity of the soft tissues. Both of these situations are common during revision procedures. Other applications include the ability to finely tune femoral neck anteversion without regard for distal femoral anatomy (Figure 8-2), which is extremely valuable in a situation where the femur has a nonanatomic morphology.

Proximally porous coated modular stems can be used in situations of minor proximal bone loss with good quality of the remaining metaphysis (type I or occasionally type II defects). They are particularly useful when neck version and leg length cannot be restored with a standard stem.

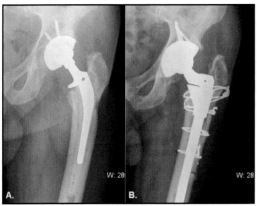

Figure 8-3. (A) Patient with a focal lateral wall deficiency but otherwise minimal bone loss with good quality seen intraoperatively. An extended trochanteric osteotomy was used to remove the distal cement plug. (B) Reconstruction with a proximally coated uncemented modular stem (S-ROM system, Depuy Orthopaedics, Warsaw, IN). The osteotomy site was repaired anatomically.

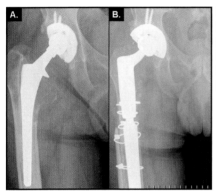

Figure 8-4. (A) Patient with severe proximal femoral bone loss in the region of the calcar. (B) Reconstruction with a distally fixed modular stem (Restoration Modular, Stryker Orthopaedics, Mahwah, NJ). The preservation of the remaining proximal bone may allow for ingrowth and decrease stresses on the modular junction.

Proximally fixed stems should not be used when severe proximal bone loss is present (types III and IV). Extended trochanteric osteotomy may be a relative contraindication for use of proximally porous-coated stems. In this situation, a proximally fixed, porous-coated stem should be used only in a Dorr type A or B femur where there is still appropriate bone stock for fixation and a tight diaphyseal fit and anatomic repair of the osteotomy can be achieved (Figure 8-3).[35]

Distally fixed modular components are indicated when substantial metaphyseal bone loss has occurred or the remaining bone is of inadequate quality to facilitate adequate ingrowth. A clear indication of long modular tapered cementless stems is with type III defects and occasionally type IV defects as long as there is enough bone to get some proximal ingrowth to relive stresses on the modular junction or a strut graft and cables are used. In type IIIA defects, either modular (Figure 8-4) or nonmodular extensively coated stems may be used with reliable results.[2,32,36] Also, when an extended trochanteric osteotomy has been used to correct proximal bone deformity and remodeling, a diaphyseal fitting stem is indicated.[2]

Massive proximal and diaphyseal bone loss (type IV) is typically best treated with a proximal femoral replacement or APC. A distally fixed fluted tapered implant may be used in select situations with this pattern of bone deficiency; however, these complex situations are probably most reliably treated with other advanced reconstructive options.

In situations where a previously placed modular component requires reintervention, a limited revision may be preferred in some circumstances. When performing an acetabular revision (thus changing the hip center) or if instability is present, the ability to increase soft tissue tension by lengthening the neck or increasing the offset without removing a distally well-fixed component or a well-fixed proximal sleeve is very useful.[23] Other applications of modular component exchange have occurred with the advent of alternative bearings. With ceramic femoral heads, the trunnion may also be changed during a head revision. Additionally, the modular necks can be used to increase femoral head length due to limitations in length options with alternative bearing heads.

Technical Tips

The S-ROM system (DePuy Orthopaedics, Warsaw, IN) and AccuMatch M-Series (Exatech, Gainesville, FL) are examples of proximally fixed modular stems. The Restoration Modular (Stryker Orthopaedics, Mahwah, NJ) and ZMR (Zimmer, Inc, Warsaw, IN) are examples of distally fixed modular designs.

Preoperative planning is essential to decide the type of implant that is best indicated for a given patient. Evaluating the quality and quantity of the remaining bone stock available for fixation is paramount to decide what type of modular stem will best establish a stable construct between the host femur and the implant. Templating assists with measuring the length and diameter of the distal stem and sleeves. If the projected implant length extends beyond the isthmus, a curved stem will likely be necessary to recreate the femoral bow and avoid anterior cortical perforation. The potential restored head height, neck length, and offset are estimated to restore kinematics and stability to the hip based on the templated acetabular reconstruction and new center of rotation. It is recommended to have different reconstructive options available at the time of surgery in case the original surgical plan cannot be accomplished.

A posterolateral, lateral, or anterolateral approach is usually recommended when choosing these types of implants as an excellent exposure of the femoral canal is necessary and the ability to extend the incision may be advantageous. If retained cement is present after component removal, all remaining cement should be removed to prevent instrument deflection. We perform all revisions using a Jackson or other type of radiolucent table to ensure the removal of all cement as well as to minimize the risk of cortical perforation. Extended trochanteric osteotomy may be necessary, and if used, careful attention should be paid to obtain good apposition of the bone to the implant when the repair is performed. If a femoral osteotomy is used, the reconstruction stem should bypass the most distal area of cortical weakness by 2 to 2.5 cortical diameters.[29,35] Double cerclage wire prophylaxis has been recommended when perforation or lytic defects are present distal to the ETO.[29]

The distal canal should be prepared by sequential reaming until good diaphyseal cortical contact is obtained. Extensively porous-coated stems are usually underreamed by 0.5 mm for a stable press-fit, although each manufacturer has its own recommendations. Intraoperative fractures can be minimized with the use of cerclage wiring to increase bone hoop strength. If a bowed stem is used, it is recommended to overream by 1.0 to 1.5 mm with flexible reamers for accommodation of the final stem. The proximal canal should then be prepared and reamed to a size based on the anterior-posterior dimension of the remaining metaphysis. When there is a significant calcar deficiency (types III), a calcar-replacing stem may be used. Otherwise, the calcar is next prepared by milling to fit the proximal sleeve component. Appropriate rotation of the trials to restore the version should be marked. When long stems (>200 mm) are used, intraoperative x-rays should be obtained to assess for unrecognized distal fractures and appropriate filling of the canal.

An appropriate closure and restoration of the soft tissue sling (abductors and vastus lateralis muscles) are important to maintain stability. A postoperative hip abduction orthosis can be used to increase stability. Heterotopic ossification can be prevented with the use of adjuvant radiation or indomethacin.

MEGAPROSTHESES

Proximal femur replacement with a modular megaprosthesis is an option for the reconstruction of severe, circumferential bone loss in the metaphysis and proximal diaphysis. First developed for use in tumor reconstructions, this technique is becoming more popular for salvage of the multiply

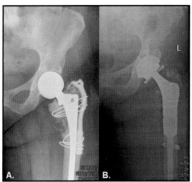

Figure 8-5. (A) Patient with multiple revisions following failed osteosynthesis of an intertrochanteric fracture and severe proximal bone deficiency. (B) Revision with cemented megaprosthesis placement with distal fixation with a constrained acetabular liner (Global Modular Replacement System, Stryker Orthopaedics, Mahwah, NJ).

revised hip arthroplasty or unreconstructable periprosthetic fractures. Because there is no reconstitution of proximal femoral bone stock for potential further revision, this implant is usually chosen in older, more sedentary patients.

Contemporary designs are modular with 3 sections: the proximal body and neck, the diaphyseal segment, and the stem. The proximal body and diaphyseal segment are typically covered with porous coating to obtain fixation with any remaining proximal bone, most importantly the greater trochanter. The proximal body has holes to which the abductors can be secured if no trochanteric bone remains. The diaphyseal segment has varying lengths to reconstruct correct leg lengths and optimize soft tissue tension. Stems can be of either cemented, noncemented, or hybrid designs and come in varying lengths depending on how much diaphyseal bone remains.

Parvizi et al[37] analyzed 43 patients with modular proximal femoral replacement at a mean of 36.5 months. They found significant improvements in Harris hip scores compared to preoperative time-points and 87% and 73% 1- and 5-year survival, respectively. The major complication was instability in 8 patients, requiring revision in 6 cases. The high prevalence of instability has also been seen in other series.[38,39] Patients are at higher risk for instability if the abductor mechanism is significantly disrupted.[40] In this case, constrained liners may be necessary to prevent dislocation, however, implantation of a constrained liner before the acetabular component is ingrown may lead to higher rates of aseptic loosening and failure of the cup.

Indications

Proximal femoral replacement is indicated in cases of massive proximal bone loss (type IV) or in situations where other reconstruction methods have poor results (Figure 8-5). Older patients who may be unable to observe the weightbearing restrictions necessary with other reconstruction methods or otherwise tolerate prohibitive postoperative precautions are ideal candidates.[40] This procedure may also be necessary in challenging Vancouver IIIB periprosthetic fractures.

Younger patients with severe bone loss may be better managed with an APC or impaction grafting to attempt to restore bone stock for subsequent revisions. If a megaprosthesis is chosen, the remaining femur must be of adequate length and quality to support the stem. If this is not the case, a total femoral replacement may be necessary. In all cases, and regardless of reconstructive method chosen, it may be advantageous to maintain as much host bone and soft tissue as possible and cable the remaining bone to the prosthesis.

Technical Tips

Examples of modular proximal femoral replacement include the GMRS (Stryker Orthopaedics) and OSS (Biomet Inc, Warsaw, IN). Preoperative planning as previously described is especially critical to this challenging procedure.

Following adequate exposure, we recommend determining the length of the femur prior to component removal by placing a pin into the pelvis and measuring to a fixed point on the intact femoral diaphysis.[40] This technique, combined with preoperative templating, will facilitate accurate restoration of leg lengths during trialing.

The old components are removed by previously discussed techniques. A transverse osteotomy is made just distal to the extent of bone loss, taking care to preserve as much length of the native femur as possible. Proximal bone may be osteotomized coronally for later reattachment to the prosthesis. Care should be especially taken to preserve any greater trochanteric bone and abductor to maximize the soft tissue function. The femoral canal is prepared by sequential reaming, and trial components are assembled and inserted. The leg length is checked by the above-mentioned method as well as clinically and can be modified by changing the diaphyseal segment length or removing more bone as needed. Component version and stability are scrutinized. If any doubts exist as to the stability of the construct, particularly in the presence of a deficient abductor mechanism, a constrained liner should be used.

The trials are then removed and the femur is prepared. If cement fixation is to be used, a cement restrictor is placed and the canal prepared according to contemporary cementation technique. The final components are then placed, taking care to maintain the same version as the trials. Stability is then rechecked and a head of appropriate size is placed.

Any remnants of proximal bone are cabled or sutured around the stem, paying particular attention to securely fix any remnants of trochanter to aid in stability. If the abductors are devoid of any trochanteric bone, they are secured to the prosthesis using heavy nonabsorbable suture. Since stability can be a major issue with these patients, a meticulous closure with attention to repairing any remaining posterior structures is required.

CEMENTED STEMS

Cemented femoral stems are infrequently used in contemporary revision THA, although they may still have utility in selected situations when revising a cemented primary stem. Survivorship for revision cemented stems is worse than primary cemented stems.[41] A biomechanical study showed decreased resistance to forces at the bone-cement interface in revision cementation.[42] Radiographic studies have indicated increased radiolucencies around the cement mantle in cemented revisions compared to primaries.[43,44] These findings have been validated in other studies, with the quality of the cement mantle predicting better long-term radiographic evidence of fixation.[44]

Early results of cemented fixation for femoral revision were poor. Multiple studies showed rerevision rates of 3% to 30% and evidence of radiographic loosening in 3% to 44% of cases at 2- to 12-year mean follow-up.[45] However, these utilized mostly first- and second-generation cementation techniques, unselected patient populations, and older prosthetic designs.

More recent studies indicate considerably better survival rates using modern cementation techniques, improved prosthetic designs, and refined indications. Haydon et al[46] analyzed long-term results of 129 cemented femoral revisions. Their main indication for cemented revision (instead of uncemented fixation) was the presence of a Dorr type C femur. Overall survivorship at 10 years was 91% and 71% with the endpoints of femoral rerevision and mechanical failure, respectively. Male gender and age less than 60 years were significant risk factors for failure. However, subgroup analysis of the patients treated with a third-generation cementation technique showed statistically better survivorship (94% versus 85% for second-generation techniques). Howie et al[47] analyzed the results of femoral revision using a cemented, polished, collarless tapered stem design with modern cementation techniques. They found a survivorship of 98% at 9 years for long stems and 93% for standard-length stems. A likely contribution to this clinical success was the cohort's mean age of 74 years. This design of cemented stems has shown excellent long-term results in primary cemented THA.[48]

Indications

Cemented femoral revision may be considered in elderly patients or those over age 60 with otherwise limited life expectancy and activity levels. Patients meeting these criteria that would benefit from the immediate full weightbearing allowed by cemented stems may be especially considered. Patients should have significant proximal bone loss and a capacious proximal femur with intact, thin cortices (ie, a Dorr type C or "stovepipe" femur).[49]

As cemented components do not have the versatility of modular components, they should be avoided in situations when offset, version, and soft tissue tension may be problematic. They should also be avoided when an ETO is necessary. Long-stem cemented components should be used with caution in patients with severe cardiopulmonary comorbidities to minimize the risk of cardiovascular collapse during implantation.

Technical Tips

We recommend using a highly polished, tapered femoral stem. This design has the best survivorship in long-term follow-up studies. Examples of this design include the Exeter (Stryker Orthopaedics), CPT (Zimmer, Inc), and C-Stem AMT (Depuy Orthopaedics) hip systems. Long-stem femoral components are preferable to bypass the previous stem by at least 2 cortical diameters.[46,49] Templating is important to ensure the options for a cemented system will restore the offset and length; if this is not the case, we recommend using a different prosthesis.

Techniques for component and cement removal are detailed in Chapter 6. The neocortex and membrane that form in the presence of a loose cemented stem must be thoroughly débrided to allow for adequate cement interdigitation with host bone.[49] The canal should be reamed and/or broached according to the specific implant system utilized, and trialing is done to ensure proper leg length and hip stability. The femoral component should be sized to leave a 2- to 3-mm cement mantle around the entire prosthesis.

The femoral canal must be meticulously prepared and modern cementation techniques should be employed. We do not recommend aggressive removal of well-fixed, well-interdigitated areas of previous cement if the reconstruction will also use cement. A cement restrictor is placed distal to the intended depth of the stem. The canal is prepared using pulsatile lavage with a canal brush. The canal is packed with epinephrine-soaked sponges to decrease bleeding and then dried. The cement is mixed under vacuum and inserted in a retrograde fashion using a cement gun to pressurize the canal. Some authors prefer antibiotic impregnated bone cement,[49] which we utilize in all revision cement cases. The prosthesis is inserted and held in the proper rotational alignment until the cement has hardened.

Tap Out-Tap In

The "tap out-tap in" (or "cement-within-cement") technique is an option for limited femoral revision in select cases. A well-fixed or loose femoral component is removed from an intact cement mantle and subsequently replaced without removing the cement. This technique has been utilized to facilitate acetabular exposure for cup revisions, for isolated femoral revision when the prosthesis has de-bonded from the cement, and possibly for changing a monoblock femoral component for reasons of leg length inequality, instability, or head size.[50]

Lieberman et al[51] reviewed 19 cases in which this technique was used and found good results at a mean of 59 months, with no revisions for loosening and all stems with stable radiographic appearance. Two patients did have cortical perforation at the time of revision while preparing the canal. Nabors and colleagues analyzed 42 hips undergoing acetabular revision with a tap out-tap in technique to enhance exposure.[52] At a mean of 67 months, 2 hips had asymptomatic radiographic loosening, and 1 solidly fixed component was revised for instability. McCallum and Hozack[50] reported on the use of ultrasonic tools to prepare the cement mantle in 15 patients. They conclude these devices may help avoid the intraoperative complication of canal perforation. Four patients were available at 2-year follow-up, with no evidence of clinical or radiographic loosening. Elting presented a series of 36 revisions over a 10-year period using smooth or polished tapered stems, with no rerevisions.[53]

The available biomechanical literature supports the viability of this technique. Greenwald[54] demonstrated little loss of shear strength when recementing into an established cement mantle. Nabors[52] also demonstrated no increase in rotational micromotion in a cadaveric study of 8 hips.

Indications

This technique should only be utilized in older sedentary patients when the cement mantle is intact. Specific indications include improving exposure for acetabular revision and replacing a loose component that has debonded from its cement mantle. Highly polished, tapered components with good long-term survivorship are the ideal candidates for this procedure.

The tap out-tap in technique should not be attempted for components with high surface roughness and irregular geometry, as the likelihood of having an intact cement mantle after stem removal is low. After prosthesis removal, if the cement mantle has more than minimal focal proximal deficiencies, a full revision should be performed.[50] Additionally, we recommend against the use of this technique in younger and physically active patients, given potential concerns with the long-term durability of the cement-cement interface.

Technical Tips

Preoperative radiographs should be scrutinized for evidence of mantle defects or lucencies at the bone-cement interface. After adequate exposure is obtained, cement is cleared from the lateral shoulder of the implant to facilitate removal and prevent disruption of the cement mantle. Tap out the component and carefully inspect the cement mantle. If a mantle fracture or mantle defects are found, proceed with full revision.

The mantle is then prepared by roughening with a bur or ultrasonic equipment depending on the surgeon's preference and equipment availability, taking care not to perforate the cement. The original stem or a new stem is then coated with a thin layer of bone cement at low viscosity and is reinserted into the cement mantle and held until the cement is bonded. Alternatively, after ensuring that the stem will fit in the old femoral component site, the canal can be refilled with cement and the new stem placed. It is important that the new cement be placed in a fairly runny state; otherwise the placement of the new stem may be difficult.

FEMORAL HEAD SIZE

There is a growing body of clinical evidence in primary THA to indicate that larger femoral head sizes are protective against dislocation, likely the result of an improved head-neck ratio.[55-57] Instability after revision THA is far more common than after primary procedures, complicating up to 15% of revision cases in a Medicare population.[58]

Studies of instability following revision THA indicate that larger femoral head sizes are beneficial to prevent dislocation. Hummel et al[59] found that when combined with a posterior capsular repair, a statistically significant improvement in dislocation rates was seen when a 32-mm femoral head was used compared to a 28-mm head (2.7% versus 10.6%, respectively). The relative contribution of the capsular repair compared to the increased head size was not analyzed. Alberton et al[60] found that in a series of 1548 revision arthroplasties, a 22-mm head size had statistically higher instability rates compared to 28- and 32-mm heads. Kung and Ries[61] compared 36- and 28-mm heads in patients with an intact abductor mechanism and also found a statistically lower rate of dislocation with the large head size (0% versus 12.7%).

It is important to note that instability after revision operations is a multifactorial problem. Compromised soft tissue tension at the time of revision is common, and a meticulous repair of any remaining capsular tissue is recommended.[59] Alberton et al[60] found that the presence of a trochanteric nonunion was highly predictive of postoperative dislocation, and Kung and Ries[61] also found that patients with an absent abductor mechanism had high rates of instability. In those patients with deficient abductors, increased femoral head size was not protective against dislocation.

Combined component positioning must also be optimized to prevent postoperative impingement, wear, and instability.[62,63] One study indicated that the biomechanical benefits of larger femoral head sizes were negated by excessive acetabular abduction (>55 degrees).[64] Therefore, isolated femoral revision is not appropriate if a well-fixed acetabular component is positioned outside of the safe zone. Other studies have indicated considerable variability in femoral component version when using cementless implants in primary THA.[65,66] This risk is likely compounded in the revision situation with aberrant anatomy of the remaining femur and when long stems extend to the diaphyseal bow. As previously discussed, modular stems with the ability to correctly independently adjust femoral anteversion are advantageous in this setting.[63] Clearly, the surgeon should not trust a large femoral head to prevent instability when suboptimal acetabular or femoral component positioning is present.

Although larger head size lessens the risk of postoperative dislocation, the relative contribution to stability is likely less than other factors including soft tissue tension and proper component alignment. In our opinion, a larger femoral head option should be utilized within the constraints of the surgeon's chosen implant system and bearing surface. This will obviously depend on the size of the acetabular shell or polyethylene and the options available with a given femoral stem. Care should be taken to ensure a polyethylene thickness of at least 6 mm to minimize the risk of failure. We routinely use 32-, 36-, 40-, and 44-mm heads in revisions.

REFERENCES

1. D'Antonio J, McCarthy JC, Bargar WL, et al. Classification of femoral abnormalities in total hip arthroplasty. *Clin Orthop Relat Res.* 1993;(296):133-139.
2. Della Valle CJ, Paprosky WG. The femur in revision total hip arthroplasty evaluation and classification. *Clin Orthop Relat Res.* 2004;(420):55-62.
3. Johnston RC, Fitzgerald RH Jr, Harris WH, Poss R, Muller ME, Sledge CB. Clinical and radiographic evaluation of total hip replacement. A standard system of terminology for reporting results. *J Bone Joint Surg Am.* 1990;72(2):161-168.
4. Cameron HU. The long-term success of modular proximal fixation stems in revision total hip arthroplasty. *J Arthroplasty.* 2002;17(4 Suppl 1):138-141.
5. Higuera CA, Capello W, Barsoum WK. Algorithmic approach for reconstruction of proximal femoral bone loss in revision total hip arthroplasty. *Orthopedics.* 2009;32(9):pii.
6. Longjohn D, Dorr, L. Bone stock loss and allografting: femur. In: Bono JV, ed. *Revision Total Hip Arthroplasty.* New York, NY: Springer; 1999:100-111.
7. Berry DJ, Harmsen WS, Ilstrup D, Lewallen DG, Cabanela ME. Survivorship of uncemented proximally porous-coated femoral components. *Clin Orthop Relat Res.* 1995;(319):168-177.
8. Malkani AL, Lewallen DG, Cabanela ME, Wallrichs SL. Femoral component revision using an uncemented, proximally coated, long-stem prosthesis. *J Arthroplasty.* 1996;11(4):411-418.
9. Woolson ST, Delaney TJ. Failure of a proximally porous-coated femoral prosthesis in revision total hip arthroplasty. *J Arthroplasty.* 1995;10(Suppl):S22-S28.
10. Engh CA Sr, Fenwick JA. Extensively porous-coated stems: avoiding modularity. *Orthopedics.* 2008;31(9):911-912.
11. Engh CA, Culpepper WJ 2nd, Kassapidis E. Revision of loose cementless femoral prostheses to larger porous coated components. *Clin Orthop Relat Res.* 1998;(347):168-178.
12. Krishnamurthy AB, MacDonald SJ, Paprosky WG. 5- to 13-year follow-up study on cementless femoral components in revision surgery. *J Arthroplasty.* 1997;12(8):839-847.
13. Moreland JR, Moreno MA. Cementless femoral revision arthroplasty of the hip: minimum 5 years followup. *Clin Orthop Relat Res.* 2001;(393):194-201.

14. Paprosky WG, Weeden SH. Extensively porous-coated stems in femoral revision arthroplasty. *Orthopedics*. 2001;24(9):871-872.

15. Hamilton WG, Cashen DV, Ho H, Hopper RH Jr, Engh CA. Extensively porous-coated stems for femoral revision: a choice for all seasons. *J Arthroplasty*. 2007;22(4 Suppl 1):106-110.

16. Engh CA Jr, Hopper RH, Jr, Engh CA Sr. Distal ingrowth components. *Clin Orthop Relat Res*. 2004;(420):135-141.

17. Engh CA Jr, Ellis TJ, Koralewicz LM, McAuley JP, Engh CA Sr. Extensively porous-coated femoral revision for severe femoral bone loss: minimum 10-year follow-up. *J Arthroplasty*. 2002;17(8):955-960.

18. Busch CA, Charles MN, Haydon CM, et al. Fractures of distally-fixed femoral stems after revision arthroplasty. *J Bone Joint Surg Br*. 2005;87(10):1333-1336.

19. Christie MJ, DeBoer DK, Tingstad EM, Capps M, Brinson MF, Trick LW. Clinical experience with a modular noncemented femoral component in revision total hip arthroplasty: 4- to 7-year results. *J Arthroplasty*. 2000;15(7):840-848.

20. Crawford SA, Siney PD, Wroblewski BM. Revision of failed total hip arthroplasty with a proximal femoral modular cemented stem. *J Bone Joint Surg Br*. 2000;82(5):684-688.

21. Schuh A, Werber S, Holzwarth U, Zeiler G. Cementless modular hip revision arthroplasty using the MRP Titan Revision Stem: outcome of 79 hips after an average of 4 years' follow-up. *Arch Orthop Trauma Surg*. 2004;124(5):306-309.

22. Wirtz DC, Heller KD, Holzwarth U, et al. A modular femoral implant for uncemented stem revision in THR. *Int Orthop*. 2000;24(3):134-138.

23. Higuera CA, Hanna G, Florjancik K, Allan DG, Robinson R, Barsoum WK. The use of proximal fixed modular stems in revision of total hip arthroplasty. *J Arthroplasty*. 2006;21(4 Suppl 1):112-116.

24. Sporer SM, Paprosky WG. Femoral fixation in the face of considerable bone loss: the use of modular stems. *Clin Orthop Relat Res*. 2004;(429):227-231.

25. Cook SD, Barrack RL, Clemow AJ. Corrosion and wear at the modular interface of uncemented femoral stems. *J Bone Joint Surg Br*. 1994;76(1):68-72.

26. Bobyn JD, Tanzer M, Krygier JJ, Dujovne AR, Brooks CE. Concerns with modularity in total hip arthroplasty. *Clin Orthop Relat Res*. 1994(298):27-36.

27. Bolognesi MP, Pietrobon R, Clifford PE, Vail TP. Comparison of a hydroxyapatite-coated sleeve and a porous-coated sleeve with a modular revision hip stem. A prospective, randomized study. *J Bone Joint Surg Am*. 2004;86-A(12):2720-2725.

28. Bono JV, McCarthy JC, Lee J, Carangelo RJ, Turner RH. Fixation with a modular stem in revision total hip arthroplasty. *Instr Course Lect*. 2000;49:131-139.

29. Jones RE. Modular revision stems in total hip arthroplasty. *Clin Orthop Relat Res*. 2004;(420):142-147.

30. Berry DJ. Femoral revision: distal fixation with fluted, tapered grit-blasted stems. *J Arthroplasty*. 2002;17 (4 Suppl 1):142-146.

31. Bircher HP, Riede U, Luem M, Ochsner PE. [The value of the Wagner SL revision prosthesis for bridging large femoral defects]. *Orthopade*. 2001;30(5):294-303.

32. Bohm P, Bischel O. Femoral revision with the Wagner SL revision stem: evaluation of one hundred and twenty-nine revisions followed for a mean of 4.8 years. *J Bone Joint Surg Am*. 2001;83-A(7):1023-1031.

33. Patel PD, Klika AK, Murray TG, Elsharkawy KA, Krebs VE, Barsoum WK. Influence of technique with distally fixed modular stems in revision total hip arthroplasty. *J Arthroplasty*. 2010;25(6):926-931.

34. Head WC, Emerson RH Jr, Higgins LL. A titanium cementless calcar replacement prosthesis in revision surgery of the femur: 13-year experience. *J Arthroplasty*. 2001;16(8 Suppl 1):183-187.

35. Mattinlgy D. Femoral revision: modular proximally porous-coated stems. In: Surgeons AAoO, ed. *Advanced Reconstruction Hip*. Rosemont, IL: American Academy of Orthopaedic Surgeons; 2005.

36. Weeden SH, Paprosky WG. Minimal 11-year follow-up of extensively porous-coated stems in femoral revision total hip arthroplasty. *J Arthroplasty*. 2002;17(4 Suppl 1):134-137.

37. Parvizi J, Tarity TD, Slenker N, et al. Proximal femoral replacement in patients with non-neoplastic conditions. *J Bone Joint Surg Am*. 2007;89(5):1036-1043.

38. Johnsson R, Carlsson A, Kisch K, Moritz U, Zetterstrom R, Persson BM. Function following mega total hip arthroplasty compared with conventional total hip arthroplasty and healthy matched controls. *Clin Orthop Relat Res*. 1985;(192):159-167.

39. Malkani AL, Settecerri JJ, Sim FH, Chao EY, Wallrichs SL. Long-term results of proximal femoral replacement for non-neoplastic disorders. *J Bone Joint Surg Br*. 1995;77(3):351-356.

40. Parvizi J, Sim FH. Proximal femoral replacements with megaprostheses. *Clin Orthop Relat Res*. 2004;(420): 169-175.

41. Alberton GM, High WA, Morrey BF. Dislocation after revision total hip arthroplasty: an analysis of risk factors and treatment options. *J Bone Joint Surg Am*. 2002;84-A(10):1788-1792.

42. Dohmae Y, Bechtold JE, Sherman RE, Puno RM, Gustilo RB. Reduction in cement-bone interface shear strength between primary and revision arthroplasty. *Clin Orthop Relat Res*. 1988;(236):214-220.

43. Barrack RL, Mulroy RD Jr, Harris WH. Improved cementing techniques and femoral component loosening in young patients with hip arthroplasty. A 12-year radiographic review. *J Bone Joint Surg Br*. 1992;74(3): 385-389.

44. Estok DM 2nd, Harris WH. Long-term results of cemented femoral revision surgery using second-generation techniques. An average 11.7-year follow-up evaluation. *Clin Orthop Relat Res*. 1994;(299):190-202.

45. Barrack RL, Folgueras AJ. Revision total hip arthroplasty: the femoral component. *J Am Acad Orthop Surg*. 1995;3(2):79-85.

46. Haydon CM, Mehin R, Burnett S, et al. Revision total hip arthroplasty with use of a cemented femoral component. Results at a mean of ten years. *J Bone Joint Surg Am*. 2004;86-A(6):1179-1185.

47. Howie DW, Wimhurst JA, McGee MA, Carbone TA, Badaruddin BS. Revision total hip replacement using cemented collarless double-taper femoral components. *J Bone Joint Surg Br*. 2007;89(7):879-886.

48. Carrington NC, Sierra RJ, Gie GA, Hubble MJ, Timperley AJ, Howell JR. The Exeter Universal cemented femoral component at 15 to 17 years: an update on the first 325 hips. *J Bone Joint Surg Br*. 2009;91(6):730-737.

49. Lieberman JR. Cemented femoral revision: lest we forget. *J Arthroplasty*. 2005;20(4 Suppl 2):72-74.

50. McCallum JD 3rd, Hozack WJ. Recementing a femoral component into a stable cement mantle using ultrasonic tools. *Clin Orthop Relat Res*. 1995;(319):232-237.

51. Lieberman JR, Moeckel BH, Evans BG, Salvati EA, Ranawat CS. Cement-within-cement revision hip arthroplasty. *J Bone Joint Surg Br*. 1993;75(6):869-871.

52. Nabors ED, Liebelt R, Mattingly DA, Bierbaum BE. Removal and reinsertion of cemented femoral components during acetabular revision. *J Arthroplasty*. 1996;11(2):146-152.

53. Elting J. Cement-within-cement femoral stem exchange facilitates acetabular revision. *Curr Orthop Pract*. 2010;21(2):190-192.

54. Greenwald AS, Narten NC, Wilde AH. Points in the technique of recementing in the revision of an implant arthroplasty. *J Bone Joint Surg Br*. 1978;60(1):107-110.

55. Peters CL, McPherson E, Jackson JD, Erickson JA. Reduction in early dislocation rate with large-diameter femoral heads in primary total hip arthroplasty. *J Arthroplasty*. 2007;22(6 Suppl 2):140-144.

56. Bystrom S, Espehaug B, Furnes O, Havelin LI; Norwegian Arthroplasty Register. Femoral head size is a risk factor for total hip luxation: a study of 42,987 primary hip arthroplasties from the Norwegian Arthroplasty Register. *Acta Orthop Scand*. 2003;74(5):514-524.

57. Berry DJ, von Knoch M, Schleck CD, Harmsen WS. Effect of femoral head diameter and operative approach on risk of dislocation after primary total hip arthroplasty. *J Bone Joint Surg Am*. 2005;87(11):2456-2463.

58. Phillips CB, Barrett JA, Losina E, et al. Incidence rates of dislocation, pulmonary embolism, and deep infection during the first six months after elective total hip replacement. *J Bone Joint Surg Am*. 2003;85-A(1): 20-26.

59. Hummel MT, Malkani AL, Yakkanti MR, Baker DL. Decreased dislocation after revision total hip arthroplasty using larger femoral head size and posterior capsular repair. *J Arthroplasty*. 2009;24(6 Suppl): 73-76.

60. Alberton GM, High WA, Morrey BF. Dislocation after revision total hip arthroplasty: an analysis of risk factors and treatment options. *J Bone Joint Surg Am*. 2002;84-A(10):1788-1792.

61. Kung PL, Ries MD. Effect of femoral head size and abductors on dislocation after revision THA. *Clin Orthop Relat Res*. 2007;465:170-174.

62. Malik A, Maheshwari A, Dorr LD. Impingement with total hip replacement. *J Bone Joint Surg Am*. 2007;89(8):1832-1842.

63. Barsoum WK, Patterson RW, Higuera C, Klika AK, Krebs VE, Molloy R. A computer model of the position of the combined component in the prevention of impingement in total hip replacement. *J Bone Joint Surg Br*. 2007;89(6):839-845.

64. Crowninshield RD, Maloney WJ, Wentz DH, Humphrey SM, Blanchard CR. Biomechanics of large femoral heads: what they do and don't do. *Clin Orthop Relat Res*. 2004;(429):102-107.

65. Pierchon F, Pasquier G, Cotten A, Fontaine C, Clarisse J, Duquennoy A. Causes of dislocation of total hip arthroplasty. CT study of component alignment. *J Bone Joint Surg Br*. 1994;76(1):45-48.

66. Wines AP, McNicol D. Computed tomography measurement of the accuracy of component version in total hip arthroplasty. *J Arthroplasty*. 2006;21(5):696-701.

Revision for Instability
Options to Consider in Challenging Cases

David C. Markel, MD; Jonathan M. Vigdorchik, MD;
and Gregory J. Golladay, MD

Dislocation is one of the most feared complications of total hip arthroplasty (THA). It causes distress for both the surgeon and the patient, and substantial costs are incurred to manage the problem.[1] Instability occurs in approximately 1% of total hip replacements in the first month after surgery, and the risk of dislocation increases at a linear rate after 1 year to a cumulative risk of 7% at 20 years.[2] A number of factors are associated with an increased risk for dislocation including female gender; obesity; cognitive dysfunction; poor general health as reflected in ASA score; diagnosis of osteonecrosis, rheumatoid arthritis, or development dysplasia of the hip; conversion from prior open reduction internal fixation or nonunion; acute femoral neck fracture; and perhaps most notably revision hip arthroplasty.[3,4] In a review of more than 10,000 THAs by Woo and Morrey, the dislocation rate doubled with revision surgery compared with primary THA.[5]

Revision surgery to treat instability is indicated when dislocations recur despite closed treatment. Loss of capsular and soft tissue restraint due to repetitive trauma creates a situation in which recurrent dislocation is more likely. For surgeons undertaking revision for recurrent dislocation, the key considerations are the etiology of dislocation and the direction of instability. Success of the revision procedure is less likely when the etiology of the dislocation is not clearly identifiable preoperatively.[6]

EVALUATION OF DISLOCATION

History

The initial evaluation of the patient with an unstable total hip must include a thorough history. This includes the activity or position that led to dislocation, the number of prior dislocations, and the treatment rendered to date. Early dislocations may be less prone to recurrence than late dislocations, as later dislocations are associated with issues such as cognitive decline and loss of neuromuscular control in addition to component wear or deformation due to use and repetitive impingement.[7] For these reasons, late dislocations are more likely to require operative intervention. Patients should be questioned and screened for historical and medical factors suggestive

Jacofsky DJ, Hedley AK.
Fundamentals of Revision Hip Arthroplasty:
Diagnosis, Evaluation, and Treatment (pp 119-142).
© 2013 SLACK Incorporated.

of infection, such as the absence of a pain-free interval, prolonged wound drainage, treatment with antibiotics, any prior or secondary procedures, and any constitutional symptoms. Screening laboratory evaluations including an erythrocyte sedimentation rate and C-reactive protein should be ordered. A preoperative aspiration is recommended if either test is abnormal or if a high index of clinical suspicion is present. Intraoperative frozen sections and a fluid cell count should be obtained in all revisions, regardless of preoperative studies due to their diagnostic accuracy.[8] Prior records, including operative notes and implant stickers, should be obtained in all cases to facilitate planning and to ensure appropriate extraction instruments and matching modular implants are available at the time of the revision procedure.

Physical Examination

Physical examination should include inspection of the surgical scar, evaluation of gait, limb length assessment, and a complete motor and sensory evaluation. Assessment of abduction strength is of particular importance. These features may give an indication of the dynamic function of the secondary hip restraints.

Surgical Approach

The surgical approach affects the risk of postoperative instability. The posterior approach historically has had a higher incidence of dislocation compared to the anterior approach. However, there is a higher incidence of limp and trochanteric pain after an anterolateral approach, due either to failure of the soft tissue repair or from injury to the superior gluteal nerve. Recent studies suggest that a posterior capsular repair reduces dislocation risk in both primary and revision surgeries.[9-13] Relative to the implant components, in general the acetabulum should be anteverted more when approaching the hip posteriorly. The hip does not tolerate neutral or retroverted components with a posterior approach. Conversely, when using an anterior or anterolateral approach, less anteversion is usually placed on the acetabular component. Newer approaches, such as the direct anterior approach, may also reduce the risk of dislocation, but further study is needed to determine the risk/benefit ratio of these alternate techniques.

Component Malposition

Component malposition is the most common cause for hip instability.[14] Unfortunately, malposition is directly related to surgical technique. Though there is no consensus regarding optimal component position, a "safe zone" acetabular component position was described as early as 1978 by Lewinnek et al.[15] The potential for this problem is higher when less invasive exposures are used as there is often limited visualization during bone preparation. There is also a learning curve associated with minimally invasive surgery. Surgeons adopting these techniques should be especially wary of the pitfall of cup malposition. Vertical inclination and inadequate anteversion are the most common errors. There are a number of techniques to more adequately ensure proper placement of components (eg, computer-aided navigation, intraoperative alignment devices, fluoroscopy), but these are evolving. To minimize positioning errors, use of a rigid pelvic positioner is recommended.[16] Attention should also be paid to the orientation of the operating table, as changes in tilt or rotation can lead the surgeon to misjudge implant position when using instrumentation with orientation guides. It is advisable during the learning curve phase of any new technique to take advantage of simple techniques like x-ray to confirm implant placement and positioning.[17]

Malposition and/or instability may be related to the surgical approach that was used. Historically, the posterior approach has had a higher incidence of dislocation when compared to the anterolateral approach. This difference has been balanced against a higher risk of limp and trochanteric pain due to inconsistent abductor healing. Over time the incidence of dislocation associated with the posterior approach has decreased significantly. The posterior dislocation issue was probably a combined problem: component position and poor reconstruction of the soft tissue. It is clear now that routine repair of the posterior capsular structures, short external rotators and quadratus (whatever was taken down during the approach), has significantly decreased the incidence of postoperative dislocation.[10,13] The cup position needs to be adjusted somewhat based on the approach that is used. In general, the acetabulum should be more anteverted when using a posterior approach compared to an anterior or anterolateral approach. The hip does not tolerate neutral or retroverted components with a posterior approach. Conversely, when using an anterior or anterolateral approach less anteversion is typically placed on the acetabulum, and the hip will not tolerate an overly anteverted cup position. It is not uncommon to find that the cup was placed in relative retroversion when an anterior-sided approach was used for the primary operation. Over time, this may lead to repetitive impingement or even posterior instability if the posterior structures have become attenuated.

Defining the correct position for the acetabular and femoral components continues to evolve as research has provided more detailed understanding of static and dynamic pelvic position. Anteversion of 15 ± 10 degrees and lateral opening of 40 ± 10 degrees has been associated with a lower risk of dislocation than in hips placed outside this range. Femoral component anteversion is also important and can be more difficult to optimize.[18] Recent modeling and clinical data suggest that combined anteversion of the femoral and acetabular components contribute to stability, and a combined anteversion of 35 degrees is a target mean.[19-21] Matching the patient's natural bony anatomy may seem intuitively ideal when implanting prosthetic components. Unfortunately, native anatomy does not always fall within a safe zone,[22] and surgeon estimation of component position is subject to error due to pelvic tilt[23] and other factors. Functional motion, as defined by a patient's particular anatomy, can be measured with navigation or other techniques and may be more applicable to the modern situation. Increased awareness of dynamic motion has gained interest, particularly as it relates to the problem of recurrent dislocation. Pelvic tilt and fixed pelvic obliquity may alter component position dynamically and should be accounted for during cup placement.[24,25]

Malposition (abduction angle or version) or abnormal cup position (eg, high hip center) may lead to impingement of the component on the component, the component on bone, the component on soft tissue, bone-on-bone, or soft tissue on soft tissue. All types of impingement may lead to and contribute to instability.[26] Usually the acetabular position is the source of the problem rather than the femoral position, although newer evidence shows that many stems are somewhat malrotated, and the surgeon's assessment of stem anteversion is inconsistent.[18] A high hip center puts the femur in a position to impinge on the pelvis. The same is true for a cup placed significantly medial, as it loses offset. On the femoral side, shortening, whether the result of implant technique or subsidence, may lead to impingement of the greater trochanter on the ilium. When offset and length are suboptimal, impingement of the lesser trochanter on the ischium may occur. The cup position may need to be adjusted based on a patient's anatomy, obliquity of the pelvis, or previous fractures to avoid impingement. In these cases using intraoperative x-ray, good preoperative planning and/or navigation techniques are important to avoid late instability. Though navigation has been shown to reduce component positioning outliers,[27] use of image-based and imageless navigation is not yet routine.

Impingement

Impingement may result in hip instability, regardless of the surgical approach or component positioning. In fact, impingement precedes dislocation in the majority of cases unless abductor deficiency is present. It is imperative during the performance of any primary or revision operation on the hip to assess stability through a wide arc of motion. Posterior stability is assessed in flexion, adduction, and internal rotation, and anterior stability is assessed with the hip in extension and external rotation. Acceptable stability has been defined as more than 45 degrees of internal rotation with the hip flexed 90 degrees.[28] Ideally, avoidance of excessive anterior placement of the socket should be sought.[29] Repetitive impingement may cause wear of the acetabular liner,

Figure 9-1. Anteroposterior radiograph of a patient who was revised for instability of the left hip. She reported to have had multiple dislocations as a result of distracting the hip by forcibly hooking her toes over the end of her bed when prone. This was apparently an unconscious habit. The components were felt to be positioned appropriately, but there was desire for increased offset and more dynamic tension. Instead of performing a trochanteric osteotomy with advancement, the surgeon revised the femoral stem to increase length and offset. While the revision surgery was successful relative to the instability and resolved the patient's complaint, the procedure resulted in a leg length discrepancy. (Note: The broken screw occurred at the index procedure.)

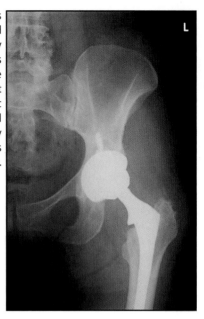

and this can create a pathway for easier dislocation. Restoration of limb length and offset is desirable from the standpoint of hip mechanical function; proper tension reduces joint reactive force, thereby decreasing wear and creating a more stable construct.[30]

As will be discussed later in this chapter, impingement may be the most significant issue relative to recurrent instability. Malposition of the cup or stem will lead to impingement between soft tissue, bone, component, or some combination.

Femoral Offset

Femoral offset, defined as the horizontal distance from the center of the femoral head to the center of the femoral shaft, affects hip stability. Increasing femoral offset increases the abductor moment arm and soft tissue tension, both of which increase hip stability by increasing muscular efficiency and decreasing impingement. As a result of these factors, hips with reduced offset can be expected to have a higher incidence of dislocation.[31] Preoperative templating is helpful in choosing components and femoral resection level to optimize offset without altering limb length (Figure 9-1).[32] One should be careful to avoid excessive offset, as this may result in trochanteric pain or bursitis and may affect the clinical outcome. Excessive offset may also limit the surgeon's ability to anatomically repair the soft tissues, which adversely affects stability. In the case of revision for instability, review of the preoperative radiographs obtained in advance of the primary operation can help guide a more anatomic reconstruction.[33]

Abnormal Wear Patterns

When instability is the result of an abnormal component wear pattern, the diagnosis can usually be made or implied from the plain radiographs. Once the dislocation is reduced, is the component shortened relative to limb length? Is there significant polyethylene wear? Has the femoral head migrated?

Substantial acetabular polyethylene wear decreases the capture of the femoral head and allows pistoning within the articulation. The conformity of the ball and socket is lost due to this wear, and as a result there is a decrease in mechanical stability. In addition, substantial wear that leads to shortening and/or loss of offset may result in impingement as well as soft tissue laxity.

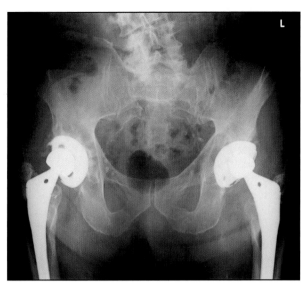

Figure 9-2. Anteroposterior radiograph showing a right total hip arthroplasty that was previously revised for instability. At the time of surgery, the polyethylene was found to have fractured as a result of wear and probably the high angle and rim loads. A piece of polyethylene was incarcerated within the joint. At the time of revision, a new polyethylene was cemented into the stable, ingrown shell and the head replaced. While the revision surgery resolved the instability problem for several years by addressing the catastrophic polyethylene failure and loss of head capture, it would have been advisable to revise the acetabular component and place it into a better anatomic position.

Unfortunately, if polyethylene wear first manifests as a prosthetic dislocation, the hip is likely quite unstable and the reduction may be difficult to maintain. In these cases a more immediate revision surgery may be necessary. At the revision, one may find that wear and oxidation-induced embrittlement combined with repetitive localized impingement has resulted in indentation or fracture of the liner, complete wear-through of the polyethylene, or signs of component-component impingement of the neck against the metal rim of the shell.

The revision surgery for instability that results from polyethylene wear is relatively straightforward and may be as simple as a polyethylene liner exchange, provided the implants are stable and in good position, have a good clinical track record, and the locking mechanism is intact. In these cases the principles that have been outlined for the treatment of acetabular osteolysis with stable components should be applied (Figure 9-2).[34]

If the implant brand/style can be identified and a new polyethylene is available, a new insert may be placed. If the shell is well fixed and well positioned but the polyethylene is not available or has less wear resistance than current materials, cementing a new liner into the existing shell is an option.[35-38] The cementing technique should also be used in cases in which the locking mechanism of the acetabular component is damaged, poor, or unreliable. However, it must be noted that the risk of dislocation in isolated acetabular insert exchange is high, and this technique has limited application in the treatment of dislocation.[39]

After thorough exposure, the well-fixed acetabular component may be retained or exchanged. Typically for a larger cementless cup, if the locking mechanism is intact, an acetabular liner with an inner diameter of 36 to 44 mm is placed within the shell. This accommodates a larger head and hopefully will provide added stability. If a compatible liner is not available or the locking mechanism is deficient, the liner may be cemented into the existing acetabular component.[36]

When cementing in a liner, it is important to texture the backside of the liner to increase the surface area for cement adhesion. A high-speed burr is used to create a "spider web" pattern on the backside of the shell. Care should be taken to prepare the liner on the back table to prevent polyethylene particles from entering the surgical field. The shell should also be textured with a carbide-tipped burr unless there are screw holes available to serve as cement anchors. These measures increase both torsional and pull-out strength.[40] The shell should be carefully dried prior to cementing, and a 2- to 4-mm cement mantle idealizes fixation of the liner. In the final construct, even when using larger heads, skirted style heads should be avoided if possible to avoid component-to-component impingement and the resultant consequence of polyethylene wear and osteolysis.[41,42]

If cementing in a liner is not an option due to cup damage, loosening, or malposition, the acetabular shell should be revised. Revision of the shell with minimal risk of bone loss is facilitated by use of special osteotomes such as the Zimmer Explant (Zimmer, Inc, Warsaw, IN) or Universal Hip Cup Removal System (Innomed Inc, Savannah, GA). Use of these devices allows efficient and safe removal of the cup by curved osteotomes attached to a spherical "head" that fits into the existing liner. A shorter and a longer osteotome are available for each 2-mm increment in cup outer diameter. Any screws in the socket will need to be removed, and if the liner has eccentric wear or other damage, a trial liner may be placed into the shell to ensure a tight fit at the bone/implant interface. Overhanging bone should be removed with a burr or osteotome, and a pencil-tip burr can be used to create an initial slot for the first osteotome. The osteotome is carefully passed circumferentially around the socket in a rocking and circular motion, first using the smaller osteotome then the larger. Care should be taken to avoid levering against the posterior column, and the socket should be completely loose of any bony attachment before any vigorous attempts are made to disimpact the shell.

It is imperative to ensure that the liner wear is not the result of, or associated with, component malposition or impingement between the components or bone. Component-component impingement is commonly encountered when the acetabular component has an elevated rim liner. Liner impingement leads to accelerated wear patterns and/or mechanical failure of the polyethylene. Due to the load burden of the polyethylene debris created by component impingement, it is common to see osteolytic changes in association with abnormal and/or accelerated wear patterns.

If osteolysis is identified by plain radiographs preoperatively, computed tomography scan can be helpful to quantify the volumetric extent of the lesion(s).[43-45] When planning for surgery in hips with osteolysis, one should be prepared to thoroughly débride the granuloma and fibrous tissue in and around the joint. This has the benefit of diminishing the burden of debris as well as allowing for bone restoration by grafting and optimizing fixation surfaces. A large amount of granulomatous tissue is frequently encountered in and around failed hip joints. The thick tissue, especially that anterior and inferior to the acetabulum, will cause impingement and postoperative instability if not excised. In contrast, adjacent to this thickened granuloma, the native dynamic soft tissue structures including the capsule and short external rotators often have become eroded or attenuated and are of poor quality. This is especially true in revisions for instability since the trauma of the dislocation(s) causes additional and significant soft tissue destruction or attenuation. In addition, adequate exposure often requires substantial soft tissue release. After débridement, there is a risk of secondary instability problems as a result of the loss of capsular tissue and/or abductor musculature.

The loss of soft tissue restraints is a major reason why even "routine" revision surgery for acetabular osteolysis and polyethylene wear with stable components and no preoperative instability (polyethylene exchange and bone grafting) has a high dislocation rate. It stands to reason, therefore, that if polyethylene wear is the primary reason for hip instability, the surgeon should be wary of an isolated poly exchange.

Wear Leading to Loosening and Component Failure

The topic of wear leading to loosening and component failure is more appropriately and extensively covered in the revision chapter covering loosening. If recurrent instability results from a change in position of the acetabular or femoral component (a stem falling into retroversion, stem subsidence, acetabulum shifting vertically or in retroversion), the treatment for the instability is clearly revision of the failed component. These are not so much an issue of instability as catastrophic component failure. Treatment of the failed component (Figure 9-3) generally resolves the instability problem.

Changes in cup position may, however, be subtle. Evaluate sequential x-rays, obtain a cross-table lateral to evaluate the acetabular version, and take films in multiple planes. There are several methods to estimate the cup version by plain radiograph.[46-51] Progression of radiolucent lines and

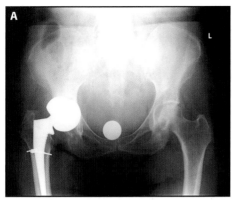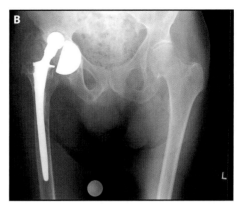

Figure 9-3. Anteroposterior pelvis radiographs depict catastrophic failure of the acetabular component. The change in position of the acetabular component led to instability in addition to the pain associated with the loosening. The pain and loosening preceded the failure and instability. Revision of the acetabular component should remedy the pain and instability.

component migration are also established indicators for loosening.[52-56] Radionuclide scans showing uptake on delayed imaging may also be diagnostic.[57,58] If it remains unclear whether the cup is stable or loose, and there is consideration of retaining the component, it is important to define the component position and the corresponding direction of the dislocations preoperatively.

These same positional and loosening issues are germane to the femur. If the instability problem is at the stem level, it may be hard to diagnose by x-ray. Much like the acetabulum, progression of lucent lines, subsidence, and other signs of loosening are indicators of stem failure.[52,59]

Sequential x-rays and physical exams are very helpful in all but obvious cases. Check the hip range of motion. As the stem falls into retroversion, a common failure mode, there will be a change in the hip motion pattern. There may be resting external rotation of the hip. The patient will externally rotate as his or her hip flexes, and internal rotation will be limited. The change in stem position may result in rotational impingement and instability particularly with hip flexion activities. Subsidence is another common failure mode. It results in decreased leg length and offset, both of which result in an abductor weakness and an increased propensity for impingement. If the abductor tension is sufficiently reduced, instability may occur. If this resulting instability is dramatic, subluxation or frank dislocation may be reproduced on physical exam.

It is common for aseptic loosening to occur in only one implant while the corresponding stem or acetabular component remains well fixed. In these circumstances, single component revision may be considered. However, the fixed position of the stable component has to be accommodated when preparing the revision construct. The concept of combined anteversion is a guiding principle in determining the placement of the revision implant.[21] Unfortunately, clinical data[60-62] demonstrate that revision of a single component has a higher dislocation rate compared to procedures in which both components are revised. If extrapolating to the instability revision situation, this is a conundrum: if the revision surgery is performed for instability and the procedure itself has an increased incidence of instability, should both components be revised in all cases of instability? Individual cases must be assessed carefully, and rigorous intraoperative assessment of stability and careful soft tissue balancing and repair must be performed.

While there is limited data to support the assertion that if a larger femoral head can be used for the single component revision the historic problems with instability would be improved, this seems to be a reasonable claim based on the mechanics of larger heads.[63,64] This concept is discussed more extensively later in this chapter.

Post-Traumatic Instability

Instability as a result of a traumatic event that causes fracture of or catastrophic failure of an implant or of the implant-bone interface should be treated according to trauma care principles. Fixing the underlying pathology will generally fix the instability problem.

If the event causes fracture of the acetabular liner, the injury may not be obvious. The behavior of the hip will be very similar to that of severe, end-stage liner wear, but may present more acutely. Liner fracture results in loss of the conformity of the head-acetabular interface and loss of head capture. In addition, pieces of the fractured liner may become trapped in the joint and prevent full relocation. Eccentricity may be apparent on post-reduction imaging. If present, this finding necessitates more urgent surgery.

When a traumatic event causes abductor rupture or trochanteric fracture, dynamic instability results. Patients who had an anterolateral approach at the time of the initial surgery may be more prone to this problem, as healing of the abduction repair is not always predictable. Patients present with a limping gait and exhibit a positive Trendelenburg sign. Generally, the surgical approach should target repair of the injury, though secondary soft tissue healing has a high failure rate. Permanent suture with or without anchors placed into decorticated bone are recommended for repair. The patient should be braced postoperatively and placed on abductor precautions for 6 to 12 weeks. When the abductors fail, they are often shortened, atrophied, and fibrotic, thus the higher failure rate of re-repair. In addition, granuloma associated with wear debris may create attritional deficiency of the surrounding bone or soft tissue. If bone stock or muscle tendon strength is compromised, it may be extremely difficult to repair the abductors securely. In order to obtain more secure fixation, extended trochanteric plates rather than suture, cables, or short fixation devices are preferred. If the repair is tenuous, use of a larger head for additional stability or use of a constrained or tripolar implant should be considered. In cases of complete abductor deficiency, use of a constrained component is strongly recommended. When a traumatic injury occurs and an occult fracture results, the missed fracture, whether acetabular, trochanteric, or femoral, may result in late positional changes of the femoral or acetabular component or dynamic changes occur relative to the abductors. The result is similar to that of the acute setting relative to aftercare and treatment. Fixing the fracture or component should fix the problem.

When trauma or surgery results in late heterotopic ossification, bony impingement may occur. Timing of removal of heterotopic bone is controversial, but historically, surgery has been delayed until the bone has matured as based on radiographs (Figure 9-4) and radionuclide imaging results. When heterotopic bone is removed, postoperative radiation or indomethacin should be used as secondary prophylaxis.[65-68]

Abductor Insufficiency

For the purposes of this chapter, abductor insufficiency is defined as a functional loss of the abductor moment arm. The insufficiency may result in dynamic hip instability. Patients with abductor weakness will have a Trendelenburg gait or positive Trendelenburg sign. Abductor weakness can be post-traumatic but is more commonly associated with failure of soft tissue repair or neurologic injury related to the initial surgical approach. Late failure may also occur in association with soft tissue loss caused by granuloma formed in response to wear debris.

After a traumatic event or as a result of wear-induced osteolysis, trochanteric fracture or nonunion may lead to abductor insufficiency with proximal or anterior migration of the trochanter. Similarly, there is a unique pattern of abductor insufficiency associated with the stress shielding and loss of the trochanteric bone seen in association with long porous-coated stems.[69] In these cases the entire trochanter and part of the lateral femur may slowly resorb over time, or thinning of the lateral cortex may result in trochanteric escape. In addition, significant osteolysis in the trochanter can be seen particularly in older hip designs that utilized polyethylene bearings with less

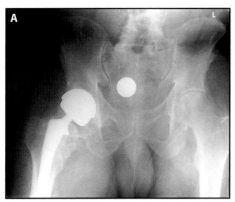
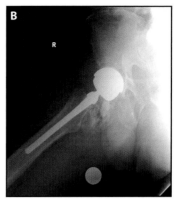

Figure 9-4. These anteroposterior and lateral radiographs show a large head metal-on-metal total hip arthroplasty with significant heterotopic ossification. The bony mass may limit range of motion and create an impingement lever arm.

wear resistance than current materials. Primary repair of the soft tissues and/or bone is very difficult in these settings due to bony deficiency and poor quality of the soft tissue. Since fixing the abductors will resolve the instability, use aggressive fixation techniques if possible. For bony problems use long cable plates rather than short trochanteric fixation devices or cables alone. For soft tissue or bony repair, protect the patient postoperatively with bracing and protected weightbearing in an attempt to unload the repair.

Adductor Tenotomy

The adductors are frequently overlooked as a contributor to hip instability. Adductor tenotomy should be considered as an adjunct in the treatment of prosthetic hip dislocation when muscle balance is adversely affected by an adduction contracture. Limited abduction of the hip causes a relative valgus moment, decreases abductor deficiency, and may allow the prosthetic head to subluxate laterally or increase risk of impingement.

Intraoperative assessment of passive abduction should be a routine step in stability testing. When adductor tightness is present, a percutaneous adductor tenotomy is performed at the conclusion of the procedure.

Behavior

Patients' behavioral issues that lead to instability are particularly difficult to handle. This is especially true for those dislocations that result from cognitive dysfunction. This is becoming more problematic with the growth of the aging population and an increasing prevalence of dementia.[3] In the past, this issue was recognized primarily in patients who had alcoholic tendencies, used drugs, or post-traumatic cases in which patients had some loss of functional motion and had problems adapting behaviorally to a new prosthesis. Some behavioral issues are not limited to cognitive dysfunction. As patients increasingly participate in high-level physical activity, high-risk behavior is becoming commonplace.[70,71] Athletic activities like skiing[71] and climbing present the risk of uncontrolled falls that lead to traumatic dislocation and/or periprosthetic fracture, both of which may ultimately lead to recurrent instability. Patients should be counseled preoperatively about acceptable activities following hip replacement and the potential risk of periprosthetic fracture or dislocation.

Explain the Whys

Usually recurrent instability is the result of a combination of factors. Be very wary of operating without an understanding of why the instability is occurring. Timing for surgery is important. In general, the first-time dislocator and usually the second-time dislocator are treated conservatively unless there is clear evidence of component failure or malposition. While closed treatment is successful in approximately two-thirds of cases,[72] recurrent dislocation beyond 3 instances is a generally accepted indication for revision ("3 strikes and you're out").

If the patient has recurrent dislocation, surgery will be required. Unfortunately, it is quite likely that even if the instability problem was the result of impingement, component malposition, or loosening, the soft tissue will have been significantly affected by the dislocation episodes. Anticipate that there will be disruption of capsular tissue and other dynamic stabilizing structures.

Reconstructive Options for Hip Instability

Constrained Liners

A constrained liner by definition "locks" the femoral head into the acetabular component. One of several different mechanisms may be used to accomplish the "locking." However, since the component is fully constrained, dislocation can only occur "catastrophically" through failure of the locking mechanism or of the implant-bone interface. If the hip is placed into an extreme position, particularly if there is impingement that creates a strong lever arm, the force may exceed the mechanical strength of the construct and the locking mechanism will fail. The loads to failure are readily available from the manufacturers. Despite case reports of closed reduction,[73-77] once dislocated these components are essentially nonreducible and will typically require open surgery. If the locking mechanism does not fail, fracture of the bone or failure of the implant bone interface must occur. Therefore, a constrained construct should, in general, be used as a last resort only when there is complete loss of the abductor function and the dynamic soft tissue sleeve or recurrent dislocation has occurred without a defined cause. These devices should not be used in primary cases, except in the most egregious situations. By keeping these warnings in mind, the use of constrained implants have been shown to have good success in the literature.[78-92]

Constrained devices necessarily decrease available range of motion, which produces component-to-component impingement. Catastrophic failure of constrained implants has been reported at all interfaces and therefore these implants should be used with caution.

One should resist the temptation to implant a constrained liner if there are any signs of impingement. This is more difficult than it seems since the stability of the constraint is seductive in the complex revision setting. However, using constraint in the face of impingement will ultimately result in late fracture or failure of the device. As the patient impinges, the lever arm created imparts very high forces to the implants and the interfaces. These forces will ultimately exceed fracture/failure threshold. The actual load to failure can be obtained from the manufacturers, but repetitive load to failure is what typically causes the implants to loosen or disengage. These forces are more likely to be exceeded in aggregate in larger patients. For this reason, the manufacturers place weight/body mass index limits on recommended patient use.

It is important to review and understand the design and method of constraint for the device one is planning to use, particularly in relation to impingement. In basic terms, the femoral head "locks" into the polyethylene. In 2-piece devices this is usually accomplished by narrowing the introitus via a locking ring (most common) or the molded shape of the polyethylene. In both cases, the polyethylene is extended laterally to deepen the capture and/or provide seating of the locking ring. The head snaps into the polyethylene under force (a similar or greater force is required to dislocate). If there is a locking ring, the ring slides into a groove that narrows or compresses the introitus (Figures 9-5 and 9-6).

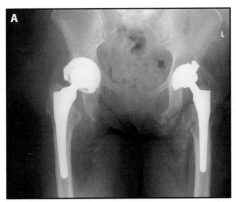
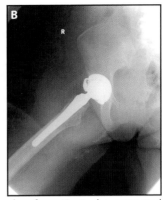

Figure 9-5. Anteroposterior and lateral radiographs of a patient who presented to the emergency room with multiple hip dislocations. Her components were able to be identified preoperatively. At the time of the revision surgery, the component position seemed appropriate but there was complete disruption of the soft tissue envelope and abductor mechanism so a modular constrained device was fit into the existing stable shell. Note the prominent locking mechanism that is prone to impingement.

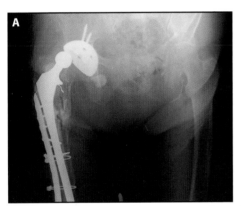
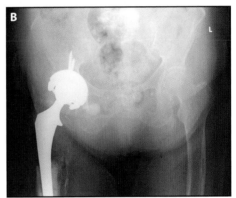

Figure 9-6. (A) Preoperative anteroposterior pelvis radiograph of a patient with a periprosthetic fracture, bone loss, abductor failure, and obvious instability. (B) Postoperative radiograph of the reconstruction. A constrained acetabular liner was placed into the stable shell to resolve the gross dynamic instability and associated bone loss.

Constrained tripolar devices have a larger bipolar head that is contained within a polyethylene liner. The manufacturer preassembles the large head/polyethylene liner combination, and the liner/head combination is size specific just as any other liner that snaps into a modular acetabular shell. A standard femoral head (size limited and specific to the bipolar implant) is snapped into the bipolar head as is traditional with hip fracture surgery. There are 2 areas of constraint: the smaller head is constrained within the bipolar head and the larger bipolar head is constrained within the polyethylene liner (Figure 9-7). Failure can occur at either interface or at the implant-bone interface if forces exceed the failure load.

In both styles of constrained device, there is a significantly decreased arc of motion before implant-implant impingement occurs. This is most notable due to the raised lips of the liner and increased depth to accommodate the locking mechanism. The diameter size of the femoral neck and the presence of a collar or skirt may further limit the range of motion. If there is obvious impingement at the time of implantation an alternate construct should be considered. In the

Figure 9-7. This anteroposterior pelvis radiograph shows a multiply revised patient with significant bone loss and loss of the abductor mechanism. His dynamic instability was addressed with a constrained liner that was placed into a stable/ingrown acetabular component. The attempted repair of the abductor mechanism was unsuccessful as demonstrated by the failed cables, but he remained located and otherwise functionally stable.

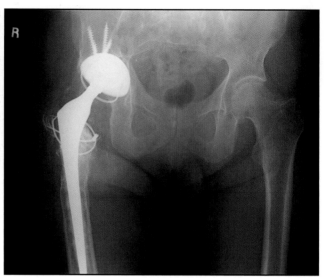

author's experience (DCM), devices that use a locking ring that slides into the plastic to narrow the introitus have a higher fracture and failure rate than the tripolar variety. The very high wall that is created to fit the locking ring significantly decreases motion. Unfortunately, older stem designs had thick femoral necks, which, when combined with the limitation of the locking mechanism (see Figure 9-5), cause an even greater risk of impingement.

It would be wise to avoid implanting a constrained device if the acetabular implant is not ingrown. If one is forced to use constraint with a newly placed acetabular component, screws should be used, and the patient should be protected weightbearing and range of motion for the first 6 to 12 weeks postoperatively. Additionally, constrained implants should be used with particular caution in association with reconstruction cages. An unfortunate example of this was noted by Khoury et al,[93] who reported high failure rates when constrained liners were cemented into cages.[94] It is clearly safer to cement into or implant a constrained device into an otherwise stable acetabular component. But even in these cases the increased forces can be problematic[86,87,95] (Figure 9-8).

As noted, the implant designs are very important. Tripolar designs tend to have increased range of motion and less impingement than constrained designs, and there is less wear as well, depending on the articulation and the materials used. In general, the tripolar devices have good locking mechanisms and can be placed into existing acetabular designs. Unfortunately the depth and shape of the constrained plastic may not allow a secure fit within certain shell geometries. In addition, there are specific limitations on head size for given acetabular diameters. Head sizes, particularly in older designs, may not match current inventories. This may present a problem in obtaining a well-mated construct utilizing implants from different manufacturers. Careful preoperative planning is essential to ensure that matching implants are available at the time of surgery.

Constrained devices are very dependent upon stem and cup design. There is a risk of early polyethylene failure due to the decreased polyethylene thicknesses required to accommodate the locking mechanisms. Older polyethylene may have been used in manufacturing of these seldom-used products, thus there is worry about increased risk of wear and mechanical failure. Shelf life is an important consideration due to the risk of polyethylene oxidation so extra vigilance is required to avoid implanting an excessively aged liner. The bottom line is that constraint is a safe and effective bailout in selected cases, but due to the high forces and loads conveyed to the construct, constrained implants should be reserved for the highest risk cases and for those in which other techniques have failed. It is expected that with the advent and availability of very large femoral heads and mobile bearing tripolar devices, the indications for a constrained implant will diminish in time.

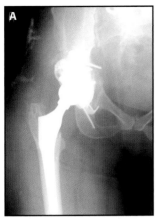
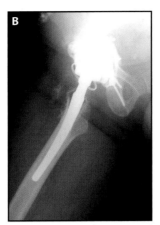
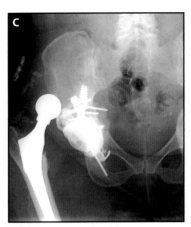

Figure 9-8. (A) Radiograph of a multiply revised patient who had been treated with a cup-cage construct. The patient had multiple dislocations beginning approximately 6 months postoperatively. (B) Radiograph depicting implantation of a constrained liner into the indwelling shell. (C) Radiograph of catastrophic failure of the reconstruction.

Indications for Use of Constrained Components

To reiterate, one must make a strong attempt to understand why the patient is dislocating. The primary indication for use of a constrained device is instability with well-positioned components. Usually this is a result of abductor insufficiency. If the components are acceptably positioned the constrained devices may be used to augment treatment of the abductor insufficiency, cognitive or behavioral issues, or when the etiology of the dislocation is not clearly identifiable either preoperatively or at the time of revision. When constrained implants are used, the decision not to revise existing components must be made carefully. Components that are not revised must be well positioned, and there must not be any impingement during a trial range of motion to have the best outcome (see Figures 9-5 through 9-7).

Contraindications to Use of Constrained Components

Impingement

Whether the impingement is implant-implant, implant-bone, or bone-bone, a lever arm is created that will repeatedly test the locking mechanism of the liner. The impingement problem is further complicated by the fact that the constrained implants decrease range of motion due to the locking mechanism mechanics. Combining preexisting impingement with an increased potential for impingement is a recipe for disaster. The increased loads from the lever arm, when combined with impingement, will lead to failure of the construct by disassociation or implant loosening.

Obesity

The manufacturers of constrained implants set weight specifications that limit use in obese patients. It is recommended that manufacturer specifications be reviewed prior to considering use of these implants. The inherent forces generated within the construct are increased by the weight of the patient, and due to hip mechanics this is a multiple of 4 or more times body weight. While obese patients tend to be at higher risk than average for dislocation, constrained implants should be utilized with extra caution in the obese.

Constrained Liners and Implant Malposition

If the femoral or acetabular component is felt to be malpositioned it needs to be exchanged at the time of the revision surgery. Despite the temptation to mitigate the instability with other techniques, failure to revise a malpositioned implant is destined to failure. While it is tempting to simply place a constrained liner into a well-fixed shell to treat an instability problem, the increased loads, wear, and impingement will ultimately lead to failure. It seems reasonable to rationalize that in cases in which the hip was stable for years prior to the onset of dislocation, the implant position must have been acceptable, especially if there is a soft tissue available for repair. However, the revision surgery for recurrent instability establishes a new starting point and without proper positioning the construct will fail. It is better to accept the risk to the bone and the complexity of implant removal in order to revise a malpositioned implant. Current implant removal devices and use of techniques such as extended trochanteric osteotomy are efficient and bone preserving in contrast to historical techniques. If the malpositioned implant is not revised, eventually impingement (which is worse with constrained liners) will lead to polyethylene fracture, failure of the locking mechanism, or catastrophic failure of the construct at the implant-bone interface.

Constrained Liners and Protrusio Cages

There are well-defined situations in which protrusio cages are required for revision surgery.[96,97] It is less clear when constrained liners should be used and combining these 2 is problematic. The early data have demonstrated that there is a high failure rate of the combined cage-constrained liner construct (see Figure 9-8).[93] While this combination technique is reserved as a bailout and last-ditch effort, it has to be emphasized that the failure rate is extraordinarily high. In these complex cases, a cup/cage/cup construct has demonstrated early clinical success. The technique involves placing the cage on top of a trabecular metal (Zimmer, Inc) ingrowth implant to maximize the ingrowth potential and minimize the loads imparted to the bone implant interface. A modular cup is then cemented within the cage, utilizing the largest inner-diameter liner available or a liner can be cemented directly into the cage. Careful cement technique and contouring of the liner backside is important to attain sufficient interfacial strength. Currently, in these high-risk cases the use of the constrained liners has been largely been supplanted by use of larger femoral heads.

Conclusions About Constrained Liners

Using a constrained acetabular implant is relatively easy whether it is cemented into a shell or designed to be assembled via a modular snap fit. Although there are some size limitations, the components are relatively well adapted to most situations and can be an easy solution to difficult problems. One should avoid use of constrained components in the morbidly obese, in the face of malpositioned implants, and in combination with acetabular cages. Use of these devices is balanced against the ability or inability to use other techniques. The risks of catastrophic failure, irreducible failure of the locking mechanism, and increased interface strain that may lead to loosening or failure of ingrowth of porous implants may make it preferable to try to employ a larger head size in most revisions for instability and to avoid constraint unless there is failure of the large head construct and/or maturation of the ingrowth bony interface.

Large Femoral Heads

There has been a recent trend toward use of larger femoral heads to decrease dislocation after total hip replacement (THR). Larger heads do allow a greater range of motion prior to impingement but this comes at the cost of greater volumetric wear. Theoretically, the use of a large femoral head and/or unconstrained tripolar device has a significant advantage over a "standard-sized" head relative to range of motion and impingement. These devices have provided a much-needed addition to the armamentarium of revision surgery and lend an added measure of security to cases where instability is a problem. Big heads are not a substitute for good implant technique or good component position. No matter what head size is used at revision, the specific cause of the dislocations needs to be addressed at the time of surgery. Thereafter, the larger head sizes will provide improved stability.

Before using a large head, it is important to review the basics. In virtually all cases of instability, impingement contributes to the initiation of the subluxation and dislocation, whether it originates from implant-implant, implant-bone, implant-soft tissue, bone-bone, bone-soft tissue, or soft tissue-soft tissue. With morbid obesity there may even be extra-articular impingement of the thigh on the abdomen in flexion that forces the hip posteriorly and inferiorly during flexion activities. Increasing the hip's functional range of motion is a key factor in dealing with these problems. Although the increased functional range of motion may not eliminate impingement, it may change the impingement point/angle. This is particularly true in cases where there is a skirted head, a thick femoral neck, elevated liner, and/or a poor head/neck ratio.

Computer models and sawbones studies have been used to demonstrate that implant design and impingement in the aforementioned areas do affect range of motion. Several different models have been designed to assess hip range of motion, but most do not take into account all of the potential initiating factors. Colwell, D'Lima, and colleagues used simulated changes in implant position such as cup angle, head size, and neck angle and applied these to a computer model that incorporated bony anatomy.[26,98] Changes in stem offset and neck diameter increased motion before impingement in identical cup positions. The findings were then validated in cadaveric models.[99-101] These authors noted that increased cup adduction led to increased flexion, extension, and abduction range, but it decreased hip adduction and rotational range. When they increased cup anteversion the result was increased flexion, but decreased abduction and extension. When the stem was placed with increased anteversion, the hip had increased flexion, but decreased adduction and extension.

When neck diameter was decreased there was an increase excursion in all positions with a generalized increased range of motion. This finding was not unexpected as the head/neck ratio increases functional motion much like increasing head size. When the neck-shaft angle decreased from 132 to 127 degrees there was increase in flexion, extension, and adduction and a concurrent decrease in abduction and external rotation. One can see that there are trade-offs based on the component design, but clearly a decreased neck size with a common head size leads to increased motion in all planes. These findings should be remembered when trying to assess the causes of instability.[102]

Component-component impingement is only a factor in some cases. When bone was added into the computer modeling, greater than 40% of the test scenarios had impingement. The bony tissue countered many of the benefits and increased motion provided by the implant alternatives. For example, with a cup abduction angle of greater than 45 degrees and anteversion of greater than 20 degrees, all components impinged in flexion. When testing was moved to the cadaver model, there were generally less differences between designs due in part to the increased episodes of bony impingement and an overall decreased range of motion.

The design of the component system is quite important and should be taken into account at the time of revision whether the implants are replaced or retained. If possible a larger head and a thinner neck should be used at revision to improve the potential motion before impingement. When only the head size is changed from 28 to 36 mm there is an increase in all planes of motion. In a report by Yamaguchi et al, using a single neck design, with a 28-mm head there was a 75-degree arc of motion, at 32-mm head size 78 degrees, and at 36-mm 81 degrees. The increased head size had a concurrent increase of jump height of 14 mm, 16 mm, and 18 mm.[103] So increasing the head size in the face of impingement gives an extra level of security, although it may not resolve the inherent problem. Burroughs, Hallstrom, and colleagues provided a very thorough algorithm evaluating hip motion relative to head size.[104] When the head size was increased to 44 mm, virtually all component-component impingement was resolved and component-bone impingement improved significantly through a defined arc of motion.

In clinical series, as head size is increased, episodes of dislocation decrease.[9,98,105,106] This was likely due to the impingement problem noted with small heads and the head-neck diameter mismatch. Clinically, instability has also been associated with the use of lipped liners that create neck-liner impingement; however, once the head size was increased to 36 mm, no further differences were noted with larger sizes.[107-109]

It appears that with current surgical technique and frequent use of larger head sizes, instability in the primary and probably in the revision setting is on the decline. In fact, Cuckler, Lombardi, and colleagues reported on a series of 616 THA cases using 38-mm heads in which no dislocations were noted at 3 months. This was compared to a 2.5% incidence when they had used 28-mm heads.[110]

Remember that there may not be an option to use a larger head at the time of revision. If the stem is stable, the surgeon is limited to use of available head sizes. For older stems, even the modular ones, the largest size is frequently 32 mm. Stable acetabular components may also have limited liner sizes available. While one could conceivably cement in a new liner with a larger inner diameter the overall dimension of the acetabulum will dictate the size of liner that can be accommodated. In addition, as head size is increased there is a significant trade-off relative to polyethylene thickness. For revision surgery, polyethylene thickness is generally not as problematic due to the frequent use of larger cup sizes. For cases in which revision is for recurrent instability, thinner polyethylene may be accepted as a trade-off for the larger head size to meet the primary goal of improved stability.

Increasing head size increases the head-neck ratio, jump height, and functional range of motion, all of which improve hip stability. Use of a larger femoral head can contribute significantly to the success of revision hip arthroplasty for instability. It is emphasized, however, that these large head features should not be used to accommodate malpositioned components.

Tripolar Constructs

In certain cases of hip instability, a tripolar construct can be useful, with successful results in more than 90% of cases.[111-113] The so-called tripolar construct is composed of a shell (one piece polished or with a large diameter polyethylene liner) and a bipolar assembly on the femoral side. There are several advantages to this technique. First, well-fixed and appropriately positioned components do not necessarily need to be removed. Second, compared to use of a constrained device, there is less load imparted to the prosthetic interface, which minimizes risk of acetabular loosening. Third, the available range of motion prior to impingement is limited by bony and soft tissue anatomy rather than by component geometry.

A tripolar device is essentially just a different way to increase the head size, the head-neck ratio, and functional range of motion. There is an inner and an outer bearing, essentially a bipolar that articulates against a polished cup or polyethylene liner. Unlike the devices discussed previously, these are not constrained and the bipolar device can dislocate freely from the acetabulum. Examples would be the ADM (Stryker Orthopaedics), Versafitcup (Medacta, Switzerland), Novae (SERF, France), or the Avantage (Biomet). The inner bearing has motion similar to a small head and acetabulum, but the outer bearing can move. As the neck hits the outer bearing, rather than "impinging," the outer bearing moves and allows additional motion within the articulation. Early data on the ADM style device is quite positive relative to actual range of motion, jump height, and in addition, it has very good wear characteristics.[114]

The lab data on the ADM showed that the jump height was better than large head metal on metal articulations.[115] The overall range of motion was not improved due to the shallow cup shape seen in the metal on metal devices (although edge loading problems were not an issue with the ADM). Data from European trials have shown that the tripolar works well relative as a clinical solution for instability.[116-120] The bipolar head requires a proper articulation, so unless the cup or matching liner can be cemented into a stable shell, the cup cemented into place, or the head fit to a stable stem, use of these devices may be limited to cases in which the acetabulum and/or stem is revised. Remember, these large head features should not be used in place of revising malpositioned components.

Much like exchanging the polyethylene in a stable shell, if implants are available and there is adequate diameter of the indwelling shell the bearing for a tripolar device can be snapped in if modular or cemented in. If cementing the liner, use the techniques previously described. Some of the tripolar devices require a specific acetabular shell (eg, ADM, Versafitcup, Novae); generally to use these devices the old acetabular component will need to be revised.

Once the new shell is implanted or the new liner bearing fixed, the bipolar head from the tripolar construct with an outer diameter matching shell/liner is then placed on the existing femoral component. The hip is taken through a trial range of motion to assess stability as per routine.

Trochanteric Advancement

Trochanteric advancement is a useful but rarely used technique in the treatment of THA instability. Its primary indication is for dynamic abductor insufficiency. The abductors must be intact and other causes of instability, such as component positioning or impingement, must be ruled out or concomitantly addressed.[121] Abductor insufficiency secondary to stretch, offset abnormality, stem-neck design, stable stem subsidence, bone loss, and/or a high hip center may be addressed with trochanteric advancement techniques. Basically, the procedure is indicated at the time of revision if there are stable well-positioned components and a lax lever arm. Remember, this is a dynamic fix. The basic concept is to move the trochanter with its abductor attachments to more distal femoral attachment and provide dynamic tension and a stronger moment arm. The trochanteric bone is advanced with the muscle-tendon unit to provide a more stable healing unit and improved ability for fixation. The implants must be stable or they need to be revised. In addition to tightening the soft tissue envelope, the distal transfer of the trochanter reduces the likelihood of trochanteric impingement on the bony pelvis (see Figure 9-1).[121]

Trochanteric advancement is ineffective if there is significant loss of the abductors. Obviously, if there is nothing of substance to advance there can be no dynamization. It is generally very difficult to get the trochanter to heal even in the primary setting. It is even more difficult to obtain healing in the revision setting in the face of osteolysis, osteoporosis, and other conditions leading to poor bone quality. When there is significant osteolysis of the trochanter, advancement will be quite demanding, healing prohibitive, and generally it should be avoided. Larger diameter revision femoral implants and the larger shoulders of many stems may make it difficult or impossible to advance the trochanter to a position where one can obtain the bone-bone contact required for healing. In these settings the concept of a trochanteric advancement will be fraught with complications. Again trabecular metal may be used to augment the repair and to enhance healing potential.

For successful trochanteric advancement, the bone-tendon unit needs to be stabilized to allow for bone-bone healing. The stem is usually in the way, there is poor seating since the trochanter has been advanced, and there are fixation challenges. By definition, the trochanter and the abductors will be fixed under tension; usually the hip is abducted at the time of the repair to shorten the lever arm and allow more advancement and secure fixation. Unfortunately, therefore, the repair is immediately placed under tension postoperatively. It is problematic and quite common that fracture of the trochanteric fragment occurs as one tightens and completes the repair. This is especially true with osteolytic bone. It is advisable to use long trochanteric plates rather than cables, wire, or sutures to avoid cantilever stresses on the bony fragment. Strongly consider using a cable plate rather than just a cable gripper for fixation. Cable grippers also tend to crush the bone and rotate the proximal fragment anteriorly as the cables are tensioned. Crushing risks failure of the repair, and malrotation may create an impingement problem that complicates the revision for the instability. It is advisable to osteotomize a long segment of bone and broadly overlap the bony fragments. Conversely, be careful not to destabilize the stem when creating the osteotomy. Consider performing an adductor release at the time of the repair to improve the dynamics and release the tension on the abductors. Similarly, release the anterior capsule to prevent impingement and increased tension on the abductors.

Postoperative bracing, a long period of protected weightbearing, and physical therapy restrictions to protect the abductors postoperatively are strongly recommended. The bottom line is that the repair must be protected, as it is frequently tenuous even with excellent surgical technique. Since advancement is performed to resolve instability, restrictions that protect the soft tissues and allow time for maturation of scar and other secondary restraints are very important.

Indications for Bracing

Hip abduction braces are frequently used after hip dislocations or postoperatively in revision surgery. The goal is to limit hip motion in flexion and adduction. A single episode of hip dislocation in which component position (positional dislocation) does not appear outside of a safe range may be treated with bracing.[122] Braces may also be employed in the postoperative management of recurrent dislocation, especially when trochanteric osteotomy or advancement has been undertaken. Most surgeons use bracing as reinforcement, to assist patient compliance with motion restrictions, and to remind ancillary caregivers to maintain precautions. While there is no clear evidence that bracing is successful in the long term, short-term bracing has a role. Range of motion of the hip abduction orthosis should be set within the stable limit defined by a trial range of motion after closed reduction. Typical settings include a flexion limit of 60 to 90 degrees and fixed abduction of 10 to 20 degrees. One should be aware that bracing allows 10 to 20 degrees of range of motion beyond the set limits, as brace fit is primarily over a mobile soft tissue envelope. In some cases, it is desirable to control rotation as well as flexion; in these circumstances, use of an HKAFO (hip-knee-ankle-foot orthosis) is necessary.

The authors recommend bracing in cases of abductor repair and/or insufficiency, trochanteric advancement or osteotomy, use of constrained liners (particularly with freshly placed components and during the period of ingrowth), and if there are patient behavioral concerns. Bracing in no way substitutes for good implant position, will not overcome impingement, and will ultimately fail if any of the direct causes for dislocation are not resolved. While there are no real contraindications to use of a brace, it is difficult to properly fit a brace to a patient who is morbidly obese or who has a very short trunk. Braces can be irritating to the soft tissue and skin and are difficult for patients to get off and on, factors that limit compliance. When the goal is simply to limit flexion, adduction, and/or to modify patient behaviors, braces do appear helpful.

SUMMARY

When performing revision surgery for instability, the best strategy is to work through the algorithm of the etiologies and to employ a stepwise approach to the underlying problem. More often than not, a combination of factors has contributed to the instability problem and a multifaceted solution is usually required. Impingement must be avoided, stable implants must be present, and soft tissue tension should be optimized with length, offset, and trochanteric fixation or advancement when needed. Available tissue or graft material may be used for capsular repair. Larger heads should be considered for most cases. Tripolar or constrained devices offer additional options in more difficult cases but should be used on a limited basis. Bracing is useful in some cases. The surgeon and patient should be aware of the potential for recurrent dislocation, and appropriate counseling is important for informed consent as well as to aid in compliance with postoperative restrictions.

REFERENCES

1. Chandler RW, Dorr LD, Perry J. The functional cost of dislocation following total hip arthroplasty. *Clin Orthop Relat Res.* 1982;(168):168-172.
2. Berry DJ, von Knoch M, Schleck CD, Harmsen WS. The cumulative long-term risk of dislocation after primary Charnley total hip arthroplasty. *J Bone Joint Surg Am.* 2004;86-A(1):9-14.
3. Paterno SA, Lachiewicz PF, Kelley SS. The influence of patient-related factors and the position of the acetabular component on the rate of dislocation after total hip replacement. *J Bone Joint Surg Am.* 1997;79(8):1202-1210.
4. Woolson ST, Rahimtoola ZO. Risk factors for dislocation during the first 3 months after primary total hip replacement. *J Arthroplasty.* 1999;14(6):662-668.

5. Woo RY, Morrey BF. Dislocations after total hip arthroplasty. *J Bone Joint Surg Am.* 1982;64(9):1295-1306.

6. Daly PJ, Morrey BF. Operative correction of an unstable total hip arthroplasty. *J Bone Joint Surg Am.* 1992;74(9):1334-1343.

7. von Knoch M, Berry DJ, Harmsen WS, Morrey BF. Late dislocation after total hip arthroplasty. *J Bone Joint Surg Am.* 2002;84-A(11):1949-1953.

8. Della Valle CJ, Bogner E, Desai P, et al. Analysis of frozen sections of intraoperative specimens obtained at the time of reoperation after hip or knee resection arthroplasty for the treatment of infection. *J Bone Joint Surg Am.* 1999;81(5):684-689.

9. Hummel MT, Malkani AL, Yakkanti MR, Baker DL. Decreased dislocation after revision total hip arthroplasty using larger femoral head size and posterior capsular repair. *J Arthroplasty.* 2009;24(6 Suppl): 73-76.

10. White RE Jr, Forness TJ, Allman JK, Junick DW. Effect of posterior capsular repair on early dislocation in primary total hip replacement. *Clin Orthop Relat Res.* 2001;(393):163-167.

11. van Stralen GM, Struben PJ, van Loon CJ. The incidence of dislocation after primary total hip arthroplasty using posterior approach with posterior soft-tissue repair. *Arch Orthop Trauma Surg.* 2003;123(5):219-222.

12. Weeden SH, Paprosky WG, Bowling JW. The early dislocation rate in primary total hip arthroplasty following the posterior approach with posterior soft-tissue repair. *J Arthroplasty.* 2003;18(6):709-713.

13. Pellicci PM, Bostrom M, Poss R. Posterior approach to total hip replacement using enhanced posterior soft tissue repair. *Clin Orthop Relat Res.* 1998;(355):224-228.

14. Parvizi J, Kim KI, Goldberg G, Mallo G, Hozack WJ. Recurrent instability after total hip arthroplasty: beware of subtle component malpositioning. *Clin Orthop Relat Res.* 2006;447:60-65.

15. Lewinnek GE, Lewis JL, Tarr R, Compere CL, Zimmerman JR. Dislocations after total hip-replacement arthroplasties. *J Bone Joint Surg Am.* 1978;60(2):217-220.

16. Morrey BF. Instability after total hip arthroplasty. *Orthop Clin North Am.* 1992;23(2):237-248.

17. Moskal JT, Capps SG. Improving the accuracy of acetabular component orientation: avoiding malposition. *J Am Acad Orthop Surg.* 2010;18(5):286-296.

18. Dorr LD, Wan Z, Malik A, Zhu J, Dastane M, Deshmane P. A comparison of surgeon estimation and computed tomographic measurement of femoral component anteversion in cementless total hip arthroplasty. *J Bone Joint Surg Am.* 2009;91(11):2598-2604.

19. Barsoum WK, Patterson RW, Higuera C, Klika AK, Krebs VE, Molloy R. A computer model of the position of the combined component in the prevention of impingement in total hip replacement. *J Bone Joint Surg Br.* 2007;89(6):839-845.

20. Dorr LD, Malik A, Dastane M, Wan Z. Combined anteversion technique for total hip arthroplasty. *Clin Orthop Relat Res.* 2009;467(1):119-127.

21. Amuwa C, Dorr LD. The combined anteversion technique for acetabular component anteversion. *J Arthroplasty.* 2008;23(7):1068-1070.

22. Murtha PE, Hafez MA, Jaramaz B, DiGioia AM 3rd. Variations in acetabular anatomy with reference to total hip replacement. *J Bone Joint Surg Br.* 2008;90(3):308-313.

23. Kalteis TA, Handel M, Herbst B, Grifka J, Renkawitz T. In vitro investigation of the influence of pelvic tilt on acetabular cup alignment. *J Arthroplasty.* 2009;24(1):152-157.

24. Babisch JW, Layher F, Amiot LP. The rationale for tilt-adjusted acetabular cup navigation. *J Bone Joint Surg Am.* 2008;90(2):357-365.

25. Zhu J, Wan Z, Dorr LD. Quantification of pelvic tilt in total hip arthroplasty. *Clin Orthop Relat Res.* 2010;468(2):571-575.

26. Kessler O, Patil S, Wirth S, Mayr E, Colwell CW Jr, D'Lima DD. Bony impingement affects range of motion after total hip arthroplasty: a subject-specific approach. *J Orthop Res.* 2008;26(4):443-452.

27. Haaker RG, Tiedjen K, Ottersbach A, Rubenthaler F, Stockheim M, Stiehl JB. Comparison of conventional versus computer-navigated acetabular component insertion. *J Arthroplasty.* 2007;22(2):151-159.

28. Toomey SD, Hopper RH Jr, McAuley JP, Engh CA. Modular component exchange for treatment of recurrent dislocation of a total hip replacement in selected patients. *J Bone Joint Surg Am.* 2001;83-A(10): 1529-1533.

29. Patel AB, Wagle RR, Usrey MM, Thompson MT, Incavo SJ, Noble PC. Guidelines for implant placement to minimize impingement during activities of daily living after total hip arthroplasty. *J Arthroplasty.* 2010;25(8):1275-1281.

30. Johnston RC, Brand RA, Crowninshield RD. Reconstruction of the hip. A mathematical approach to determine optimum geometric relationships. *J Bone Joint Surg Am.* 1979;61(5):639-652.

31. Fackler CD, Poss R. Dislocation in total hip arthroplasties. *Clin Orthop Relat Res.* 1980;(151):169-178.

32. Barrack RL, Burnett RS. Preoperative planning for revision total hip arthroplasty. *Instr Course Lect.* 2006;55:233-244.

33. Ritter MA. Dislocation and subluxation of the total hip replacement. *Clin Orthop Relat Res.* 1976;(121): 92-94.

34. Maloney WJ, Paprosky W, Engh CA, Rubash H. Surgical treatment of pelvic osteolysis. *Clin Orthop Relat Res.* 2001;(393):78-84.

35. Callaghan JJ, Liu SS, Schularick NM. Shell retention with a cemented acetabular liner. *Orthopedics.* 2009;32(9):pii.

36. Haft GF, Heiner AD, Callaghan JJ, et al. Polyethylene liner cementation into fixed acetabular shells. *J Arthroplasty.* 2002;17(4 Suppl 1):167-170.

37. Springer BD, Hanssen AD, Lewallen DG. Cementation of an acetabular liner into a well-fixed acetabular shell during revision total hip arthroplasty. *J Arthroplasty.* 2003;18(7 Suppl 1):126-130.

38. Mauerhan DR, Peindl RD, Coley ER, Marshall A. Cementation of polyethylene liners into well-fixed metal shells at the time of revision total hip arthroplasty. *J Arthroplasty.* 2008;23(6):873-878.

39. Blom AW, Astle L, Loveridge J, Learmonth ID. Revision of an acetabular liner has a high risk of dislocation. *J Bone Joint Surg Br.* 2005;87(12):1636-1638.

40. Haft GF, Heiner AD, Dorr LD, Brown TD, Callaghan JJ. A biomechanical analysis of polyethylene liner cementation into a fixed metal acetabular shell. *J Bone Joint Surg Am.* 2003;85-A(6):1100-1110.

41. Kusaba A, Kuroki Y. Wear of bipolar hip prostheses. *J Arthroplasty.* 1998;13(6):668-673.

42. Kim KJ, Rubash HE. Large amounts of polyethylene debris in the interface tissue surrounding bipolar endoprostheses. Comparison to total hip prostheses. *J Arthroplasty.* 1997;12(1):32-39.

43. Leung S, Naudie D, Kitamura N, Walde T, Engh CA. Computed tomography in the assessment of periacetabular osteolysis. *J Bone Joint Surg Am.* 2005;87(3):592-597.

44. Claus AM, Totterman SM, Sychterz CJ, Tamez-Pena JG, Looney RJ, Engh CA Sr. Computed tomography to assess pelvic lysis after total hip replacement. *Clin Orthop Relat Res.* 2004;(422):167-174.

45. Puri L, Wixson RL, Stern SH, Kohli J, Hendrix RW, Stulberg SD. Use of helical computed tomography for the assessment of acetabular osteolysis after total hip arthroplasty. *J Bone Joint Surg Am.* 2002;84-A(4): 609-614.

46. Widmer KH. A simplified method to determine acetabular cup anteversion from plain radiographs. *J Arthroplasty.* 2004;19(3):387-390.

47. Liaw CK, Hou SM, Yang RS, Wu TY, Fuh CS. A new tool for measuring cup orientation in total hip arthroplasties from plain radiographs. *Clin Orthop Relat Res.* 2006;451:134-139.

48. Pradhan R. Planar anteversion of the acetabular cup as determined from plain anteroposterior radiographs. *J Bone Joint Surg Br.* 1999;81(3):431-435.

49. Markel DC, Andary JL, Pagano P, Nasser S. Assessment of acetabular version by plain radiograph. *Am J Orthop (Belle Mead NJ).* 2007;36(1):39-41.

50. Stem ES, O'Connor MI, Kransdorf MJ, Crook J. Computed tomography analysis of acetabular anteversion and abduction. *Skeletal Radiol.* 2006;35(6):385-389.

51. Wines AP, McNicol D. Computed tomography measurement of the accuracy of component version in total hip arthroplasty. *J Arthroplasty.* 2006;21(5):696-701.

52. DeLee JG, Charnley J. Radiological demarcation of cemented sockets in total hip replacement. *Clin Orthop Relat Res.* 1976;(121):20-32.

53. Carlsson AS, Gentz CF. Radiographic versus clinical loosening of the acetabular component in noninfected total hip arthroplasty. *Clin Orthop Relat Res.* 1984;(185):145-150.

54. O'Neill DA, Harris WH. Failed total hip replacement: assessment by plain radiographs, arthrograms, and aspiration of the hip joint. *J Bone Joint Surg Am.* 1984;66(4):540-546.

55. Stauffer RN. Ten-year follow-up study of total hip replacement. *J Bone Joint Surg Am.* 1982;64(7):983-990.

56. Harris WH, McGann WA. Loosening of the femoral component after use of the medullary-plug cementing technique. Follow-up note with a minimum five-year follow-up. *J Bone Joint Surg Am.* 1986;68(7):1064-1066.

57. Williamson BR, McLaughlin RE, Wang GW, Miller CW, Teates CD, Bray ST. Radionuclide bone imaging as a means of differentiating loosening and infection in patients with a painful total hip prosthesis. *Radiology.* 1979;133(3 Pt 1):723-725.

58. Temmerman OP, Raijmakers PG, Berkhof J, Hoekstra OS, Teule GJ, Heyligers IC. Accuracy of diagnostic imaging techniques in the diagnosis of aseptic loosening of the femoral component of a hip prosthesis: a meta-analysis. *J Bone Joint Surg Br.* 2005;87(6):781-785.

59. Gruen TA, McNeice GM, Amstutz HC. "Modes of failure" of cemented stem-type femoral components: a radiographic analysis of loosening. *Clin Orthop Relat Res.* 1979;(141):17-27.

60. Amstutz HC, Ma SM, Jinnah RH, Mai L. Revision of aseptic loose total hip arthroplasties. *Clin Orthop Relat Res.* 1982;(170):21-33.

61. Berger RA, Quigley LR, Jacobs JJ, Sheinkop MB, Rosenberg AG, Galante JO. The fate of stable cemented acetabular components retained during revision of a femoral component of a total hip arthroplasty. *J Bone Joint Surg Am*. 1999;81(12):1682-1691.

62. Hamlin BR, Rowland C, Morrey BF. Retention of all-polyethylene acetabular components after femoral revision of a cemented total hip replacement. *J Bone Joint Surg Am*. 2001;83-A(11):1700-1705.

63. Beaule PE, Schmalzried TP, Udomkiat P, Amstutz HC. Jumbo femoral head for the treatment of recurrent dislocation following total hip replacement. *J Bone Joint Surg Am*. 2002;84-A(2):256-263.

64. Amstutz HC, Le Duff MJ, Beaule PE. Prevention and treatment of dislocation after total hip replacement using large diameter balls. *Clin Orthop Relat Res*. 2004;(429):108-116.

65. Matta JM, Siebenrock KA. Does indomethacin reduce heterotopic bone formation after operations for acetabular fractures? A prospective randomised study. *J Bone Joint Surg Br*. 1997;79(6):959-963.

66. Vavken P, Castellani L, Sculco TP. Prophylaxis of heterotopic ossification of the hip: systematic review and meta-analysis. *Clin Orthop Relat Res*. 2009;467(12):3283-3289.

67. Fransen M, Neal B. Non-steroidal anti-inflammatory drugs for preventing heterotopic bone formation after hip arthroplasty. *Cochrane Database Syst Rev*. 2004(3):CD001160.

68. Iorio R, Healy WL. Heterotopic ossification after hip and knee arthroplasty: risk factors, prevention, and treatment. *J Am Acad Orthop Surg*. 2002;10(6):409-416.

69. Bugbee WD, Culpepper WJ 2nd, Engh CA Jr, Engh CA Sr. Long-term clinical consequences of stress-shielding after total hip arthroplasty without cement. *J Bone Joint Surg Am*. 1997;79(7):1007-1012.

70. Yun AG. Sports after total hip replacement. *Clin Sports Med*. 2006;25(2):359-364, xi.

71. McGrory BJ. Periprosthetic fracture of the femur after total hip arthroplasty occurring in winter activities: report of two cases. *J Surg Orthop Adv*. 2004;13(2):119-123.

72. Sanchez-Sotelo J, Haidukewych GJ, Boberg CJ. Hospital cost of dislocation after primary total hip arthroplasty. *J Bone Joint Surg Am*. 2006;88(2):290-294.

73. Flint JH, Phisitkul P, Callaghan JJ. Closed reduction of a dislocated constrained total hip arthroplasty using a novel technique with a peg board. *Orthopedics*. 2010;10:201-203.

74. Harman MK, Hodge WA, Banks SA. Closed reduction of constrained total hip arthroplasty. *Clin Orthop Relat Res*. 2003;(414):121-128.

75. Miller CW, Zura RD. Closed reduction of a dislocation of a constrained acetabular component. *J Arthroplasty*. 2001;16(4):504-505.

76. McPherson EJ, Costigan WM, Gerhardt MB, Norris LR. Closed reduction of dislocated total hip with S-ROM constrained acetabular component. *J Arthroplasty*. 1999;14(7):882-885.

77. Birdwell S, Wilke E. Closed reduction of constrained total hip arthroplasty in the ED. *J Emerg Med*. 2011;40(2):162-166.

78. Fricka KB, Marshall A, Paprosky WG. Constrained liners in revision total hip arthroplasty: an overuse syndrome: in the affirmative. *J Arthroplasty*. 2006;21(4 Suppl 1):121-125.

79. McCarthy JC, Lee JA. Constrained acetabular components in complex revision total hip arthroplasty. *Clin Orthop Relat Res*. 2005;(441):210-215.

80. Berend KR, Lombardi AV Jr, Mallory TH, Adams JB, Russell JH, Groseth KL. The long-term outcome of 755 consecutive constrained acetabular components in total hip arthroplasty examining the successes and failures. *J Arthroplasty*. 2005;20(7 Suppl 3):93-102.

81. Etienne G, Ragland PS, Mont MA. Use of constrained acetabular liners in total hip arthroplasty. *Orthopedics*. 2005;28(5):463-469; quiz 470-461.

82. Callaghan JJ, O'Rourke MR, Goetz DD, Lewallen DG, Johnston RC, Capello WN. Use of a constrained tripolar acetabular liner to treat intraoperative instability and postoperative dislocation after total hip arthroplasty: a review of our experience. *Clin Orthop Relat Res*. 2004;(429):117-123.

83. Goetz DD, Bremner BR, Callaghan JJ, Capello WN, Johnston RC. Salvage of a recurrently dislocating total hip prosthesis with use of a constrained acetabular component. A concise follow-up of a previous report. *J Bone Joint Surg Am*. 2004;86-A(11):2419-2423.

84. Callaghan JJ, Parvizi J, Novak CC, et al. A constrained liner cemented into a secure cementless acetabular shell. *J Bone Joint Surg Am*. 2004;86-A(10):2206-2211.

85. Su EP, Pellicci PM. The role of constrained liners in total hip arthroplasty. *Clin Orthop Relat Res*. 2004;(420):122-129.

86. Shrader MW, Parvizi J, Lewallen DG. The use of a constrained acetabular component to treat instability after total hip arthroplasty. *J Bone Joint Surg Am*. 2003;85-A(11):2179-2183.

87. Bremner BR, Goetz DD, Callaghan JJ, Capello WN, Johnston RC. Use of constrained acetabular components for hip instability: an average 10-year follow-up study. *J Arthroplasty*. 2003;18(7 Suppl 1):131-137.

88. Shapiro GS, Weiland DE, Markel DC, Padgett DE, Sculco TP, Pellicci PM. The use of a constrained acetabular component for recurrent dislocation. *J Arthroplasty.* 2003;18(3):250-258.

89. Burroughs BR, Golladay GJ, Hallstrom B, Harris WH. A novel constrained acetabular liner design with increased range of motion. *J Arthroplasty.* 2001;16(8 Suppl 1):31-36.

90. Goetz DD, Capello WN, Callaghan JJ, Brown TD, Johnston RC. Salvage of total hip instability with a constrained acetabular component. *Clin Orthop Relat Res.* 1998;(355):171-181.

91. Goetz DD, Capello WN, Callaghan JJ, Brown TD, Johnston RC. Salvage of a recurrently dislocating total hip prosthesis with use of a constrained acetabular component. A retrospective analysis of fifty-six cases. *J Bone Joint Surg Am.* 1998;80(4):502-509.

92. Anderson MJ, Murray WR, Skinner HB. Constrained acetabular components. *J Arthroplasty.* 1994;9(1):17-23.

93. Khoury JI, Malkani AL, Adler EM, Markel DC. Constrained acetabular liners cemented into cages during total hip revision arthroplasty. *J Arthroplasty.* 2010;25(6):901-905.

94. Klein GR, Rapuri V, Hozack WJ, Parvizi J, Purtill JJ. Caution on the use of combined constrained liners and cages in revision total hip arthroplasty. *Orthopedics.* 2007;30(11):970-971.

95. Cooke CC, Hozack W, Lavernia C, Sharkey P, Shastri S, Rothman RH. Early failure mechanisms of constrained tripolar acetabular sockets used in revision total hip arthroplasty. *J Arthroplasty.* 2003;18(7):827-833.

96. Paprosky WG, Sporer SS, Murphy BP. Addressing severe bone deficiency: what a cage will not do. *J Arthroplasty.* 2007;22(4 Suppl 1):111-115.

97. Sporer SM, Paprosky WG, O'Rourke MR. Managing bone loss in acetabular revision. *Instr Course Lect.* 2006;55:287-297.

98. Padgett DE, Lipman J, Robie B, Nestor BJ. Influence of total hip design on dislocation: a computer model and clinical analysis. *Clin Orthop Relat Res.* 2006;447:48-52.

99. D'Lima DD, Chen PC, Colwell CW Jr. Optimizing acetabular component position to minimize impingement and reduce contact stress. *J Bone Joint Surg Am.* 2001;83-A(Suppl 2 Pt 2):87-91.

100. Malik A, Maheshwari A, Dorr LD. Impingement with total hip replacement. *J Bone Joint Surg Am.* 2007;89(8):1832-1842.

101. Charles MN, Bourne RB, Davey JR, Greenwald AS, Morrey BF, Rorabeck CH. Soft-tissue balancing of the hip: the role of femoral offset restoration. *Instr Course Lect.* 2005;54:131-141.

102. Barrack RL, Butler RA, Laster DR, Andrews P. Stem design and dislocation after revision total hip arthroplasty: clinical results and computer modeling. *J Arthroplasty.* 2001;16(8 Suppl 1):8-12.

103. Yamaguchi M, Akisue T, Bauer TW, Hashimoto Y. The spatial location of impingement in total hip arthroplasty. *J Arthroplasty.* 2000;15(3):305-313.

104. Burroughs BR, Hallstrom B, Golladay GJ, Hoeffel D, Harris WH. Range of motion and stability in total hip arthroplasty with 28-, 32-, 38-, and 44-mm femoral head sizes. *J Arthroplasty.* 2005;20(1):11-19.

105. Shon WY, Baldini T, Peterson MG, Wright TM, Salvati EA. Impingement in total hip arthroplasty: a study of retrieved acetabular components. *J Arthroplasty.* 2005;20(4):427-435.

106. Bartz RL, Nobel PC, Kadakia NR, Tullos HS. The effect of femoral component head size on posterior dislocation of the artificial hip joint. *J Bone Joint Surg Am.* 2000;82(9):1300-1307.

107. Hall RM, Siney P, Unsworth A, Wroblewski BM. Prevalence of impingement in explanted Charnley acetabular components. *J Orthop Sci.* 1998;3(4):204-208.

108. Hedlundh U, Ahnfelt L, Hybbinette CH, Wallinder L, Weckstrom J, Fredin H. Dislocations and the femoral head size in primary total hip arthroplasty. *Clin Orthop Relat Res.* 1996;(333):226-233.

109. Peters CL, McPherson E, Jackson JD, Erickson JA. Reduction in early dislocation rate with large-diameter femoral heads in primary total hip arthroplasty. *J Arthroplasty.* 2007;22(6 Suppl 2):140-144.

110. Cuckler JM, Moore KD, Lombardi AV Jr, McPherson E, Emerson R. Large versus small femoral heads in metal-on-metal total hip arthroplasty. *J Arthroplasty.* 2004;19(8 Suppl 3):41-44.

111. Grigoris P, Grecula MJ, Amstutz HC. Tripolar hip replacement for recurrent prosthetic dislocation. *Clin Orthop Relat Res.* 1994;(304):148-155.

112. Levine BR, Della Valle CJ, Deirmengian CA, et al. The use of a tripolar articulation in revision total hip arthroplasty: a minimum of 24 months' follow-up. *J Arthroplasty.* 2008;23(8):1182-1188.

113. Beaule PE, Roussignol X, Schmalzried TP, Udomkiat P, Amstutz HC, Dujardin FH. [Tripolar arthroplasty for recurrent total hip prosthesis dislocation]. *Rev Chir Orthop Reparatrice Appar Mot.* 2003;89(3):242-249.

114. Dong N, Nevelos J, Thakore M, Wang A, Manley M, Morris H. Dislocation potential in conventional and dual mobility hip joint couples. Poster presented at: 56th Annual Meeting of the Orthopaedic Research Society 2010; New Orleans, LA.

115. Nevelos J, Bhimji S, Dong N, MacIntyre J, Coustance A, Mont M. Acetabular bearing design has a greater influence on jump distance than head diameter. Poster presented at: 56th Annual Meeting of the Orthopaedic Research Society 2010; New Orleans, LA.

116. Hamadouche M, Biau DJ, Huten D, Musset T, Gaucher F. The use of a cemented dual mobility socket to treat recurrent dislocation. *Clin Orthop Relat Res.* 2010;468(12):3248-3254.

117. Massin P, Besnier L. Acetabular revision using a press-fit dual mobility cup. *Orthop Traumatol Surg Res.* 2010;96(1):9-13.

118. Philippot R, Adam P, Reckhaus M, et al. Prevention of dislocation in total hip revision surgery using a dual mobility design. *Orthop Traumatol Surg Res.* 2009;95(6):407-413.

119. Langlais FL, Ropars M, Gaucher F, Musset T, Chaix O. Dual mobility cemented cups have low dislocation rates in THA revisions. *Clin Orthop Relat Res.* 2008;466(2):389-395.

120. Philippot R, Camilleri JP, Boyer B, Adam P, Farizon F. The use of a dual-articulation acetabular cup system to prevent dislocation after primary total hip arthroplasty: analysis of 384 cases at a mean follow-up of 15 years. *Int Orthop.* 2009;33(4):927-932.

121. Dennis DA, Lynch CB. Trochanteric osteotomy and advancement: a technique for abductor related hip instability. *Orthopedics.* 2004;27(9):959-961.

122. Dorr LD, Wolf AW, Chandler R, Conaty JP. Classification and treatment of dislocations of total hip arthroplasty. *Clin Orthop Relat Res.* 1983;(173):151-158.

Management of Infection in Total Hip Arthroplasty
Fundamentals of Hip Arthroplasty

Bryan D. Springer, MD; Raymond H. Kim, MD; and Douglas A. Dennis, MD

INTRODUCTION AND INCIDENCE OF INFECTION

Total hip arthroplasty (THA) is one of the most successful operations in orthopedic surgery with dramatic functional improvement and excellent reported long-term survivorship.[1-3] Improvements in methods of fixation and bearing surfaces have expanded the indications to include younger and more active patients. Projections indicate that by the year 2030, the demand for primary THA and revision THA will increase by 174% and 137%, respectively.[4]

Infection after THA remains one of the most dreaded and difficult complications to treat. The incidence of infection ranges between 1% and 2% for primary THA and 2% to 4% for revision THA.[5-7] Despite improvements in infection control protocols and standardization of antibiotic regimes, between 1990 and 2004, a nearly 2-fold increase was observed in the incidence of infection for both hip and knee arthroplasties in the United States.[8] In 69,663 Medicare patients undergoing elective total knee arthroplasty, 1400 total knee arthroplasty infections were identified. Infection incidence within 2 years was 1.55%. The incidence between 2 and up to 10 years was 0.46%.[9] The economic impact of treating a patient with an infection after total hip replacement is staggering. It is associated with extremely high costs, ranging from $60,000 to well over $100,000 dollars per episode, longer hospital stays, and a higher complication rate.[10,11] Managing a patient with an infected total joint arthroplasty is among the most resource consumptive procedures in all of orthopedic surgery.

This chapter will focus on the risk factors and prevention of infection in patients undergoing THA as well as the diagnosis and treatment of the patient with an infected THA. It is important to develop a rational algorithmic approach to the patient with an infected THA. This includes a thorough clinical history and exam, laboratory evaluation, radiographic assessment, and formulation of a treatment plan. Due to the complexity of these patients, a team approach is favored and should involve not only the orthopedic surgeon, but also an infectious disease specialist with experience in the management of orthopedic hardware infections. The most recent data would indicate that the majority of patients with infection following THA are being referred for treatment to urban tertiary treatment centers.[10]

Jacofsky DJ, Hedley AK.
Fundamentals of Revision Hip Arthroplasty:
Diagnosis, Evaluation, and Treatment (pp 143-158).
© 2013 SLACK Incorporated.

TABLE 10-1. RISK FACTORS FOR INFECTION IN PATIENTS UNDERGOING TOTAL JOINT ARTHROPLASTY

- Rheumatoid arthritis
- Homologous blood
- Duration of hospitalization
- Superficial wound infection
- Wound drainage
- Wound hematoma
- Wound dehiscence
- Decubitus ulcers
- >4 hospital stays prior to total joint replacement
- Steroid therapy
- Diabetes mellitus
- Prior septic arthritis
- Prior arthroplasty
- Malignancy
- Lymphocytes <1.5 x 109

RISK FACTORS AND PREVENTION OF INFECTION

Because of the devastating effects that infection can have on a patients following THA, the hallmark of treatment is prevention. Prevention begins with identifying those patients that are at increased risk for the development of deep periprosthetic infection prior to undergoing surgery. Risk factors can be categorized into those that are controllable or modifiable and those that are not modifiable. Table 10-1 lists the risk factors that have been shown to place patients at increased risk for infection following total joint arthroplasty.

Nonmodifiable risk factors include those patients with a prior history of infection or sepsis, immune deficiency, inflammatory arthropathy, such as rheumatoid arthritis and lupus, and prior malignancy. It is important that these patients are counseled regarding the increasing risk of periprosthetic infection following THA, and every effort should be made to improve the modifiable risk factors prior to surgery. Although no specific guidelines exist, it is generally recommended that patients discontinue immunosuppressants prior to surgery and restart them after wound healing has occurred postoperatively (4 to 6 weeks). Patients with a prior history of institutionalization and carriers of methicillin-resistant *Staphylococcus aureus* (MRSA) have been shown to be at increased risk for development of deep periprosthetic infection.[12,13] Screening protocols and decolonizations regimes exist to identify and treat these patients prior to surgery.[14,15] Several studies have evaluated the efficacy of these protocols and have shown a reduction in the incidence of periprosthetic infection.[15] The routine use and screening of all patients prior to total joint arthroplasty, however, remains controversial. Additionally, 2 of the most commonly encountered modifiable risk factors are obesity and diabetes mellitus.

Obesity has reached epidemic proportions in the United States. Over one-third of the US population is considered obese (body mass index [BMI] >30).[16] Obesity has been shown to be a risk factor for the development of osteoarthritis, and these patients frequently require total joint arthroplasty. Several studies have shown that obese patients have as good of an outcome and comparable survivorship to a normal weight cohort of patients undergoing total joint arthroplasty.[17-19] However, obesity does increase the patient's risk for perioperative morbidity and surgery. To perform total joint arthroplasty on these patients is often more technically challenging.

Despite successful overall outcomes in terms of survivorship, several studies document an overwhelmingly increased risk for deep periprosthetic infection in obese patients. Choong et al reported that patients with BMI greater than 30 (obese) and 2 additional comorbidities were at elevated risk for infection.[20] Recently, Malinzak et al demonstrated a staggering 18-fold increase in deep infection in patients with a BMI >50 (super obese).[21] With these data, it is difficult to justify total joint arthroplasty in this patient population. Patients must understand that their weight can directly influence the outcome of infection, and steps should be taken to maximize weight loss prior to surgery. Additionally, because most studies show that patients do not lose weight following total joint arthroplasty, weight reduction should take place prior to surgery.[22,23]

The number of patients diagnosed with diabetes mellitus is expected to increase and so too will the number of patients with diabetes that will require total joint arthroplasty. Currently, approximately 8% of patients undergoing total joint arthroplasty in the United States have diabetes.[24] Patients with poor glycemic control (HGB A1c >7) have been shown to be at increased risk for perioperative morbidity and mortality following total joint arthroplasty.[25] Compared to a cohort with well-controlled diabetes or no diabetes, the poorly controlled group had higher odds of stroke, urinary tract infection, transfusion requirements, wound infection, and death. Malinzak et al demonstrated that diabetic patients were 3 times more likely to become infected than non-diabetic patients.[21] It is important that the surgeon work with the patient and his or her medical doctors or endocrinologist to ensure adequate glycemic control is obtained both preoperatively and in the postoperative period.

In addition to the aforementioned patient risk factors, there are several factors that are under the control of the surgeon and hospital that must be considered. These include the appropriate use of prophylactic antibiotics and the operating room environment. Current antibiotic prophylaxis guidelines recommend a single dose of a first-generation cephalosporin (cefazolin or cefuroxime) within 1 hour of surgical incision. Patients with a true allergy to these antibiotics should be given an alternative, such as clindamycin or vancomycin. Patients with a history of MRSA or those at high risk (immunocompromised patients, patients who reside in skilled care facilities, etc) should be dosed with vancomycin within 2 hours of surgical incision due to its slower infusion rate. Postoperatively, antibiotics should be continued for 24 hours after surgery. Table 10-2 lists the AAOS recommendations for the use of intravenous antibiotic prophylaxis in primary total joint arthroplasty.[26]

Infection after THA may be directly related to operating room contamination. It must be realized that the operating room personnel are a major source of the bacteria. This has been proven, as evidenced by the documented increase in bacterial colony-forming units per square foot per hour from 13 units in an empty operating room to greater than 400 units during actual surgery.[27] Longer operative time and increased traffic from operating room personnel increase the risk for the development of periprosthetic infection. Therefore, to reduce environmental bacteria contamination, the number of personnel in the operating room, traffic, and the length of time for the actual surgery should be reduced, because wound contamination occurs first by direct fall out from the environment and second by contaminated equipment and gloved hands that initially were contaminated by the environment.

Environmental control in the operating room, such as the use of laminar air flow, body exhaust suits, and ultraviolet lights, can be helpful in reducing infection. Laminar airflow or ultraviolet light have shown greater than 90% reduction of airborne bacteria at the wound and 60% reduction of airborne bacteria in the operating room.[28] Over a 19-year period, Ritter et al showed a 3.1 times higher rate of infection for total hip and knee arthroplasty when the surgery was performed without the use of ultraviolet light.[28] Additionally, controversy exists regarding the optimum skin preparation to be used prior to surgery, with chlorhexadine alcohol and providone-iodine skin solutions being the most common. Darouiche et al reported on a prospective randomize trial of 849 subjects (409 in the chlorhexidine-alcohol group and 440 in the povidone-iodine group) qualified for the intention-to-treat analysis. The overall rate of surgical site infection was

---

TABLE 10-2. AMERICAN ACADEMY OF ORTHOPAEDIC SURGEONS RECOMMENDATIONS FOR THE USE OF INTRAVENOUS ANTIBIOTIC PROPHYLAXIS IN PRIMARY TOTAL JOINT ARTHROPLASTY

RECOMMENDATION 1

- The antibiotic used for prophylaxis should be carefully selected and consistent with current recommendations in the literature, taking into account the issues of resistance and patient allergies.
- Currently, cefazolin and cefuroxime are the preferred antibiotics for patients undergoing orthopedic procedures. Clindamycin or vancomycin may be used for patients with a confirmed beta-lactam allergy.
- Vancomycin may be used in patients with known colonization with methicillin-resistant Staphylococcus aureus (MRSA) or in facilities with recent MRSA outbreaks. In multiple studies, exposure to vancomycin is reported as a risk factor in the development of vancomycin-resistant enterococcus colonization and infection. Therefore, vancomycin should be reserved for the treatment of serious infection with beta-lactam–resistant organisms or for the treatment of infection in patients with life-threatening allergy to beta-lactam antimicrobials.

RECOMMENDATION 2

- Timing and dosage of antibiotic administration should optimize the efficacy of the therapy.
- Prophylactic antibiotics should be administered within 1 hour before skin incision. Due to an extended infusion time, vancomycin should be started within 2 hours before incision. When a proximal tourniquet is used, the antibiotic must be completely infused before inflation of the tourniquet. Dose amount should be proportional to patient weight; for patients more than 80 kg, the doses of cefazolin should be doubled. Additional intraoperative doses of antibiotic are advised when the duration of the procedure exceeds 1 to 2 times the antibiotic's half-life or when there is significant blood loss during the procedure. The general guidelines for frequency of intraoperative antibiotic administration are as follows: cefazolin every 2 to 5 hours, cefuroxime every 3 to 4 hours, clindamycin every 3 to 6 hours, vancomycin every 6 to 12 hours.

RECOMMENDATION 3

- Duration of prophylactic antibiotic administration should not exceed the 24-hour postoperative period.
- Prophylactic antibiotics should be discontinued within 24 hours of the end of surgery. The medical literature does not support the continuation of antibiotics until all drains or catheters are removed, and provides no evidence of benefit when they are continued past 24 hours.

Recommendations available at: http://www.aaos.org/about/papers/advistmt/1027.asp

significantly lower in the chlorhexidine-alcohol group than in the povidone-iodine group (9.5% versus 16.1%; P = 0.004; relative risk, 0.59; 95% confidence interval, 0.41 to 0.85). Chlorhexidine-alcohol was significantly more protective than povidone-iodine against both superficial incisional infections (4.2% versus 8.6%, P = 0.008) and deep incisional infections (1% versus 3%, P = 0.05).[29]

DIAGNOSIS OF INFECTION

There are several tools that can be utilized to assist in the diagnosis of a patient with a suspected infected THA. These include plain radiographs, laboratory tests, joint aspiration, advanced imaging techniques, and intraoperative testing. A thorough clinical history and physical exam, however, are the mainstay in the initial evaluation. As a general rule every patient with a painful THA should be suspected as having an infection until proven otherwise.

It is important to ascertain in the clinical history the location of the pain. Patients may often present with other sources of referred pain to the hip, particularly the lumbar spine. If concern arises, it is important to investigate these possible sources of referred pain. The timing of onset of the patient's pain is important. Has it been persistent since surgery or did he or she have a pain-free interval? Patients that have had pain since the time of surgery or no relief of pain with the surgery may indicate an infection that developed early or pathology other than the hip as a source of pain. Late development of pain, with a pain-free interval, may indicate a late acute hematogenous infection. It is also important to ascertain whether or not they had any wound healing issues or drainage problems at the time of the initial surgery. Did they return to the operating room for any additional procedure on the hip? Were they ever placed on antibiotics for a suspected infection and have they undergone any procedures that would have caused a bacteremic episode, such as dental work, colonoscopy, or urologic procedures without appropriate antibiotic prophylaxis?

A description of the severity and the character of the pain can be helpful. Patients with infection often have pain at rest and at night in addition to activity-related pain. If the infection is deep, patients may not notice any warmth or redness around the joint, and contrary to patients' popular belief, they often do not feel sick as a result of prosthetic infection. Any suspicion for infection on the history or clinical exam should warrant a full evaluation.

Plain radiographs may provide useful information in the diagnosis of infection. Most importantly, obtaining initial x-rays and comparing them to the most recent will provide the most help. Early loosening of the prosthesis or failure of ingrowth may be attributed to infection. Plain radiographs in the setting of infection may show periosteal lamination, subchondral bony resorption, progressive radiolucencies or localized osteolysis. It is important to remember, however, that bony destruction may not be seen until up to 3 weeks after the start of an infection, and lytic lesions are typically only seen after there has been 30% to 50% loss of bone.

Hematologic tests include systemic white blood cell count, erythrocyte sedimentation rate (ESR), C-reactive protein (CRP), and more recently, interleukin-6 (IL-6). No one test is 100% specific or sensitive for infection. These tests generally have a high sensitivity and a low specificity, making them good screening tests rather than accurate predictors of infection.[30-32] Therefore, while a negative result may lower the suspicion for infection it should not preclude good sound clinical judgment. In addition, positive inflammatory markers should not be used as the sole criteria for the diagnosis and treatment of infection after THA, but should prompt the surgeon to use additional, more specific tests to make the diagnosis.

The systemic white blood cell count is not a reliable indicator in the face of infected total joint arthroplasty. Studies have shown that up to 70% of patients with infection may have a normal white blood cell count.[33,34] The ESR generally peaks 5 to 7 days after surgery and will return to normal slowly in about 3 months. The CRP rises within 6 hours of surgery, generally peaks in 2 to 3 days, and will return to normal by 3 weeks. Neither of these tests alone is sufficient to make a diagnosis of infection with a specificity of only 56%.[35] Both tests, however, when used in combination, can accurately rule out the presence of infection with a sensitivity of 96% and a negative predictive value of 95%. It is important to remember that other systemic inflammatory conditions, such as rheumatoid arthritis and lupus, may cause an elevated ESR and CRP. In these patients, a high index of suspicion and the liberal use of joint aspiration is important to evaluate these patients for suspected infection.

Serum IL-6 has recently gained popularity. It generally peaks within 6 hours of surgery, but can return to normal in 72 hours after surgery and has been shown to have a sensitivity of 100% and a specificity of 95%.[36] Because of its more rapid return to normal, it may be more useful as a tool to follow a patient's response to treatment for infection. It is not readily available in all clinical settings, however.

Radionucleotide scanning may be useful in assisting with the diagnosis of infection particularly in equivocal cases. These tests, however, are expensive, cumbersome for the patients, and suffer from a lack of specificity for the diagnosis of infection. A technetium-labeled scan is a measure of osteoblastic activity, and while it may be positive in the presence of infection, there are also several other factors that may result in a positive result including trauma, stress fracture, degenerative joint disease, and tumor. Most importantly, these scans may stay positive for up to 12 months following surgery, and even longer at the tip of the trochanter, tip of the stem, and the acetabulum.[37] They have a sensitivity and a positive predictive value in the range of 30% to 38%.[38,39] An indium-labeled leukocyte scan accumulates in areas of white blood cells in an area of interest. It has been shown to have a sensitivity of 77% and a specificity of 86%.[40] Combining these 2 techniques will improve the specificity and is generally recommended when using radionucleotide scanning to combine these tests to improve their specificity.[41] The addition of a sulfur colloid marrow scan to these test has shown improved accuracy in the diagnosis of infection. Palestro et al demonstrated the accuracy of combined labeled leukocyte and sulfur colloid marrow imaging (95%) was higher than that of labeled leukocyte scintigraphy alone (78%), bone scintigraphy alone (74%), or combined labeled leukocyte and bone scintigraphy (75%).[42] In general, these tests are not used routinely as a test for infection but rather may be most helpful when there are equivocal results from laboratory work or aspiration, and the additional information that these tests provide may be useful in ruling out infection.

The gold standard for the diagnosis of deep prosthetic infection remains arthrocentesis. It can be done preoperatively as part of the infection work-up and also at the time of surgery, obtaining a fluid aspirate before entering the hip capsule with the approach. It can be associated with false-negatives, and the patient should be instructed to be off of antibiotics for at least 3 weeks prior to aspiration.[43] Additionally, because of the technique required to aspirate a THA, false-positive rates have been reported in up to 13% of patients.[44,45] The exact number of white blood cells and their differential remains somewhat open to debate. What is clear, however, is that total number of white blood cells present on an aspirate is quite low, and is substantially lower than that reported for a native hip.

Mason et al showed that a white blood cell count of greater than 2500 with greater than 60% polymorphonuclear leukocytes had a sensitivity of 98%, a specificity of 95%, and a positive predictive value of 91% in the diagnosis of infection in total knee arthroplasty.[46] Della Valle et al reported when both the ESR and the CRP were elevated, a synovial fluid white blood cell count of 3,000 and a differential of 80% polymorphonuclear leukocytes had the highest sensitivity, specificity, and positive and negative predictive values.[47] Leone et al showed that in patients with an aspirate of less than 2,000 white blood cells with a differential of less than 50%, there was a 98% negative predictive value in ruling out infection.[48] Ghanem et al reported cut-off values for optimal accuracy in the diagnosis of infection were greater than 1100 cells/1023 cm^3 for the fluid leukocyte count and greater than 64% for the neutrophil differential. When both tests yielded results below their cut-off values, the negative predictive value of the combination increased to 98.2% (95% confidence interval, 95.5% to 99.5%), whereas when both tests yielded results greater than their cut-off values, infection was confirmed in 98.6% (95% confidence interval, 94.9% to 99.8%) of the cases.[49]

Intraoperative testing includes the use of gram stain and frozen section histopathology. The gram stain suffers from a lack of sensitivity and is unreliable in ascertaining the presence or absence of infection. Individually it should not be used in the evaluation, and some question its role at all in the diagnosis of infection.[50] The accuracy of frozen section is technique dependent.

In general, a sample or multiple samples should be taken from areas around the hip that look suspicious for infection. These generally include the synovium that is adjacent to the process. The results are dependent on the experience and interest of the pathologist. Often times, samples may have the presence of osteolytic debris or metal staining that may be mistaken for infection. Depending on the criteria used to make the diagnosis of infection, frozen section histopathology has variable results.[51-53] Various tests show that somewhere between 5 and 10 white blood cells per high power field has adequate sensitivity and specificity when making the diagnosis of infection. This number should, however, be used in the context of the clinical picture and preoperative evaluation done prior to surgery.

Recently, there has been much interest in the use of molecular genetic markers for the diagnosis of infection. This can include polymerase chain reaction techniques for the detection of bacterial DNA.[54,55] In addition, it appears that white blood cells in the presence of infection may secrete specific markers that may be useful in the diagnosis of infection. Many of these tests allow for rapid processing within 4 to 6 hours and can even be effective in the presence of antibiotics. The disadvantages include that they do not provide any antibiotic sensitivity results and may have higher false-positive results if any contamination, even from recently killed bacteria, occurs. The technology, as of now, is complex, limited in scope, and somewhat expensive.

It is important that the treating physician develops a consistent and algorithmic approach to the evaluation of a patient with a painful THA. This should begin with a high index of suspicion. Because the treatment of infection is so dramatically different, one should assume that every patient with a painful total joint is infected until proven otherwise. The clinical history, physical exam, ESR, and CRP should serve as a low-cost screening panel in these patients. If the inflammatory markers are normal, this essentially rules out infection with 95% to 100% certainty. If either of these tests are positive, or clinical suspicion still remains high, the patient's hip should be aspirated. Radionucleotide scanning should be reserved for equivocal cases, and when ordered, combining a technetium scan with a white blood cell scan will improve specificity. Intraoperatively, a frozen section analysis is used to assist in making the diagnosis in combination with the previously obtained tests.

CLASSIFICATIONS, TREATMENT OPTIONS, AND OUTCOME

The treatment of a patient with an infected total hip can include retention of the prosthesis and antibiotic suppression, open irrigation and débridement with polyethylene liner exchange, or prosthesis removal. Prosthesis removal includes definitive resection arthroplasty (girdlestone) (Figure 10-1), arthrodesis, amputation, single-stage exchange arthroplasty, or two-stage exchange arthroplasty. There are several treatment variables when deciding which treatment option is most appropriate. These include the depth and timing of the infection, the soft tissue status, the fixation of the prosthesis, the pathogenic organism, the ability of the host to fight the infection, the physician resources, and patient expectations.

Tsukayama et al have provided a classification system for patients with infected total joint arthroplasty (Table 10-3).[56] A type I infection involves a patient who has had a positive culture from the time of surgery, but was not known to be infected until postoperatively. A type II infection is an early infection that occurs within the first 4 weeks after surgery. A type III infection is a late, acute, hematogenous infection that occurs after the hip arthroplasty has been in place in which the patient presents with less than 4 weeks of symptoms and a definitive event that appears to have led to the infection (eg, dental cleaning). A type IV infection is a late, chronic infection where the patient has had symptoms for greater than 4 weeks.

Figure 10-1. Girdlestone resection arthroplasty for a chronically infected hip.

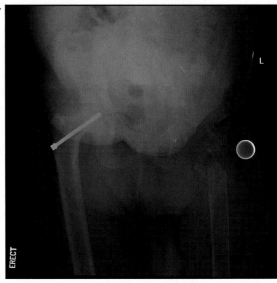

TABLE 10-3. CLASSIFICATION OF PERIPROSTHETIC INFECTION AND TREATMENT RECOMMENDATIONS

TYPE	DEFINITION	TIMING	TREATMENT
Type I	+ Intraoperative cultures	Surgery	Antibiotic therapy
Type II	Early	<4 weeks from surgery	Irrigation and débridement*
Type III	Late, acute	<4 weeks symptoms	Irrigation and débridement
Type IV	Chronic	>4 weeks symptoms	Prosthetic removal* (two-stage exchange)

*Treatment depends on host, isolated bacteria, and clinical situation.

PROSTHETIC RETENTION

Antibiotic suppression should only be reserved for a patient who is so debilitated medically that he or she is unable to undergo surgery. The patient should have a low virulence organism; stable, well-fixed components; and be able to be treated with a suitable oral antibiotic agent that has a low toxicity and side effect profile. The literature would suggest that the success rate of antibiotic suppression is only approximately 20%.[57] The emergence of resistant organisms will only continue to hinder any success with this treatment option.

Open débridement and retention is generally indicated for patients who present with symptoms of less than 4 weeks' duration. This includes patients who present within the first 4 weeks of the index operation or those patients who have had their replacement for some time but develop acute symptoms. These will often arise from an inciting bacteremic episode, such as dental work or sepsis from another source. If the patient does not have an inciting event, then the acuity of the infection should be questioned and it is important to determine whether the patient had any prior symptoms or previous concerns for infection. The success of an open irrigation, débridement, and retention is dependent on several factors that must be taken into consideration. The patient should be healthy enough to fight the infection; have stable, well-fixed components; and the organism should be of low virulence to allow for appropriate antibiotic therapy. Contraindications to irrigation and débridement should include duration of symptoms greater than 4 weeks, an open draining sinus tract, and the presence of polymicrobial or resistant organisms.

Results in the literature are variable and success ranges from 0% to 71%. Tsukayama et al reported on 35 early postoperative infections treated with irrigation and débridement. The overall success rate was 71%.[56] The success of patients with late acute hematogenous infections was only 50%, however. Crockarell et al reported success in only 4 of 19 patients treated with irrigation and débridement for infection in the early postoperative period.[58] In addition, all patients treated with irrigation and débridement with prosthetic retention that had chronic infection (>4 weeks symptoms) failed, and there is little, if any, role for irrigation and débridement with prosthetic retention in the patient that has a chronically infected total joint replacement (>4 weeks symptoms).

Recently published multicentered data have shown high failure rates for irrigation and débridement in patients with total knee arthroplasty with resistant organisms such as MRSA.[59] In this study there was an 89% failure of irrigation and débridement with polyethylene exchange in patients who had MRSA, regardless of the timing of presentation of their infection and cast a doubt on the role and indications for irrigation and débridement in the face of a resistant organism. Whether or not this data translates into THA remains to be seen, but clearly caution should be used in these situations when a resistant organism is present. Some surgeons now advocate a longer course of oral antibiotics after intravenous antibiotics are completed, but these trials remain largely unpublished.

Primary exchange arthroplasty involves removal of all components and foreign material (cement), a thorough débridement, and reinsertion of another prosthesis at the same setting. The main advantage of a single-stage procedure is less morbidity to the patient as only one surgery is required. Likewise, as a result of a single surgery, there is less cost associated with treating the infection. Several studies have reported on the result of single-stage exchange.

Between 1977 and 1983, Callaghan et al reported on 24 single-stage revision surgeries for septic failure of a THA.[60] Twelve patients died, and none were lost to follow-up at a minimum of 10 years after the procedure. Infection recurred around 2 hips (8.3%). If the selected criteria (patients without draining sinuses, without immune-compromise, and with adequate bone quality after débridement) and the standard approach (meticulous débridement, use of antibiotic-impregnated cement, a course of intravenous antibiotics, and use of 3 to 6 months postoperative oral antibiotic therapy) used in this study were implemented, direct exchange of an infected THA construct was deemed a reasonable and cost-effective alternative for some patients with infection after THA. Raut et al reported on 183 THAs that were revised for deep infection in a single-stage procedure using antibiotic containing acrylic cement and systemic perioperative antibiotics.[61] At an average follow-up of 7 years 9 months, 154 (84.2%) patients were free of infection. The remaining 29 (15.8%) patients had evidence of persistent infection

In 2000, Jackson et al performed a literature review to determine when direct exchange was most likely to be successful.[62] Twelve reports provided outcome data on infected hip replacements treated with direct exchange. The average duration of follow-up was 4.8 years. Of the 1299 infected hip replacements treated with direct exchange, 1077 (83%) were thought to be free of infection at the last follow-up. Antibiotic-impregnated bone cement was used in 1282 of the cases (99%). There was wide variability in the duration of parenteral antibiotic therapy, ranging from just 24 hours to as many as 8 weeks.

Factors associated with a successful direct exchange have been shown to be the following:

- Absence of wound complications after the initial total hip replacement
- Good general health of the patient

TABLE 10-4. RESULTS OF TWO-STAGE EXCHANGE ARTHROPLASTY FOR TREATMENT OF INFECTED TOTAL HIP ARTHROPLASY

AUTHOR	YEAR	# OF POINTS	AVERAGE FOLLOW-UP	SUCCESS
Lieberman[70]	1994	46	40 months	91%
Hoffman[67]	2005	27	76 months	94%
Masri[71]	2007	29	24 months	90%
Biring[68]	2009	99	12 years	89%
Sanchez-Sotelo[72]	2009	168	7 years	93%

- Methicillin-sensitive *Staphylococcus epidermidis*, *Staphylococcus aureus*, and *Streptococcus* species
- An organism that was sensitive to the antibiotic mixed into the bone cement

Factors associated with failure included the following:

- Polymicrobial infection
- Gram-negative organisms, especially *Pseudomonas* species
- Certain gram-positive organisms such as methicillin-resistant *Staphylococcus epidermidis* and Group D *Streptococcus*

In addition, the need for cemented revision in order to use antibiotics in the cement has been associated with a higher mechanical failure rate compared to cementless revisions.[63] Most importantly, with a failure rate reported at 8% to 17%, the sequelae of recurrence of infection with this technique is formidable and will require the extraction of a long cemented femoral stem. In early acute infections, when the implants are not yet fixed, some surgeons advocate a single-stage exchange instead of a single femoral head and liner exchange, as removal of components at this early stage is relatively easy and may improve results. Little exists in the literature, however, regarding this specific scenario.

PROSTHETIC REMOVAL

A two-stage exchange arthroplasty involves removal of the infected prosthesis, placement of a high-dose antibiotic cement spacer, and treatment with an average of 6 weeks of intravenous antibiotics prior to a second stage surgery to reimplant the prosthesis. The success of two-stage exchange in the literature ranges from 90% to 95%, and this procedure remains the gold standard for the treatment of a patient with a chronic infected total hip replacement. Table 10-4 lists the current result reported in the literature on the two-stage exchange arthroplasty. There are several variables, however, that need to be taken into consideration with this procedure. These include the amount and type of antibiotics and cement used in the procedure, the use of static versus articulating spacers, the duration of antibiotic treatment, and the interval between resection and reimplantation.

The purpose of antibiotics in cement at the time of resection for infection is to treat the infection. Therefore, local levels of antibiotics in cement should be at or above the minimal inhibitory concentration. Recently, the US Food and Drug Administration has approved commercially

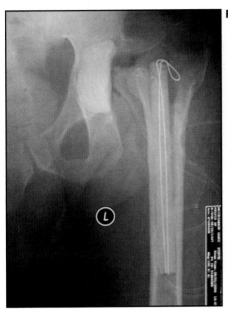

Figure 10-2. Static nonarticulating antibiotic cement spacer.

available premixed antibiotic-loaded cement. It is important to understand that this type of cement contains only 0.5 to 1 g of antibiotic per pack of cement and should be considered a prophylactic dose, not a treatment dose. In order to achieve treatment doses of antibiotics in cement, the surgeon must mix the antibiotic into the cement at the time of surgery. In order for the antibiotic to be effective, it should be thermostable to withstand the exothermic reaction of cement polymerization, and generally, in its powdered form. The most commonly used antibiotics that meet this criteria are vancomycin, gentamicin, and tobramycin. Currently between 2 to 4 g of vancomycin and 2.4 to 4.8 g of tobramycin are recommended per 40-g pack of cement in order to achieve treatment doses. It is important to remember that different cements elute antibiotics differently and this should be taken into consideration when preparing the antibiotic spacer. While there are variable case reports of systemic toxicity from antibiotics in cement, in general, high local concentrations of antibiotics in cement are generally well tolerated with minimal systemic risk.[64-66]

There are 2 types of described antibiotic spacers that may be used in dealing with infection or articulating spacers. A static antibiotic hip spacer generally involves placing a hand-made fabricated tube of antibiotic cement down the femoral canal and a bolus of cement in the acetabulum (Figure 10-2). The spacer is not articulated, and the patient is left with a flail leg during the interval until reimplantation. The main advantages of a static spacer include no risk of dislocation and less interval bone loss in the absence of an articulation with motion. The main disadvantages are limited functional ability for the patient to ambulate during the resection period. In addition, the patient often develops a contracted and shortened leg during the interval, making the reimplantation procedure difficult as a larger exposure with soft tissue dissection is required in order to relocate the hip and restore leg length during reimplantation, possibly leading to a higher rate of dislocation.

The articulating spacer involves the use of an antibiotic-coated prosthesis that articulates with the acetabulum (Figure 10-3). These types of spacers come prefabricated or can be fashioned via a mold at the time of surgery. The main advantage of an articulating spacer is that the length and soft tissue tension of the leg is maintained during the interval period, making the patient more comfortable and functional. The disadvantages of an articulating spacer include the risk of dislocation. In addition, the fully prefabricated molded spacers contain inadequate doses of antibiotics for treatment.

Figure 10-3. Articulating antibiotic-loaded cement spacer.

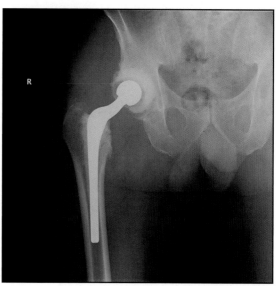

Between June 1991 and December 2001, Hofmann et al reported on 42 patients treated for chronically infected THA using a two-stage articulating antibiotic hip spacer technique.[67] Of the 27 patients available for review, 26 (94%) remain clinically free of infection at an average 76 months (range: 28 to 148 months) postoperatively. All patients received a minimum of 6 weeks of intravenous antibiotics and the Harris hip scores improved from 53 (range: 36 to 68) to 92 (range: 81 to 99) postoperatively. The authors noted the advantage of the articulating hip spacer included improved patient function, maintenance of bone stock and soft tissue tension, and an easier reimplantation. Biring et al reported the outcome at 10 to 15 years of two-stage revision for hip infection in 99 patients using the PROSTALAC articulated hip spacer system.[68] The mean follow-up was 12 years (range: 10 to 15). The long-term success rate was 89% and with additional surgery improved to 96%. The mean global Western Ontario and McMaster University Osteoarthritis Index score was 80.6 (SD = 18.3). The mean satisfaction score was 90.5 (SD = 15.3).

The length of antibiotic therapy is variable; no single study has confirmed the appropriate duration of therapy. It is generally accepted that 6 weeks of intravenous therapy with an appropriate antibiotic, ideally based on culture results, is adequate for the treatment of infection. Intravenous antibiotic therapy, however, is no substitute for a thorough débridement and removal of all foreign material at the time of surgery. If the patient still has retained foreign debris, particularly cement, he or she should still be considered infected and a second débridement should be performed. Equally important to the length of antibiotic therapy is the time the patient is off antibiotics prior to reimplantation. This "antibiotic holiday" ensures that eradication of the infection, rather than temporary suppression of the infection, has taken place. During this holiday period of generally 3 to 6 weeks, the patient should be monitored clinically, as well as with serological markers. There should be an ongoing downward trend in the ESR and CRP from the preresection values. Any increase in these values, or sign and symptoms of recurrence of infection, should prompt further evaluation with a joint aspiration.

Reimplantation is contraindicated in patients who show evidence of persistent infection. Relative contraindications include patients with poor bone stock and inadequate soft tissue to allow for appropriate coverage. Prior to reimplantation, patients should be evaluated for the presence of persistent infection. Normalization of blood serology and joint aspiration can be used to assist with the decision-making process.

Definitive resection arthroplasty (girdlestone without reimplantation) is indicated for failure to eradicate infection or when no reconstruction option exists due to bone or soft tissue compromise (see Figure 10-3). The reported results on girdlestone resection indicate an overall acceptable rate of infection eradication, but poor functional results due to a limited walking tolerance and leg length discrepancy. Ballard et al reported a 98% infection eradication rate with girdlestone resection, but only 73% patient satisfaction.[69] Amputation or hip disarticulation is generally reserved for patients with life-threatening fulminant infections where rapid life-saving measures are required. Additionally, amputation may be indicated in patients with severe bony or soft tissue compromise or patients with vascular injury to the affected extremity. Arthrodesis may be indicated in younger patients but is often difficult to achieve in the face of compromised bone stock, and the use of hardware required for fusion may be contraindicated in the face of active ongoing infection.

SUMMARY

Despite the overall success of THA, infection still remains one of the most common and devastating modes of failure. Projections indicate an increasing demand for primary and revision THA over the next 20 years and an increasing number of infections. Prevention and the identification of high-risk patients remains the most important part of treatment.

All patients with a painful THA should be considered infected until proven otherwise. The timing of the infection is critical in the determination of appropriate treatment. It is important in these situations to have a multidisciplinary team approach to these often complex patients. Two-stage exchange arthroplasty with the use of a high-dose antibiotic cement spacer remains the gold standard for chronic, periprosthetic infection. It is clear, however, that newer emerging technology is needed to continue to improve diagnosis and treatment success in infection following THA.

REFERENCES

1. Callaghan JJ, Albright JC, Goetz DD, Olejniczak JP, Johnston RC. Charnley total hip arthroplasty with cement. Minimum twenty-five-year follow-up. *J Bone Joint Surg Am*. 2000;82(4):487-497.
2. Georgiades G, Babis GC, Hartofilakidis G. Charnley low-friction arthroplasty in young patients with osteoarthritis: outcomes at a minimum of twenty-two years. *J Bone Joint Surg Am*. 2009;91(12):2846-2851.
3. Mallory TH, Lombardi AV Jr, Leith JR, et al. Minimal 10-year results of a tapered cementless femoral component in total hip arthroplasty. *J Arthroplasty*. 2001;16(8 Suppl 1):49-54.
4. Kurtz S, Mowat F, Ong K, Chan N, Lau E, Halpern M. Prevalence of primary and revision total hip and knee arthroplasty in the United States from 1990 through 2002. *J Bone Joint Surg Am*. 2005;87(7):1487-1497.
5. Poss R, Thornhill TS, Ewald FC, Thomas WH, Batte NJ, Sledge CB. Factors influencing the incidence and outcome of infection following total joint arthroplasty. *Clin Orthop Relat Res*. 1984;(182):117-126.
6. Salvati EA, Gonzalez Della Valle A, Masri BA, Duncan CP. The infected total hip arthroplasty. *Instr Course Lect*. 2003;52:223-245.
7. Spangehl MJ, Younger AS, Masri BA, Duncan CP. Diagnosis of infection following total hip arthroplasty. *Instr Course Lect*. 1998;47:285-295.
8. Kurtz SM, Lau E, Schmier J, Ong KL, Zhao K, Parvizi J. Infection burden for hip and knee arthroplasty in the United States. *J Arthroplasty*. 2008;23(7):984-991.
9. Kurtz SM, Ong KL, Lau E, Bozic KJ, Berry D, Parvizi J. Prosthetic joint infection risk after TKA in the Medicare population. *Clin Orthop Relat Res*. 2010;468(1):52-56.
10. Kurtz SM, Ong KL, Schmier J, et al. Future clinical and economic impact of revision total hip and knee arthroplasty. *J Bone Joint Surg Am*. 2007;89(Suppl 3):144-151.
11. Bozic KJ, Ries MD. The impact of infection after total hip arthroplasty on hospital and surgeon resource utilization. *J Bone Joint Surg Am*. 2005;87(8):1746-1751.
12. Garvin KL, Hinrichs SH, Urban JA. Emerging antibiotic-resistant bacteria. Their treatment in total joint arthroplasty. *Clin Orthop Relat Res*. 1999;(369):110-123.
13. Bongartz T, Halligan CS, Osmon DR, et al. Incidence and risk factors of prosthetic joint infection after total hip or knee replacement in patients with rheumatoid arthritis. *Arthritis Rheum*. 2008;59(12):1713-1720.

14. Hacek DM, Robb WJ, Paule SM, Kudrna JC, Stamos VP, Peterson LR. *Staphylococcus aureus* nasal decolonization in joint replacement surgery reduces infection. *Clin Orthop Relat Res.* 2008;466(6):1349-1355.

15. Rao N, Cannella B, Crossett LS, Yates AJ Jr, McGough R 3rd. A preoperative decolonization protocol for *Staphylococcus aureus* prevents orthopaedic infections. *Clin Orthop Relat Res.* 2008;466(6):1343-1348.

16. Flegal KM, Carroll MD, Ogden CL, Curtin LR. Prevalence and trends in obesity among US adults, 1999-2008. *JAMA.* 2010;303(3):235-241.

17. Jackson MP, Sexton SA, Walter WL, Walter WK, Zicat BA. The impact of obesity on the midterm outcome of cementless total knee replacement. *J Bone Joint Surg Br.* 2009;91(8):1044-1048.

18. Jackson MP, Sexton SA, Yeung E, Walter WL, Walter WK, Zicat BA. The effect of obesity on the midterm survival and clinical outcome of cementless total hip replacement. *J Bone Joint Surg Br.* 2009;91(10): 1296-1300.

19. Yeung E, Jackson M, Sexton S, Walter W, Zicat B. The effect of obesity on the outcome of hip and knee arthroplasty. *Int Orthop.* 2011;35(6):929-934.

20. Choong PF, Dowsey MM, Carr D, Daffy J, Stanley P. Risk factors associated with acute hip prosthetic joint infections and outcome of treatment with a rifampinbased regimen. *Acta Orthop.* 2007;78(6):755-765.

21. Malinzak RA, Ritter MA, Berend ME, Meding JB, Olberding EM, Davis KE. Morbidly obese, diabetic, younger, and unilateral joint arthroplasty patients have elevated total joint arthroplasty infection rates. *J Arthroplasty.* 2009;24(6 Suppl):84-88.

22. Dowsey MM, Liew D, Stoney JD, Choong PF. The impact of pre-operative obesity on weight change and outcome in total knee replacement: a prospective study of 529 consecutive patients. *J Bone Joint Surg Br.* 2010;92(4):513-520.

23. Zeni JA Jr, Snyder-Mackler L. Most patients gain weight in the 2 years after total knee arthroplasty: comparison to a healthy control group. *Osteoarthritis Cartilage.* 2010;18(4):510-514.

24. Bolognesi MP, Marchant MH Jr, Viens NA, Cook C, Pietrobon R, Vail TP. The impact of diabetes on perioperative patient outcomes after total hip and total knee arthroplasty in the United States. *J Arthroplasty.* 2008;23(6 Suppl 1):92-98.

25. Marchant MH Jr, Viens NA, Cook C, Vail TP, Bolognesi MP. The impact of glycemic control and diabetes mellitus on perioperative outcomes after total joint arthroplasty. *J Bone Joint Surg Am.* 2009;91(7):1621-1629.

26. Holtom PD. Antibiotic prophylaxis: current recommendations. *J Am Acad Orthop Surg.* 2006;14(10):98-100.

27. Ritter MA. Operating room environment. *Clin Orthop Relat Res.* 1999;(369):103-109.

28. Ritter MA, Olberding EM, Malinzak RA. Ultraviolet lighting during orthopaedic surgery and the rate of infection. *J Bone Joint Surg Am.* 2007;89(9):1935-1940.

29. Darouiche RO, Wall MJ Jr, Itani KM, et al. Chlorhexidine-alcohol versus povidone-iodine for surgical site antisepsis. *N Engl J Med.* 2010;362(1):18-26.

30. Ghanem E, Antoci V Jr, Pulido L, Joshi A, Hozack W, Parvizi J. The use of receiver operating characteristics analysis in determining erythrocyte sedimentation rate and C-reactive protein levels in diagnosing periprosthetic infection prior to revision total hip arthroplasty. *Inter J Infect Dis.* 2009;13(6):e444-e449.

31. Greidanus NV, Masri BA, Garbuz DS, et al. Use of erythrocyte sedimentation rate and C-reactive protein level to diagnose infection before revision total knee arthroplasty. A prospective evaluation. *J Bone Joint Surg Am.* 2007;89(7):1409-1416.

32. Shih LY, Wu JJ, Yang DJ. Erythrocyte sedimentation rate and C-reactive protein values in patients with total hip arthroplasty. *Clin Orthop Relat Res.* 1987;(225):238-246.

33. Della Valle CJ, Sporer SM, Jacobs JJ, Berger RA, Rosenberg AG, Paprosky WG. Preoperative testing for sepsis before revision total knee arthroplasty. *J Arthroplasty.* 2007;22(6 Suppl 2):90-93.

34. Della Valle CJ, Zuckerman JD, Di Cesare PE. Periprosthetic sepsis. *Clin Orthop Relat Res.* 2004;(420):26-31.

35. Austin MS, Ghanem E, Joshi A, Lindsay A, Parvizi J. A simple, cost-effective screening protocol to rule out periprosthetic infection. *J Arthroplasty.* 2008;23(1):65-68.

36. Di Cesare PE, Chang E, Preston CF, Liu C-J. Serum interleukin-6 as a marker of periprosthetic infection following total hip and knee arthroplasty. *J Bone Joint Surg Am.* 2005;87(9):1921-1927.

37. Utz JA, Lull RJ, Galvin EG. Asymptomatic total hip prosthesis: natural history determined using Tc-99m MDP bone scans. *Radiology.* 1986;161(2):509-512.

38. Kraemer WJ, Saplys R, Waddell JP, Morton J. Bone scan, gallium scan, and hip aspiration in the diagnosis of infected total hip arthroplasty. *J Arthroplasty.* 1993;8(6):611-616.

39. Bernay I, Akinci M, Kitapci M, Tokgozoglu N, Erbengi G. The value of Tc-99m Nanocolloid scintigraphy in the evaluation of infected total hip arthroplasties. *Ann Nucl Med.* 1993;7(4):215-222.

40. Scher DM, Pak K, Lonner JH, Finkel JE, Zuckerman JD, Di Cesare PE. The predictive value of Indium[111] leukocyte scans in the diagnosis of infected total hip, knee, or resection arthroplasties. *J Arthroplasty.* 2000;15(3):295-300.

41. Joseph TN, Mujtaba M, Chen AL, et al. Efficacy of combined technetium-99m sulfur colloid/Indium[111] leukocyte scans to detect infected total hip and knee arthroplasties. *J Arthroplasty*. 2001;16(6):753-758.

42. Palestro CJ, Swyer AJ, Kim CK, Goldsmith SJ. Infected knee prosthesis: diagnosis with In-111 leukocyte, Tc-99m sulfur colloid, and Tc-99m MDP imaging. *Radiology*. 1991;179(3):645-648.

43. Barrack RL, Harris WH. The value of aspiration of the hip joint before revision total hip arthroplasty. *J Bone Joint Surg Am*. 1993;75(1):66-76.

44. Lachiewicz PF, Rogers GD, Thomason HC. Aspiration of the hip joint before revision total hip arthroplasty. Clinical and laboratory factors influencing attainment of a positive culture. *J Bone Joint Surg Am*. 1996;78(5):749-754.

45. Schinsky MF, Della Valle CJ, Sporer SM, Paprosky WG. Perioperative testing for joint infection in patients undergoing revision total hip arthroplasty. *J Bone Joint Surg Am*. 2008;90(9):1869-1875.

46. Mason JB, Fehring TK, Odum SM, Griffin WL, Nussman DS. The value of white blood cell counts before revision total knee arthroplasty. *J Arthroplasty*. 2003;18(8):1038-1043.

47. Della Valle CJ, Sporer SM, Jacobs JJ, Berger RA, Rosenberg AG, Paprosky WG. Preoperative testing for sepsis before revision total knee arthroplasty. *J Arthroplasty*. 2007;22(6 Suppl 2):90-93.

48. Leone JM, Hanssen AD. Management of infection at the site of a total knee arthroplasty. *Instr Course Lect*. 2006;55:449-461.

49. Ghanem E, Parvizi J, Burnett RS, et al. Cell count and differential of aspirated fluid in the diagnosis of infection at the site of total knee arthroplasty. *J Bone Joint Surg Am*. 2008;8:1637-1643.

50. Chimento GF, Finger S, Barrack RL. Gram stain detection of infection during revision arthroplasty. *J Bone Joint Surg Br*. 1996;78(5):838-839.

51. Banit DM, Kaufer H, Hartford JM. Intraoperative frozen section analysis in revision total joint arthroplasty. *Clin Orthop Relat Res*. 2002;(401):230-238.

52. Della Valle CJ, Bogner E, Desai P, et al. Analysis of frozen sections of intraoperative specimens obtained at the time of reoperation after hip or knee resection arthroplasty for the treatment of infection. *J Bone Joint Surg Am*. 1999;81(5):684-689.

53. Fehring TK, McAlister JA Jr. Frozen histologic section as a guide to sepsis in revision joint arthroplasty. *Clin Orthop Relat Res*. 1994;(304):229-237.

54. Gallo J, Sauer P, Dendis M, et al. [Molecular diagnostics for the detection of prosthetic joint infection]. *Acta Chir Orthop Traumatol Cech*. 2006;73(2):85-91.

55. Patel R, Osmon DR, Hanssen AD. The diagnosis of prosthetic joint infection: current techniques and emerging technologies. *Clin Orthop Relat Res*. 2005;(437):55-58.

56. Tsukayama DT, Estrada R, Gustilo RB. Infection after total hip arthroplasty. A study of the treatment of one hundred and six infections. *J Bone Joint Surg Am*. 1996;78(4):512-523.

57. Hanssen AD, Rand JA. Evaluation and treatment of infection at the site of a total hip or knee arthroplasty. *Instr Course Lect*. 1999;48:111-122.

58. Crockarell JR, Hanssen AD, Osmon DR, Morrey BF. Treatment of infection with débridement and retention of the components following hip arthroplasty. *J Bone Joint Surg Am*. 1998;80(9):1306-1313.

59. Bradbury T, Fehring TK, Taunton M, et al. The fate of acute methicillin-resistant *Staphylococcus aureus* periprosthetic knee infections treated by open débridement and retention of components. *J Arthroplasty*. 2009;6:101-104.

60. Callaghan JJ, Katz RP, Johnston RC. One-stage revision surgery of the infected hip. A minimum 10-year followup study. *Clin Orthop Relat Res*. 1999;(369):139-143.

61. Raut VV, Siney PD, Wroblewski BM. One-stage revision of total hip arthroplasty for deep infection. Long-term followup. *Clin Orthop Relat Res*. 1995;(321):202-207.

62. Jackson WO, Schmalzried TP. Limited role of direct exchange arthroplasty in the treatment of infected total hip replacements. *Clin Orthop Rel Res*. 2000;381:101-105.

63. Estok DM 2nd, Harris WH. Long-term results of cemented femoral revision surgery using second-generation techniques. An average 11.7-year follow-up evaluation. *Clin Orthop Relat Res*. 1994;(299):190-202.

64. Dovas S, Liakopoulos V, Papatheodorou L, et al. Acute renal failure after antibiotic-impregnated bone cement treatment of an infected total knee arthroplasty. *Clin Nephrol*. 2008;69(3):207-212.

65. van Raaij TM, Visser LE, Vulto AG, Verhaar JA. Acute renal failure after local gentamicin treatment in an infected total knee arthroplasty. *J Arthroplasty*. 2002;17(7):948-950.

66. Springer BD, Lee GC, Osmon D, Haidukewych GJ, Hanssen AD, Jacofsky DJ. Systemic safety of high-dose antibiotic-loaded cement spacers after resection of an infected total knee arthroplasty. *Clin Orthop Relat Res*. 2004;(427):47-51.

67. Hofmann AA, Goldberg TD, Tanner AM, Cook TM. Ten-year experience using an articulating antibiotic cement hip spacer for the treatment of chronically infected total hip. *J Arthroplasty*. 2005;20(7):874-879.

68. Biring GS, Kostamo T, Garbuz DS, Masri BA, Duncan CP. Two-stage revision arthroplasty of the hip for infection using an interim articulated Prostalac hip spacer: a 10- to 15-year follow-up study. *J Bone Joint Surg Br.* 2009;11:1431-1437.

69. Ballard WT, Lowry DA, Brand RA. Resection arthroplasty of the hip. *J Arthroplasty.* 1995;10(6):772-779.

70. Lieberman JR, Callaway GH, Salvati EA, Pellicci PM, Brause BD. Treatment of the infected total hip arthroplasty with a two-stage reimplantation protocol. *Clin Orthop Relat Res.* 1994;(301):205-212.

71. Masri BA, Panagiotopoulos KP, Greidanus NV, Garbuz DS, Duncan CP. Cementless two-stage exchange arthroplasty for infection after total hip arthroplasty. *J Arthroplasty.* 2007;22(1):72-78.

72. Sanchez-Sotelo J, Berry DJ, Hanssen AD, Cabanela ME. Midterm to long-term followup of staged reimplantation for infected hip arthroplasty. *Clin Orthop Relat Res.* 2009;467(1):219-224.

11

Minimizing Complications

James Cashman, MD; Justin Brothers, MD; and Javad Parvizi, MD, FRCS

Revision total hip arthroplasty (THA) is a successful procedure that both restores function and relieves pain. Although uncommon, complications of this surgery do occur and can be devastating. Consequences can vary from nuisances that prolong hospital stay to serious, life-threatening situations. Studies have reported total postoperative complication rates from revision hip arthroplasty to be as high as 20%.[1,2]

Periprosthetic infection, discussed in a different chapter, is a popular subject for research and discussion, but should not overshadow other complications. Recognition of deep vein thrombosis (DVT), nerve injury, limb length inequality, and dislocation as potential complications is critical to patient outcomes, and steps should be taken to minimize their occurrence.

DEEP VEIN THROMBOSIS

Etiology

DVT is a disease state in which blood clots form intravascularly. Normal feedback mechanisms usually prevent formation of clots in the absence of vascular injury and hemorrhage. However, this system can be disturbed by a number of states present during and after surgery. Although the presence of DVT alone can cause local edema, discomfort, and possibly late post-phlebitic syndrome, the most consequential adverse effect is the potential for development of pulmonary emboli (PE). Historically it is believed that PE commonly arise from limb DVT. In recent years this dogma has been reexamined. A study looking at DVT and PE in orthopedic patients did not demonstrate this expected association. Only 10.8% of patients with either DVT or PE had both complications.[3] In light of emerging data, the significance of DVT in the extremity, particularly the distal limb, is being reexamined. The American College of Chest Physicians (ACCP) has, however, issued guidelines for prevention of thromboembolic disease that uses prevention of distal DVT as the outcome parameter.[4] The rationale behind the ACCP guidelines is that prevention of DVT is likely to reduce the incidence of PE. The latter has not been to be the case in the orthopedic literature as there has been no change in the incidence of PE despite administration of

Jacofsky DJ, Hedley AK.
Fundamentals of Revision Hip Arthroplasty:
Diagnosis, Evaluation, and Treatment (pp 159-174).
© 2013 SLACK Incorporated.

aggressive anticoagulation to prevent DVT.[5] The American Academy of Orthopaedic Surgeons issued their set of guidelines with this proviso in mind.[6] This dichotomy has stimulated much debate between the medical and orthopedic communities.

Risk Factors

Initially described by German physician Rudolf Virchow and known as Virchow's Triad, the most common predisposing factors for DVT are hypercoagulability, endothelial damage, and venous stasis. All of these states are present in some form during revision hip arthroplasty.

Hypercoagulability is described as an imbalance of the coagulation/thrombolysis pathway that favors clotting. Many local and systemic factors are associated with hypercoagulability. Inflammatory diseases such as rheumatoid arthritis, systemic lupus erythematosus, and AIDS are procoagulant states. The stress from severe trauma, burns, and surgery has a similar systemic effect. Elevated levels of coagulation factors from estrogen in oral contraceptives or obesity can also tilt the balance in favor of DVT formation. Conversely, depressed levels or efficacy of anticoagulation factors, as seen in nephritic syndrome, factor V Leiden or antithrombin III, factor S, or factor C deficiency can have the same effect.[7]

Endothelial damage from trauma or surgery activates coagulation pathways to aid with hemostasis. However, this damage and activation lasts into the postoperative period, putting THA patients at risk for DVT. Finally, stasis allows for blood components to settle and coagulate. This is seen during periods of immobilization such as long flights or hospitalization with minimal mobilization. Venous stasis may also occur during hip dislocation in surgery, where positioning of the dislocated leg may stretch or kink the femoral vein (Table 11-1).

Although risk factors for DVT are well described, the weight and cumulative effects of multiple factors has only recently been reported. The Caprini risk assessment model developed at the University of Michigan Health System in 2005 is an easy scoring method for DVT and PE risk stratification.[8] By adding the assigning point values for each risk factor, surgeons can determine individual patient risk for venous thromboembolism (VTE) and select an appropriate regime for anticoagulation. Furthermore, the Caprini scoring method was validated recently by a study of 8216 surgical patients. Those patients who were scored as highest risk were significantly more likely to suffer VTE within 30 days than the high risk group (1.94% versus 0.97%).[9]

Techniques to Minimize

Due to the high prevalence, often clinically silent nature, and potential severity of complications from DVT, steps must be taken to reduce its incidence. By recognizing contributing factors, physicians can take a multipronged approach to minimizing occurrence of DVT.

Several nonpharmocologic interventions are often implemented as prophylactic measures. Elastic stockings, intermittent pneumatic compression, and early mobilization have been shown to be effective in reducing the incidence of DVT. Although the reduction in risk is minor, these techniques can be implemented in conjugation with pharmacologic treatments to further reduce incidence without risk of bleeding.[10-13]

Inferior vena cava filters can be surgically placed and used, along with stockings and intermittent pneumatic compressions in a select group of patients in whom anticoagulation is not an option. This protocol has been shown to reduce early postoperative PE. However, due to clogging of the filter and subsequent resistance to venous flow, inferior vena cava filters can actually increase risk of late DVT formation.[14]

Pharmacologic correction of the hypercoagulable postsurgical state with anticoagulant agents is the mainstay of DVT prophylaxis. The use of many families of drugs has been proven to decrease the incidence of DVT in elective hip surgery patients[15-19] (Table 11-2).

Aspirin and low-dose unfractionated heparin prophylaxis alone provide relative risk reduction of 26% and 45%, respectively.[20-23] However, these drugs are not as effective as other

TABLE 11-1. CONDITIONS THAT PLACE PATIENTS AT INCREASED RISK OF PULMONARY EMBOLISM AND/OR MAJOR BLEEDING* (COMPARED TO OTHER PATIENTS HAVING TOTAL HIP ARTHROPLASTY)

	PREOPERATIVE CONDITIONS	PERIOPERATIVE EVENTS
Increased risk of pulmonary embolism	■ Previous documented history of pulmonary embolism ■ Previous documented history of other thromboembolic events ■ Maintenance treatment with anticoagulants ■ Limitations to mobility that would impair early adequate mobilization postsurgery ■ Known hypercoagulable states (malignancy, estrogen use, protein C and S deficiency, antiphospholipid antibodies, antithrombin deficiency, factor V Leiden, acquired or congential thrombophilias, prothrombin mutation 20210A, hyperhomocystinemia) ■ Documented family history of pulmonary embolism ■ Obesity, smoking, venous stasis, IDDM, concomitant fracture ■ Hormone replacement therapy or continuing on oral contraceptive (other than low dose progesterone only)	Any event that limits mobilization, including but not limited to: ■ Cardiac events ■ Infections ■ Severe pain ■ Ileus
Increased risk of major bleeding	■ Known bleeding disorder ■ History of documented bleeding on chemoprophylaxis agents ■ History of documented major gastrointestinal bleeding ■ History of documented hemorrhagic stroke ■ History of other documented major bleeding event	■ Revision THA/TKA ■ Major surgical site bleeding ■ Other major bleeding episode

*In general, the definitions of a major bleed include life threatening, intraocular, intracerebral, or a bleed requiring more than a specified number of transfusions.

IDDM indicates insulin dependent diabetes mellitus; THA, total hip arthroplasty; TKA, total knee arthroplasty.

TABLE 11-2. SELECTION OF THE MOST APPROPRIATE CHEMOTHERAPEUTIC PROPHYLAXIS BASED ON PATIENTS' RISK OF BLEEDING AND RISK OF DEVELOPING VENOUS THROMBOEMBOLISM*

		BLEEDING	
		Standard Risk	High Risk
VTE	Standard risk	a. Aspirin b. LMWH c. Synthetic pentasaccharides d. Warfarin	a. Aspirin b. Warfarin c. None
	High risk	a. LMWH b. Synthetic pentasaccharides c. Warfarin	a. Aspirin b. Warfarin c. None

*Patients should receive one of the chemoprophylactic agents evaluated in this guideline.

VTE indicates venous thromboembolism; LMWH indicates low molecular weight heparins.

anticoagulation regimes and should be avoided in revision THA. Use of both these agents in conjugation is also not advised, as synergistic anticoagulation may produce greater than expected bleeding adverse effects.

The 2 most popular anticoagulation protocols used by orthopedic surgeons include adjusted-dose oral anticoagulation with warfarin sodium and low molecular weight heparins (LMWH) such as enoxaparin. Anticoagulation with warfarin is popular due to the oral route of administration, which is easily continued after discharge. However, achieving adequate anticoagulation with oral warfarin can be a challenge. This can be difficult due to the lag in response after dosing which often leaves patients subtherapeutic until postoperative day 3. For this reason, the first dose should be given immediately after surgery.[24,25] Warfarin also has innumerable drug interactions, and its effect can be modulated by changes in a patient's diet after discharge. Another problem with warfarin is the need for monitoring of the international normalized ratio (INR) by performing blood tests. Conversely, LMWH is administered subcutaneously, does not require dose adjustment, and has a rapid onset of action. Fondaparinux is a synthetic pentasaccharide factor Xa inhibitor, closely related to LMWH. In contrast to heparin, it does not inhibit thrombin. Unlike direct factor Xa inhibitors, it mediates its effects indirectly through antithrombin III, but unlike heparin, it is selective for factor Xa. Currently oral anticoagulants (factor Xa and direct thrombin inhibitors) that do not require monitoring are in use outside the United States for primary hip and knee arthroplasty and being considered for approval by the US Food and Drug Administration.

Initial studies evaluating LMWH for elective hip surgery prophylaxis found it to be much superior to aspirin and unfractionated heparin prophylaxis. In one study, incidence of DVT in the control group was 51.3% while the LMWH group enjoyed a rate of 10.8% with minimal risk of hemorrhage.[10,26] Many studies comparing LMWH against adjusted-dose oral warfarin have found the 2 provide similar risk reduction.[17,18] Meta-analysis of this data has shown THA patients given prophylaxis with LMWH experience lower incidence of DVT (13.7%) when compared to those on warfarin (20.7%). However, the LMWH group also experiences higher rates of bleeding

TABLE 11-3. THE DOSAGE AND TIMING OF CHEMOPROPHYLACTIC AGENTS THAT SHOULD BE CONSIDERED*

DRUG	DOSE	START TIME	DURATION OF TREATMENT
Aspirin	325 mg[†] 2 times per day	Day of surgery	6 weeks
LMWH	Per package	12 to 24 hours postoperation[‡]	7 to 12 days**
Fondaparinux	Per package	12 to 24 hours postoperation[‡]	7 to 12 days**
Warfarin	INR ≤2.0	Night before/after	3 to 6 weeks
Combination			Unclear (no data)

*The duration for the administration of chemoprophylactic agents has not been clearly established. The older literature notes that most postoperative pulmonary embolism occurred within the first 6 weeks. Therefore, many regimens were established to encompass that experience.

**There are some data, with the heparin-like drugs, that show that it is not necessary to prolong the administration beyond the first 8 to 12 days. These recommendations reflect those practices.

[†]Can adjust down to 81 mg 1 time per day for gastrointestinal symptoms

[‡]Or after indwelling epidural catheter removed

LMWH indicates low molecular weight heparins; INR, international normalized ratio.

complications (5.3% versus 3.3%). These data suggest LMWH is more effective than warfarin for prevention of DVT but at the risk of increasing surgical site bleeding and hematoma formation.[17,19,25,27]

Timing and duration of prophylaxis has been another variable of debate. Although most surgeons implement DVT prophylaxis while the patient is hospitalized, continued anticoagulation after discharge is variable. Some believe the hypercoagulable state induced by surgery persists for weeks after discharge. In fact, 10% to 20% of patients will develop a new DVT within 1 month of discharge if not on home prophylaxis. Furthermore, a study looking at LMWH anticoagulation versus placebo for 35 days after discharge found a decrease in incidence of DVT from 36.7% in the placebo group to 19.7% in the LMWH group.[28] Another study compared timing of anticoagulation. Two groups of THA patients received LMWH prophylaxis either started before or after surgery and incidence of DVT was recorded. They concluded that this variable had little effect on DVT development (Table 11-3).[27]

Finally, the risks of anticoagulation should not be disregarded. Bleeding complications such as hematoma can predispose patients to devastating periprosthetic infection. Patients with recent vascular surgery, recent hemorrhagic stroke, and history of liver failure should not be anticoagulated. Also, some argue elderly patients with unsteady gait should receive prophylaxis only after evaluation on a case by case basis. One recent study evaluated the available literature and found that the incidence of all-cause mortality was in fact higher after administration of chemoprophylaxis compared to mechanical compression devices and aspirin.[29] In addition, It appears that despite administration of various chemoprophylactic agents the orthopedic community has made little impact on the incidence of fatal and nonfatal pulmonary embolus over the last 10 to 15 years.[30]

Figure 11-1. T1-weighted axial magnetic resonance imaging through the hips. Injudicious placement of retractors can cause compression of the sciatic nerve posteriorly (blue circle) or compression of the femoral neurovascular bundle (red circle). The lateral femoral cutaneous nerve of the thigh (yellow circle) can be injured in a direct anterior approach.

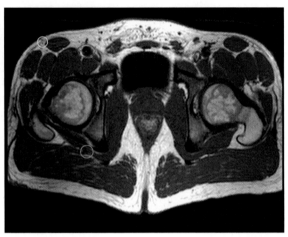

NERVE INJURY

Etiology

Nerve injury following revision hip arthroplasty can range from an annoying sensory loss to devastating motor dysfunction. Injury can occur via direct ligation, thermal damage, and neuropraxia from stretching or compression. Most studies report neurologic complications in 0% to 7.6% for revision THA. Clinical exam alone has been found to underestimate this number while electromyography has shown nearly 70% of cases to have detectable but not clinically evident nerve injury. The sciatic nerve is most commonly injured due to proximity to the hip joint (Figure 11-1). However, femoral, lateral cutaneous, and obturator nerves may all be injured. For mild injury, recovery may take weeks while severe cases with axonal damage could take 1 to 2 years.[31-33]

Risk

Several studies have retrospectively reviewed large samples of patients undergoing THA and delineated risk factors for postoperative nerve palsy. A preoperative diagnosis of developmental dysplasia of the hip or post-traumatic arthritis is independently associated with nerve injury. Revision arthroplasty, female sex, and history of diabetes are also predictors.[34,35]

Correctable factors associated with nerve injury include surgery through the posterior approach, intraoperative limb lengthening, and postoperative hematoma. One study found that in cases of peroneal palsy the average limb lengthening was 2.7 cm (range: 1.9 to 3.7 cm) while lengthening of 4.4 cm (range: 4.0 to 5.1 cm) was correlated with sciatic nerve palsies. If diagnosed, the nerve should be immediately relieved of tension by flexing the knee and extending the hip.[36] Another study found 1.69% of THA cases developed sciatic nerve palsy secondary to postoperative hematoma in the area of the nerve. In this series, cases diagnosed and evacuated early enjoyed rapid improvement of symptoms while delayed diagnosis was associated with little or no recovery.[37]

Less commonly, the branches of the femoral nerve, including the lateral femoral cutaneous nerve, can be injured during an anterior approach. Most frequently, excessive or poorly placed retractors can impinge the nerve. Finally, at least one paper has reported an iliacus hematoma causing femoral nerve palsy after a revision hip arthroplasty.[38] More commonly, however, the inciting event that caused nerve injury is never identified with certainty.

Techniques to Minimize

Due to the often long-lasting and debilitating consequences of nerve injury, care should be taken to prevent their development. This can be accomplished primarily through disciplined surgical technique.

Although not directly related to the operative field, nerve injury can occur throughout the body from poor patient positioning. The common peroneal nerve is particularly susceptible to compression injury due to its subcutaneous course near the fibular head.

In general, surgeons should use the approach with which they feel most comfortable and that they deem necessary to obtain appropriate visualization for the revision. However, included in the approach should be identification and protection of nerves at risk. Care should be taken to place retractors in safe locations and avoid vigorous retraction.

When cemented components are used, thermal damage can occur to soft tissues during the exothermic curing of solidifying methyl methacrylate cement. Any cement that is extruded during implantation should be removed from the field.

Maintenance of meticulous hemostasis is also imperative to prevent formation of postoperative hematoma. Similarly, levels of postoperative anticoagulation should be kept within the target range. Surgical exploration is warranted in patients that develop acute neurologic deficits or signs of hematoma, as evacuation will improve outcomes.

Although correction of limb length discrepancy is important part of THA to improve ambulation, care should be taken to avoid excessive stretching of the soft tissues. Although a threshold length for injury has not been described, some authors have found sciatic nerve injury at greater than 4 cm.[36,39] If diagnosed, the nerve should be immediately relieved of tension by flexing the knee and extending the hip to prevent further damage. Surgical exploration with limb shortening by exchanging the modular prosthetic head and neck may also be necessary. Early relief of any potentially reversible etiology has been shown to reduce duration and severity of nerve injury.[34]

LIMB LENGTH INEQUALITY

Etiology

One of the important aspects of revision THA is the restoration of limb length, which besides its importance to the patient, can influence soft tissue balancing and joint stability and the overall outcome of revision THA with regard to gait and potential for low back pain. In addition, limb length combined with offset directly influences the biomechanics of the joint and can affect the long-term outcome of revision arthroplasty. Limb length differences are often present in the healthy population and postoperative discrepancies of less than 1 cm are generally well tolerated.[40] However, acute or large changes in limb length can have drastic consequences.[41-43] Furthermore, patient dissatisfaction with leg length discrepancy following THA is the most common reason for legal action against orthopedic joint surgeons.[44]

Resulting gait abnormalities can be particularly disturbing, as it can be both annoying to the patient and make ambulation difficult. A recent study, in which healthy subjects were given artificial limb length inequality of 2 cm with shoe lifts, showed markedly increased oxygen and caloric consumption as well as heart rate.[45] Electromyographic studies have shown increases in the erector spinae muscle activity with as little as 3 cm of leg-length discrepancy.[46]

Pelvic asymmetry and structural misalignment of the spine is a well-documented source of chronic low back pain. Biomechanical studies show that leg length inequality imposes structural alignment changes on the lumbar spine, which is associated with pain.[47,48] Conversely, several studies report relief of this asymmetry with shoe lifts, which reduced low back pain scores.[49,50]

As discussed previously, changes in limb length can stretch the sciatic nerve causing sometimes permanent nerve palsies. Acting synergistically with changes in biomechanics, loss of muscle strength severely interferes with comfortable, smooth ambulation.

Risk

Although already quite prevalent in the general population, certain factors put patients at increased risk for leg length inequality.[40] Any disease process affecting the pelvic girdle or lower extremities can alter normal biomechanics and both create leg length inequality and make assessment challenging. Muscle contracture may create an apparent discrepancy in leg length. Furthermore, scoliosis, developmental dysplasia of the hip, lumbar degenerative disk disease, previous spinal surgery, and poliomyelitis can have an effect on pelvic tilt and leg length. Finally, shorter patients are more likely to report functionally significant leg length inequality.[40]

Techniques to Minimize

A firm understanding of the various components of leg length and their relation to revision hip arthroplasty is required to prevent postoperative leg length inequality and its accompanying complications. Both preoperative planning and intraoperative techniques are imperative.

Preoperative assessment and planning is an easy way to help prevent leg length inequality. Asking the patient's perception of any leg length inequality or use of a shoe lift are simple ways to screen in the clinic. Apparent leg length inequality is measured from the umbilicus to medial malleolus. Since muscle contracture can cause an apparent leg length inequality, a thorough physical exam evaluating range of motion is important. Next, determination of true limb length can be measured from the anterior superior iliac spine to the medial malleolus. However, this method can be difficult in obese patients with soft tissue obscuring bony landmarks. Furthermore, it does not assess abduction or adduction contracture at the hip.

Next, physical exam should assess for spinal deformity and pelvic obliquity. Correction of leg length inequality with shoe lifts will resolve pelvic asymmetry compensating for true leg length inequality due to bony or prosthetic differences. It will not correct pelvic tilt in cases of leg length inequality secondary to soft tissue contracture at the hip. Finally, realistic expectations and risks should be discussed in detail with the patient before surgery.

Preoperative radiographic assessment is an excellent way to confirm physical exam findings. Anteroposterior pelvic radiographs with legs held in 20 degrees of internal rotation help visualize landmarks. A common measurement is from the lesser trochanters to a horizontal line tangent to the ischial tuberosities. Similarly, measurement from the tip of the greater trochanters may be useful. In revision surgery, identification of metaphyseal and diaphyseal landmarks can be difficult due to osteolysis or bone deficiency from the primary arthroplasty. Any available landmarks that can be identified intraoperatively should be noted to help guide restoration of balanced leg length.[51]

Preoperative templating of the prosthesis also helps determine what to expect intraoperatively. The acetabular template should be placed in contact with host bone, and the acetabular component determines the hip center of rotation. The femoral component template determines femoral offset and leg lengths. After planning appropriate offset, the height of the osteotomy and neck length may be measured to match the nonoperative leg. These measurements will guide surgery but should also be combined with intraoperative assessment. Although very useful for planning, preoperative templates may be inaccurate when extent of acetabular reaming is poorly estimated[43] (Figure 11-2).

Intraoperative assessment relies both on proper patient positioning and on the ability to reliably find anatomic landmarks used previously in radiographic templating. Surgeons can determine the osteotomy height by measuring the distance from the lesser trochanter calculated preoperatively. The top of the femoral head to the osteotomy is a more accurate intraoperative measurement for

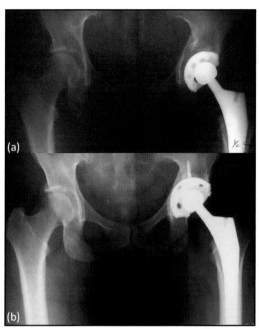

Figure 11-2. Leg length discrepancy can be multifactorial. The surgeon can influence leg length discrepancy intraoperatively by appropriate component position. The patient's leg length discrepancy seen in (A) will be corrected if the cup is seated in the correct position relative to the teardrop (B).

primary cases.[52] This technique can be mimicked in revision cases by measuring distance of the components to an anatomic landmark. Similarly, calculating the distance between the center of trial heads and the lesser trochanter and selecting the appropriate neck length has shown promising results.[53]

Intraoperative radiographs are useful when compared to preoperative films and measurements. In revision surgeries, where anatomic landmarks are hard to identify, different trial components can be fitted until the desired measurement is achieved. Physical measurements using Steinman pins placed in the pelvis and the greater trochanter have also been described. Recently, computer-assisted navigation has been used to guide arthroplasty. So far, these studies have shown no improvement over freehand methods with regards to leg length inequality.[54]

DISLOCATION

Etiology

Dislocation is a leading and underemphasized cause of failure in revision hip arthroplasty. Dislocation is defined as the complete loss of contact between the acetabular and femoral components. Dislocation occurs after 0.3% to 10% of primary THAs and some studies have reported dislocation rates in revision THA patients as high as 14% to 20%.[55-58] The risk of dislocation is multifactorial, with risk factors consisting of surgical approach, previous hip surgery, component malposition, component design, and postoperative range of motion, among others (Table 11-4). Additional risks can arise over time, such as with neurologic decline of the patient, wear of the components, infection, and trauma. An improved understanding of the etiology of dislocation and refinements in surgical techniques have led to a decrease in the rate of dislocation over time. Although most dislocations occur in the early postoperative period while the soft tissue envelope is healing, there is still risk throughout the life of the prosthesis. Furthermore, revision surgeries are much more likely to dislocate than primary THA due to more soft tissue dissection, poorer quality tissue, and bone loss.

TABLE 11-4. FACTORS ASSOCIATED WITH DISLOCATION IN REVISION HIP ARTHROPLASTY

	FACTORS AFFECTING STABILITY	NOTES	SOURCE
Patient	Age	Not significant	Conroy et al. *J Arthroplasty*. 2008;23(6):867-872.
	Gender		
	Cognitive impairment	Increased risk of dislocation	Khatod et al. *Clin Orthop Relat Res*. 2006.447:19-23.
	Neuromuscular disorders		
	Abductor function	Increased risk of dislocation applies to cognitive impairment and neuromuscular disorders	Kung et al. *Clin Orthop Relat Res*. 2007;465:170-174.
Surgeon	Approach	While significant in primary THA, no difference in revision THA	Paterno et al. *J Bone Joint Surg Am*. 1997;79(8):1202-1210
	Experience	Less revisions if >50 done per year versus <5 per year	Katz et al. *J Bone Joint Surg Am*. 2001; 83-A(11):1622-1629.
Implant	Head size	↑head size = ↓dislocation rate	Alberton at al. *J Bone Joint Surg Am*. 2002;84:1788-1792.
	Linear	Lipped or offset liner associated with impingement	*J Orthop Res*. 2007 Nov;25(11):1401-1407.
	Version	Malposition increases risk of dislocation	Lewinnik et al. *J Bone Joint Surg Am*. 1978;60(2):217-220.

Risk

Many factors have been reported to increase incidence of dislocation following THA. Unlike the experience with dislocation after primary procedures, age and gender were not found to be significant risk factors for dislocation after revision hip surgery in the present study. Prosthesis size has been consistently associated with dislocation. Large femoral head size provides a larger bearing surface and subsequently increases the jump distance required for the head to dislocate. Conversely, a small prosthesis head is associated with greater rate of dislocation.[59,60] Large head size does not completely obliterate the risk, as the benefit of head size decreases once acetabular version or abduction increase beyond the safe zone[61] or once bone-bone impingement occurs. Skirted necks are often used to augment neck length and offset to provide adequate soft tissue tension. However, they can have an adverse affect on head-neck ratio and can lead to impingement.[62]

Lewinnek et al described the "ideal" position for acetabular version as 15 degrees of anteversion and 45 degrees of abduction.[63] As the primary concern in seating the acetabular implant is getting adequate host bone contact, the version of the component may stray from this ideal. This can increase the risk of dislocation, and indeed, many studies have found dislocations to occur more frequently if the cup is retroverted or in greater than 55 degrees of abduction.[64-66]

Several studies have shown the posterior approach in primary THA to be associated with higher rates of dislocation when compared to the anterolateral approach due to soft tissue damage.[67] This risk is reduced with repair of the posterior structures.[68] However, this risk is not seen in the revision setting.[69] Presumably, this is because the soft tissue mass is dissected and heals as one solid tissue mass.

Furthermore, surgeons performing higher volume THA experience lower rates of dislocation. One study reported those who perform fewer than 10 THAs annually suffer a dislocation rate 3 times higher than the average.[70] While this could be extrapolated to the revision setting, it has not been yet documented in the literature.

Many patient factors have been associated with dislocation, although few are universally agreed upon. Age has been a suggested risk factor and several studies have found increased rates in patients over 80 years of age. One study reported greater than twice the incidence of dislocation in patients over 80 years old, while another found a 4.5 times greater dislocation risk in patients over 85 years of age.[60,70,71] Female gender is a well-documented risk factor for dislocation after a primary arthroplasty.[72] The compromised muscle function that exists in both male and female patients following revision surgery may be a factor that overrides the gender difference.

High preoperative American Association of Anesthesiologist (ASA) score, even after controlling for confounding factors, baseline cognitive dysfunction, and neuromuscular dysfunction have all been associated with dislocation. A study reported 10 times more frequent dislocation in patients with an elevated ASA score.[73] Patients with neuromuscular diseases, such as cerebrovascular or Parkinson's disease, seizure disorders, or patients who abuse alcohol have poor control of their limbs. Loss of balance and proprioception leading to falls contribute to their high rates of dislocation.

Preoperative diagnosis of rheumatoid arthritis or developmental dysplasia of the hip also predisposes to dislocation.[73] This is likely due to mechanical properties of the deformed joint. Furthermore, history of subtrochanteric osteotomy is associated with higher dislocation rates than is seen in developmental dysplasia of the hip alone.[74]

Techniques to Minimize

Although many of the demographic risk factors cannot be avoided, many strategies can be implemented during and after surgery to prevent dislocation. The use of large femoral heads provides better articulating bearing surfaces and stability. Femoral offset and acetabular version are 2 surgeon-dependent factors for dislocation. Careful preoperative planning with templates and meticulous intraoperative assessment as described above will ensure few technical errors. Some surgeons also report it easier to achieve appropriate anteversion with an anterior approach. If using the posterior approach, some surgeons have found reconstruction of the posterior capsule and external rotators to help reduce incidence of postoperative dislocation. One study out of China reported zero dislocations in 47 revision THAs using this procedure.[75] Despite the higher rate of dislocation with the posterior approach, surgeons should use whichever method with which they are most comfortable in order to avoid other unseen complications.

In some cases, use of highly cross-linked polyethylene bearings allows for larger articulating surface, alleviating some of the risk of small femoral heads. Also, ceramic-on-ceramic or metal-on-metal can be used to increase the head-to-neck ratio. This way the use of a skirted neck may be avoided.[76] Early studies evaluating the French dual mobility cups have been promising. An ultrahigh molecular weight polyethylene dual articulation bearing is inserted between the head and cup. The design allows minimal motion on the concave side and great mobility on the convex side. One study experienced a dislocation rate of only 3.7% in revision patients using this implant.[77] Whichever is used, surgeons should always assess for instability after components are in place.[67] Modular femoral stems, where femoral version can be independently adjusted after placement of the stem, may also allow for improved stability.

Postoperative care plays an important role in preventing dislocation in the early postoperative period. Many surgeons implement hip precautions that prevent patients from putting excessive strain on the new joint. Limited adduction, flexion, and internal rotation are allowed at the hip joint and certain motions are prohibited. However, a recent study has shown the removal of hip precautions did not adversely affect dislocation rates in a large population.[78]

SUMMARY

The burden of revision hip arthroplasty is projected to increase. By 2030, the annual demand for primary THAs is estimated to grow by 174% to 572,000.[79] An awareness of the potential complications of revision hip arthroplasty is necessary in order to counsel patients and reduce the risk of their occurrence. The more common risk factors for failure in revision hip arthroplasty, leg length inequality, nerve injury, dislocation, and thromboembolic disorders can all be minimized with due consideration and care.

REFERENCES

1. Stavrev VP, Stavrev PV. Complications in total hip replacement. *Folia Med (Polydiv)*. 2004;46(2):25-30.
2. Kavanagh BF, Ilstrup DM, Fitzgerald RH Jr. Revision total hip arthroplasty. *J Bone Joint Surg Am*. 1985;67:517-526.
3. Parvizi J, Jacovides CL, Bican O, et al. Is DVT a good proxy for pulmonary embolus? *J Arthroplasty*. 2010;25(3):e14.
4. Geerts WH, Berggvist D, Pineo GF, et al. Prevention of venous thromboembolism: American College of Chest Physicians evidence-based clinical practice guidelines. 8th ed. *Chest*. 2008;133(6 Suppl):381S-453S.
5. Gillespie W, Murray D, Gregg PJ, Warwick D. Risks and benefits of prophylaxis against venous thromboembolism in orthopaedic surgery. *J Bone Joint Surg Br*. 2000;82(4):475-479.
6. Haas SB, Barrack RL, Westrich G, Lachiewicz PF. Venous thromboembolic disease after total hip and knee arthroplasty. *J Bone Joint Surg Am*. 2008;90(12):2764-2780.
7. Guan ZP, Chen YZ, Song YN, Qin XL, Jiang J, Clinical risk factors for deep vein thrombosis after total hip and knee arthroplasty. *Zhonghua Wai Ke Za Zhi*. 2005;43(20):1317-1320.
8. Caprini J. Thrombosis risk assessment as a guide to quality patient care. *Dis Mon*. 2005;51:70-78.
9. Bahl V, Hu HM, Henke PK, Wakefield TW, Campbell DA Jr, Caprini JA. A validation study of retrospective venous thromboembolism risk scoring method. *Ann Surg*. 2010;251(2):344-350.
10. Lassen MR, Borris LC, Christiansen HM, et al. Prevention of thromboembolism in 190 hip arthroplasties: comparison of LMW heparin and placebo. *Acta Orthop Scand*. 1991;62(1):33-38.
11. Samama CM, Clergue F, Barre J, Montefiore A, Ill P, Samii K. Low molecular weight heparin associated with spinal anestheisa and gradual compression stockings in total hip replacement surgery. *Arar Study Group Br J Anaesth*. 1997;78:660-665.
12. Fordyce MJ, Ling RS. A venous foot pump reduces thrombosis after total hip replacement. *J Bone Joint Surg*. 1992;74-B:45-49.
13. Francis CW, Pellegrini VD Jr, Marder VJ, et al. Comparison of warfarin and external pneumatic compression in prevention of venous thrombosis after total hip replacement. *JAMA*. 1992;267:2911-2915.
14. Vaughn BK, Knezevich S, Lombardi AV Jr, Mallory TH. Use of the Greenfield filter to prevent fatal pulmonary embolism associated with total hip and knee arthroplasty. *J Bone Joint Surg*. 1989;71:1542-1548.
15. Xing KH, Morrison G, Lim W, Douketis J, Odueyungbo A, Crowther M. Has the incidence of deep vein thrombosis in patients undergoing total hip/knee arthroplasty changed over time? A systematic review of randomized controlled trials. *Thromb Res*. 2008;123:24-34.
16. Geerts WH, Heit JA, Clagett GP, et al. Prevention of venous thromboembolism. *Chest*. 2001;119 (1 Suppl):132S-175S.

17. Hull R, Raskob G, Pineo G, et al. A comparison of subcutaneous low-molecular-weight heparin with war-farin sodium for prophylaxis against deep-vein thrombosis after hip or knee implantation. *N Engl J Med.* 1993;329:1370-1376.

18. [No authors listed]. RD heparin compared with warfarin for prevention of venous thromboembolic disease following total hp or knee arthroplasty. *J Bone Joint Surg.* 1994;76:1174-1185.

19. Hamulyák K, Lensing AW, van der Meer J, Smid WM, van Ooy A, Hoek JA. Subcutaneous low-molecular weight heparin or oral anticoagulants for the prevention of deep-vein thrombosis in elective hip and knee replacement? *Thromb Haemost.* 1995;74:1428-1431.

20. Collins R, Scrimgeour A, Yusuf S, Peto R. Reduction in fatal pulmonary embolism and venous thrombosis by perioperative administration of subcutaneous heparin: overview of results of randomized trials in general, orthopaedic, and urologic surgery. *N Engl J Med.* 1988;318:1162-1173.

21. Leyvraz PF, Richard J, Bachmann F, et al. Adjusted versus fixed-dose subcutaneous heparin in the preven-tion of deep-vein thrombosis after total hip replacement. *N Engl J Med.* 1983;309:954-958.

22. Siragusa S, Vicentini L, Carbone S, Barone M, Beltrametti C, Piovella F. Intermittent pneumatic leg com-pression (IPLC) and unfractionated heaprin (UFH) in the prevention of post-operative deep vein thrombosis in hip surgery. *Blood.* 1994;84(Suppl 1):70a.

23. Antiplatelet Trialists' Collaboration. Collaborative overview of randomised trials of antiplatelet therapy: III. Reduction in venous thrombosis and pulmonary embolism by antiplatelet prophylaxis among surgical and medical patients. *BMJ.* 1994;308:235-246.

24. Heit JA, Berkowitz SD, Bona R, et al. Efficacy and safety of low molecular weight heparin (ardeparin sodi-um) compared to warfarin for the prevention of VTE after total knee replacement surgery: a double-blind, dose-ranging study. *Thromb Haemost.* 1997;77:32-38.

25. Francis CW, Pellegrini VD Jr, Totterman S, et al. Prevention of deep-vein thrombosis after total hip arthroplasty: comparison of warfarin and dalteparin. *J Bone Joint Surg.* 1997;79:1365-1372.

26. Turpie AG, Levine MN, Hirsh J, et al. A randomized controlled trial of low-molecular-weight heparin (enoxaparin) to prevent deep-vein thrombosis in patients undergoing elective hip surgery. *N Engl J Med.* 1986;315(15):925-929.

27. Hull RD, Pineo GF, Francis C, et al. Low-molecular-weight heparin prophylaxis using dalteparin in close proximity to surgery versus warfarin in hip arthroplasty patients: a double-blind, randomized comparison. *Arch Intern Med.* 2000;160:2199-2207.

28. Hull RD, Pineo GF, Francis C, et al. Low-molecular-weight heparin prophylaxis using dalteparin extended out-of-hospital vs in-hospital warfarin/out-of-hospital placebo in hip arthroplasty patients: a double-blind, randomized comparison. North American Fragmin Trial Investigators. *Arch Intern Med.* 2000;160(14): 2208-2215.

29. Sharrock NE, Gonzalez Della Valle A, Go G, Lyman S, Salvati EA. Potent anticoagulants are associated with a higher all-cause mortality rate after hip and knee arthroplasty. *Clin Orthop Relat Res.* 2008;466(3): 714-721.

30. Howie C, Hughes H, Watts AC. Venous thromboembolism associated with hip and knee replacement over a ten-year period: a population-based study. *J Bone Joint Surg Br.* 2005;87(12):1675-1680.

31. Weber ER, Daube JR, Coventry MB. Periperpheral neuropatheis associated with total hip arthroplasty. *J Bone Joint Surg.* 1976;58:66-69.

32. Solheim LF, Hagen R. Femoral and sciatic neuropathies after total hip arthroplasty. *Acta Orthop Scand.* 1980;51:531-534.

33. Brown GD, Swanson EA, Nercessian OA. Neurologic injuries after total hip arthroplasty. *Am J Orthop.* 2008;37(4):191-197.

34. Farrell CM, Springer BD, Haidukewych GJ, Morrey BF. Motor nerve palsy following primary total hip arthroplasty. *J Bone Joint Surg.* 2005;87(12):2619-2625.

35. Schmalzried TP, Amstutz HC, Dorey FJ. Nerve palsy associated with total hip replacement. Risk factors and prognosis. *J Bone Joint Surg.* 1991;73(7):1074-1080.

36. Edwards BN, Tullos HS, Noble PC. Contributory factors and etiology of sciatic nerve palsy in total hip arthroplasty. *Clin Orthop Relat Res.* 1987;218:136-141.

37. Butt AJ, McCarthy T, Kelly IP, Glynn T, McCoy G. Sciatic nerve palsy secondary to postoperative haema-toma in primary total hip replacement. *J Bone Joint Surg Br.* 2005;11(87-B):1465-1467.

38. Nakamura Y, Mitsui H, Toh S, Hayashi Y. Femoral nerve palsy associated with iliacus hematoma following pseudoaneurysm after revision hip arthroplasty. *J Arthroplasty.* 2008;23(8):1240.e1-e4.

39. Wasielewski RC, Crossett LS, Rubash HE. Neural and vascular injury in total hip arthroplasty. *Orthop Clin North Am.* 1992;23:219-235.

40. Ranawat CS, Rodriguez JA. Functional leg-length inequality following total hip arthroplasty. *J Arthroplasty.* 1997;12:359-364.

41. Friberg O. Clinical symptoms and biomechanics of lumbar spine and hip joint in leg length inequality. *Spine*. 1983;8:643-651.

42. Parvizi J, Sharkey PF, Bissett GA, Rothman RH, Hozack WJ. Surgical treatment of limb-length discrepancy following total hip arthroplasty. *J Bone Joint Surg*. 2003;85(12):2310-2317.

43. Clark CR, Huddleston HD, Schoch EP 3rd, Thomas BJ. Leg-length discrepancy after total hip arthroplasty. *J Am Acad Orthop Surg*. 2006;14:38-45.

44. White AB. AAOS Committee on Professional Liability: study of 119 malpractice claims involving hip replacement. *AAOS Bulletin*. July 1994.

45. Gurney B, Mermier C, Robergs R, Gibson A, Rivero D. Effects of limb-length discrepancy on gait economy and lower-extremity muscle activity in older adults. *J Bone Joint Surg*. 2001;83-A(6):907-915.

46. Vink P, Huson A. Lumbar back muscle activity during walking with a leg inequality. *Acta Morphol Neerl Scand*. 1987;25:261-271.

47. Giles LGF, Taylor JR. Lumbar spine structural changes associated with leg length inequality. *Spine*. 1982;7:159-162.

48. Giles LGF, Taylor JR. Low-back pain associated with leg length inequality. *Spine*. 1981;6:510-521.

49. Brady RJ, Dean JB, Skinner TM, Gross MT. Limb length inequality: clinical implications for assessment and intervention. *J Orthop Sports Phys Ther*. 2003;33(5):221-234.

50. Grofton J. Persistent low back pain and leg length inequality. *J Rheumatol*. 1985;12:747-750.

51. Maloney WJ, Keeney JA. Leg length discrepancy after total hip arthroplasty. *J Arthroplasty*. 2004;19(4 Suppl 1):108-110.

52. Woolson ST, Hartford JM, Sawyer A. Results of a method of leg-length equalization for patients undergoing primary total hip replacement. *J Arthroplasty*. 1999;14:159-164.

53. Matsuda K, Nakamura S, Matsushita T. A simple method to minimize limb-length discrepancy after hip arthroplasty. *Acta Orthop*. 2006;77(3):375-379.

54. Manzotti A, Cerveri P, De Momi E, Pullen C, Confalonieri N. Does computer-assisted surgery benefit leg length restoration in total hip replacement? Navigation versus conventional freehand. *Int Orthop*. 2011;35(1):19-24.

55. Woo RY, Morrey B. Dislocations after total hip arthroplasty. *J Bone Joint Surg*. 1982;64-A:1295-1306.

56. Fackler CD, Poss R. Dislocation in total hip arthroplasties. *Clin Orthop*. 1980;151:169-178.

57. Turner RS. Postoperative total hip prosthetic femoral head dislocations: incidence, etiologic factors and management. *Clin Orthop*. 1994;119:263-266.

58. Phillips CB, Barrett JA, Losina E, et al. Incidence rates of dislocation, pulmonary embolism and deep infection during the first six months after elective total hip replacement. *J Bone Joint Surg*. 2003;85:20-26.

59. Bartz RL, Nobel PC, Kadakia NR, Tullos HS. The effect of femoral component head size on posterior dislocation of the artificial hip joint. *J Bone Joint Surg*. 2000;82:1300-1307.

60. Byström S, Espehaug B, Furnes O, Havelin LI; Norwegian Arthroplasty Register. Femoral head size is a risk factor for total hp luxation: a study of 42,987 primary hip arthroplasties from the Norwegian Arthroplasty Register. *Acta Orthop Scand*. 2003;74:514-524.

61. Blumenfeld TJ, Bargar WL. Use of larger femoral heads in revision total hip arthroplasty: will this solve dislocation? *Orthopedics*. 2008;31(10).

62. Krushell RJ, Burke DW, Harris WH. Elevated-rim acetabular components: effect on range of motion and stability in total hip arthroplasty. *J Arthroplasty*. 1991;6(Suppl):S53-S58.

63. Lewinnek GE, Lewis JL, Tarr R, Compere CL, Zimmerman JR. Dislocations after total hip-replacement arthroplasties. *J Bone Joint Surg Am*. 1978;60(2):217-220.

64. Biedermann R, Tonin A, Krismer M, Rachbauer F, Eibl G, Stöckl B. Reducing the risk of dislocation after total hip arthroplasty. *J Bone Joint Surg Br*. 2005;87-B:762-769.

65. Lewinnek GE, Lewis JL, Tarr R, Compere CL, Zimmerman JR. Dislocations after total hip replacement arthroplasties. *J Bone Joint Surg*. 1978;60-A:217-220.

66. Dorr LD, Wan Z. Causes of and treatment protocol for instability of total hip replacement. *Clin Orthop*. 1998;355:144-151.

67. Ritter MA, Harty LD, Keating ME, Faris PM, Meding JB. A clinical comparison of the anterolateral and posterolateral approaches to the hip. *Clin Orthop Relat Res*. 2001;385:95-99.

68. Pellicci PM, Bostrom M, Poss R. Posterior approach to total hip replacement using enhanced posterior soft tissue repair. *Clin Orthop Relat Res*. 1998;(355):224-228.

69. Alberton GM, High WA, Morrey BF. Dislocation after revision total hip arthroplasty: an analysis of risk factors and treatment options. *J Bone Joint Surg Am*. 2002;84-A(10):1788-1792.

70. Hedlundh U, Ahnfelt L, Hybbinette CH, Weckstrom J, Fredin H. Surgical experience related to dislocations after total hip arthroplasty. *J Bone Joint Surg Br*. 1996;78:206-209.

71. Hedlundh U, Fredin H. Patient characteristics in dislocations after primary total hip arthroplasty: 60 patients compared with a control group. *Acta Orthop Scand*. 1995;66:225-228.

72. Woo RY, Morrey BF. Dislocations after total hip arthroplasty. *J Bone Joint Surg Am*. 1982;64(9):1295-1306.

73. Khatod M, Barber T, Paxton E, Namba R, Fithian D. An analysis of the risk of hip dislocation with a contemporary total joint registry. *Clin Orthop Relat Res*. 2006;447:19-23.

74. Masonis JL, Patel JV, Miu A, et al. Subtrochanteric shortening and derotational osteotomy in primary total hip arthroplasty for patients with severe hip dysplasia: 5-year follow-up. *J Arthroplasty*. 2003;18:68-73.

75. Li YJ, Zhang LC, Yang GJ, et al. Prevention of prothesis dislocation after the revision of total hip arthroplasty. *Zhongguo Gu Shang*. 2008;21(3):173-175.

76. Meek RM, Allan DB, McPhillips G, Kerr L, Howie CR. Epidemiology of dislocation after total hip arthroplasty. *Clin Orthop*. 2006;447:9-18.

77. Philippot R, Adam P, Reckhaus M, et al. Prevention of dislocation in total hip revision surgery usign a dual mobility design. *Orthop Traumatol Surg Res*. 2009;95(6):407-413.

78. Restrepo C, Mortazavi SM, Brothers J, Parvizi J, Rothman RH. Hip dislocation: are hip precautions necessary? Eastern Orthopaedic Association 2009; Paradise Island, Bahamas.

79. Kurtz S, Ong K, Lau E, Mowat F, Halpern M. Projections of primary and revision hip and knee arthroplasty in the United States from 2005 to 2030. *J Bone Joint Surg Am*. 2007;89(4):780-785.

12

Special Topic
Osteolysis and Stress Shielding

Michael T. Manley, FRSA, PhD; Steven M. Kurtz, PhD; and Kevin L. Ong, PhD

Approximately 40,000 revision hip arthroplasty procedures are performed annually in the United States.[1] The prognosis for revision joint replacement is generally worse than in primary surgery; revision patients are approximately 5 times more likely of undergoing a subsequent revision compared to patients undergoing their first revision.[2] Furthermore, due to the cost of revision surgery,[3,4] there is great incentive to not only increase the longevity of initial primary joint replacement, but also to reduce the incidence of subsequent revisions for revision patients.

The most commonly reported indications for revision surgery are instability/dislocation, mechanical loosening, and infection, while periprosthetic osteolysis and/or wear accounts for up to 16% of the reasons for revision.[5,6] Although there is significant discussion of osteolysis, bone remodeling, and stress shielding following primary hip arthroplasty, the outcomes of revision surgery, as it pertains to these complications, has not been well studied. Mechanical loosening may be due to a loss of fixation due to periprosthetic bone remodeling or stress shielding. Osteolysis may be further complicated by the need for significant reconstruction during revision surgery, particularly when extensive bone loss is encountered or substantial trabecular bone resection is required during implant removal. The quality of treatment of pre-existing osteolytic lesions or reconstruction with bone graft can affect the risk of subsequent osteolysis, bone remodeling, and stress shielding.

The purpose of this chapter is to provide a comprehensive review of the scientific evidence regarding the prevalence, etiology, prevention, and treatment of osteolysis, bone remodeling, and stress shielding following revision hip arthroplasty.

INCIDENCE

Osteolysis

The incidence of pelvic osteolysis for historical cup designs using conventional polyethylene may be as high as 40%[7] and is related to the quality of polyethylene, the design of the cup, the type of fixation, and implant positioning. Schmalzried et al[8] reported on the incidence of

Jacofsky DJ, Hedley AK.
Fundamentals of Revision Hip Arthroplasty:
Diagnosis, Evaluation, and Treatment (pp 175-188).
© 2013 SLACK Incorporated.

Figure 12-1. Localized/expansive pattern of osteolysis around an uncemented cup. (Reprinted with permission from Zicat B, Engh CA, Gokcen E. Patterns of osteolysis around total hip components inserted with and without cement. *J Bone Joint Surg Am.* 1995;77(3):432-439.)

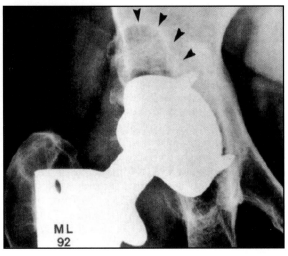

osteolysis following the use of an uncemented acetabular component with conventional polyethylene in 113 hips (93 patients). At an average of 64 months after implantation, although no components were revised for loosening or were radiographically loose, the prevalence of balloon-like pelvic osteolysis was 17% (19 hips). Zicat et al[7] reviewed the radiographs of patients who had been implanted with an extensively porous-coated femoral component, in conjunction with either a cementless acetabular component (74 patients) or cemented component (63 patients). At a mean follow-up of 105 months (range: 54 to 142 months), the rate of pelvic osteolysis in unrevised hips with a cemented acetabular component was 37% (19 of 51) and was most frequently of the linear type. With cementless components, the osteolysis rate was 18% (13 of 71) and tended to be localized and expansive with correspondingly more bone loss (Figure 12-1). However, the linear-type osteolysis found with the cemented cups was associated with a high prevalence of loosening (30%).

Osteolysis with conventional polyethylene bearings seems to depend as much on the quality of fixation of the implants to bone (debris access pathways) as it does to the bearing material itself. Hellman et al[9] followed 76 hips in young active patients implanted with Omnifit-HA femoral and acetabular components (Stryker Orthopaedics, Mahwah, NJ) for 10 years (average). Twenty-five (35.7%) hips showed proximal osteolysis at the femoral resection level or in the acetabulum. Of these, 13 had reoperation with bone graft for large progressive proximal femoral osteolytic lesions independent of stem loosening. However, there were no cases (0%) of intramedullary osteolysis in the series. This finding suggests that the quality of fixation provided by the hydroxyapatite coating prevented debris ingress to the femoral fixation interface. The suggestion that the quality of femoral fixation prevents debris ingress to the femur was confirmed in a different series with the same stem at up to 13 years follow-up.[10] Three-hundred eighty Omnifit-HA stems implanted in patients with an average age of 51 years had a mechanical failure rate of 0.5% at 10 to 13 years after primary surgery. All survivors had bone stable fixation and no patient had distal endosteal osteolysis.

As highly cross-linked polyethylene has become the most common acetabular articulation surface used for total hip arthroplasty (THA), it is expected that the lower wear rates of highly cross-linked polyethylene compared with conventional polyethylene[11] will lead to lower incidence of osteolysis. This has been documented by researchers such as Leung et al,[12] who reported the rate of polyethylene wear and osteolysis in 40 hips implanted with conventional polyethylene and 36 hips implanted with cross-linked polyethylene after a minimum of 5 years postsurgery. The incidence of osteolysis was significantly greater for patients with conventional polyethylene (11/40, 28%) compared to those with cross-linked material (3/36, 8%; p = 0.04). The average lesion volume for hips with conventional polyethylene was also significantly greater (7.5 ± 6.7 cm^3 versus

1.2 ± 0.1 cm^3; p = 0.01). Highly cross-linked polyethylene has also been paired with large diameter femoral heads (>32 mm) in patients considered to be at high risk for dislocation. Geller et al[13] conducted a prospective study of 42 patients (45 hips) who had total hip replacement using large diameter cobalt-chrome femoral heads articulating with a highly cross-linked polyethylene after a minimum of 3 years follow-up. At final follow-up, there were no radiographic failures or episodes of loosening, nor any evidence of pelvic or femoral osteolysis. Lachiewicz et al[14] also reported no incidence of pelvic or femoral osteolysis for 90 patients (102 hips) who were implanted with highly cross-linked polyethylene, after at least 5 years of follow-up (average 5.7 years). The median linear wear rate was 0.028 mm/year (mean 0.04 mm/year), and the median volumetric wear rate was 25.6 mm^3/year (mean 80.5 mm^3/year). These researchers also investigated the effects of head size and found that while the linear wear rate of polyethylene was not related to femoral head diameter, there was greater volumetric wear (156.6 mm^3/year) with the 36- and 40-mm heads.

In addition to highly cross-linked polyethylene, alternative hard-on-hard bearings have also become more widely adopted in the patient population.[15] The predicted 10 to 100 times lower wear rates of ceramic-on-ceramic (COC) and metal-on-metal (MOM) hip bearings compared to conventional polyethylene lead to reductions in the rate of osteolysis. Particle-induced osteolysis with hard-hard hip bearings is thought to be a rare complication.[16,17] According to limited intermediate clinical follow-up, the prevalence of osteolysis in COC and MOM hips is substantially lower compared to that of conventional ultrahigh-molecular-weight polyethylene. Recent reports have suggested noise with some COC bearings, with squeaking rates ranging from 0.7% to 20.9% in different series.[18] In a few instances, the noise may be severe enough for the patient to contemplate revision.[19]

In MOM implants, revisions are linked to early osteolysis due to an apparent delayed hypersensitivity to metal.[17,20] This association is not completely understood. Park et al[20] performed a retrospective review of 165 patients (169 hips) who had undergone primary cementless total hip replacement with a contemporary MOM total hip design in the early 2000s. After a minimum follow-up of 2 years, 9 patients (10 hips) developed an osteolytic lesion localized to the greater trochanter. Based on skin-patch tests, these 9 patients had a significantly higher rate of hypersensitivity reaction to cobalt compared with total hip patient controls (p=0.031). It remains unclear if a causal relationship between metal hypersensitivity and osteolysis exists.

More recently, the risk of pseudotumors in MOM hips have also been reported[21-26] and may cause pain and lead to revision surgery. The outcome of revision for pseudotumor is poor; the incidence of major complications after revision for pseudotumor has been reported to be significantly higher than for revisions due to other causes (50% versus 14%) in some series.[26] The tissue reactions can be caused by high implant wear, but may also occur with low implant wear. The cause of these reactions is not well understood but could be due to excessive wear, metal hypersensitivity, or an as-yet unknown cause.

Stress Shielding

Due to the removal of host bone and use of bone graft during the revision procedure, revision joints may be susceptible to postoperative bone remodeling changes. The extent of periprosthetic bone remodeling following revision hip surgery has been generally reported for the femur, but is not as well documented for the acetabulum. In the femur, most of the changes in bone mineral density (BMD) occur in Gruen zones I and VII, so-called proximal stress shielding, regardless of revision stem design. Furthermore, to reduce the risk of loosening, extensively coated femoral implants or distally anchored stems may be used, which could potentially unload the proximal bone.

Adolphson et al[27] reported on the BMD changes following revision THA with a proximally porous and hydroxyapatite-coated stem (Bi-Metric stem; Biomet Inc, Warsaw, IN) in 22 hips. At a mean follow-up of 6 years, there was a marked reduction in BMD on the reoperated femur in all regions compared to the unoperated side. The largest reduction of 36% to 45% occurred in zones

Figure 12-2. Proximal femoral stress shielding at 4-years postsurgery. The 55-year-old female had preoperative bone loss of grade 3. (Reprinted with permission from Kimura H, Kaneuji A, Sugimori T, Matsumoto T. Revision total hip arthroplasty by nonmodular short and long cementless stems. *J Orthop Sci.* 2008;13(4):335-340.)

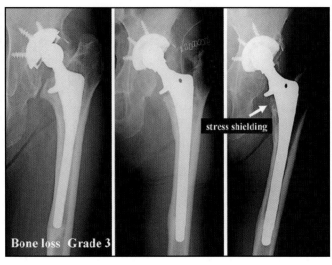

stress shielding

Bone loss Grade 3

I, II, VI, and VII. Hydroxyapatite-ceramic coated stems (JRI-Furlong stem; JRI Instrumentation Ltd, London, UK) were implanted by Raman et al[28] in 82 consecutive revision hip patients (86 hips). In 81 hips with radiological follow-up (12.6 years mean follow-up), major signs of osseointegration were observed in 76 femoral components (94%). Stress shielding was seen around 23 femoral components (28%) in the proximal metaphysis with minimal amounts of resorption in 15 hips (18.5%) and moderate bone loss in 8 hips (10%). No proximal femur showed complete cortical resorption and the stress shielding did not progress after the first 3 years.

In the revision situation, Mahoney et al[29] performed a retrospective analysis of 40 patients who underwent revision THA with extensively hydroxyapatite-coated long stem (Restoration HA stem, Stryker Orthopaedics), 39 of whom had severe bone destruction and were classified as grade 3 or 4 using either Paprosky or Endo-Klinic classification systems. Calcar resorption was observed in 44% of the femurs at 1 year and 72% at 5 years, but further clinically significant stress shielding was only observed in one hip. Although the rate of clinically significant stress shielding was low, the authors noted that this finding may have been confounded by the severity of femoral destruction seen in most of these patients before the revision procedure (ie, stress shielding could not be exhibited because they contained too little intact bone). All femurs demonstrated bone ingrowth in multiple zones by approximately 1 year postoperatively. At a minimum of 5 years postoperatively (average 7.4 years), bone ingrowth was observed in 80% of the femurs in zones I and VII.

Proximally porous-coated short stems or fully porous-coated long stems were implanted in 20 patients that were followed for 2 to 6 years (mean 4.3 years).[30] Proximally porous-coated short stems (HA/TCP Anatomic Hip Prosthesis, Zimmer, Inc, Warsaw, IN) were used in 5 femurs with minimal bone loss, while fully porous-coated long stems (Versys Beaded Fullcoat Plus, Zimmer, Inc) were used in the remaining femurs with metaphyseal bone loss. The incidence of stress shielding was 45% (9 hips: 7 with the fully porous-coated long stem and 2 with the proximally porous-coated short stem) (Figure 12-2). Two hips with calcar rounding had first-degree stress shielding, while 4 hips with isolated calcar loss had second-degree stress shielding and 3 hips with loss of cortical density proximal to the diaphysis had third-degree stress shielding. However, none of these patients had symptoms related to stress shielding and stress shielding did not have an effect on the clinical results.

In addition to monoblock stems, modular revision stems have also been widely used, some of which have a long clinical history. The versatility of the modular systems enables accommodation of patients with different bony deficiencies and anatomic features such as offset and stem length. McCarthy et al[31] retrospectively reviewed the outcomes for 67 hips (57 uncemented, 10 cemented) using a proximally coated, modular femoral component (S-ROM, DePuy, Warsaw, IN). These stems were used in complex revision cases with 52 (78%) of these hips classified as Paprosky class III and IV, 19 of which were class IIIB or IV. With a mean follow-up of 14 years (minimum 8 years), bone ingrowth was observed in 47 (82%) of the 57 uncemented hips. Thirty-three (57%) of the uncemented hips also exhibited endosteal hypertrophy. Nonbridging pedestals also occurred in 50% of cases from the distal stem abutting the anterior cortex. There was mild calcar resorption in 28% of the hips, while proximal lysis resulted in 4 hips (all went on to revision) and no distal lysis was found.

Koster et al[32] reported on the outcomes for 48 patients (49 hips) who were implanted with the Profemur-R modular revision stem (Wright Medical Technology, Arlington, TN) at an average of 6.2 years post-surgery. Persistent periprosthetic defects were evident in 43 (88%) of the 49 femurs immediate post-surgery, but at the last follow-up examination, these defects were no longer radiologically visible in 30 (70%) of the 43 hips, while partial restoration of defects could be observed in the remaining 13 hips (30%). The number of osteolysis in a given area was also markedly reduced, decreasing from 39 to 8 in Gruen zone VII, from 30 to 4 in zone VI, from 34 to 9 in zone I, and from 37 to 8 in zone II. Stress shielding was also observed around 7 stems, but only 2 showed generalized atrophy. The remaining 5 developed atrophy only proximally, with the implant distally fixed.

In contrast, there is very limited information regarding periacetabular bone remodeling following revision hip surgery. In a radiographic analysis of 59 revision hip patients using a hydroxyapatite-coated threaded cup or a nonthreaded hydroxyapatite-cup with augmented screw fixation (JRI-Furlong), Raman et al[28] found bone ingrowth in at least 52 (88%) acetabular components, indicating stable fixation. Eighty-six percent of the cups produced ingrowth in DeLee-Charnley zone I, while 39% and 66% of the cups had ingrowth in zones II and III, respectively. Studies involving bone remodeling around primary acetabular components have shown that, in the presence of an uncemented cup, the load bypasses the periacetabular trabecular bone in most regions around the implant and is transferred instead through the superior cortical bone. This may be due to the elasticity mismatch that focuses stresses to the peripheral cortical regions. The presence of a cementless cup appears to shift the proximal stress distribution from the central cancellous bone to the peripheral cortical bone.[33,34] Although an increase in proximal cortical bone density may result, an overall decrease in combined cancellous and cortical bone density has been observed,[34] which indicates an altered stress pattern due to cup implantation. Wright et al also reported similar bone remodeling phenomenon in 26 patients who underwent hybrid THA with uncemented hemispherical Ti-alloy cup.[35] These patients experienced decreases in cancellous bone mineral density of 20% to 33%, superior to the cup, at 1.3 years postoperatively.

Cancellous bone density has been reported to decline progressively by as much as 30% cranially, 49% anteriorly, and 66% posteriorly at 3 years post-surgery in uncemented acetabuli.[36] Concurrently, cortical bone density remained relatively stable superior to the cup, increasing by 7%, but bone loss was progressive in the anterior (-12%) and posterior (-22%) regions. Korovessis et al also measured no significant bone changes in DeLee-Charnley zone I for 33 uncemented Zweymueller hips after mean 25 months follow-up.[37] However, there was a combined cortical and cancellous BMD reduction of 19% and 24% in the medial (zone II) and caudal (zone III) regions compared to the contralateral hip. In a study of 50 patients undergoing bilateral uncemented THA with an alumina liner on one side and polyethylene liner on the other side, Kim et al observed significant regional changes in BMD in all zones for both liner groups after 5 years postoperatively.[38] BMD increased in both groups by 20% in DeLee-Charnley zone I (p = 0.003), but decreased by 24% and 25% in zone II (p = 0.001) for the alumina and polyethylene groups, respectively. Although both groups exhibited progressive bone loss in zone III in the first 3 years (24%: alumina; 17%: polyethylene), these were restored to baseline levels at final follow-up. Interestingly, the study also concluded that the change in stiffness of the liner was insufficient to affect density changes, which indicates that the choice of liner material could not overcome the stiffness of the metal backing. Similar lack of influence of soft and hard liners have also been reported by others.[33]

By comparison, the cemented cup often preserves bone quality and may produce bone gain in some isolated periprosthetic regions. Mueller et al were one of the few to report bone loss following computed tomography (CT) evaluation of 3 sites (anterior, posterior, and cranial) in cemented acetabular patients (n = 15) after 26 months postsurgery.[39] They found that the mean cortical and cancellous BMD decreased significantly by 16% and 31%, respectively, in the anterior region, though these were relatively unchanged in the posterior and cranial regions. In contrast, the bone around 19 cemented Mueller cups exhibited 27% higher BMD in DeLee-Charnley zone I,[37] compared with the contralateral hip. Digas et al did not find significant proximal BMD changes at 2 years follow-up, but instead measured 14% BMD increase in the distal region over the ischial tuberosity.[40] Digas and coworkers also conducted another DEXA study comparing the relative changes in BMD around cemented all-polyethylene cups with either conventional or highly cross-linked polyethylene.[41] At 2 years postoperatively, the conventional polyethylene and highly cross-linked polyethylene groups had significant increases in BMD distally over the ischial tuberosity (+11.7%) and proximally above the cup (+12.0%), respectively.

From these studies, one may conclude that the bone loss around cementless cups is generally greater than around cemented prostheses. Due to the short follow-up in many of the studies, it is presently unclear if the reported bone changes may progress and lead to complications such as implant loosening.

ETIOLOGY

The generation of prosthetic implant wear in total joint arthroplasty patients is widely recognized as the major initiating event in development of periprosthetic osteolysis and aseptic loosening. Linear and expansive bone resorption around total joint prostheses was initially attributed to "cement disease" or fragmented cement around loosened cemented implants.[42] However, focal areas of bone resorption were later noted around uncemented implants that were believed to be mechanically stable, whereby focal aggregates of macrophages with particulate polyethylene and metallic debris were identified in histological samples.[43] This led to the identification of the inflammatory response of cells to wear debris as the most important underlying cause of osteolysis.

Several different cell types have been implicated in the development of periprosthetic osteolysis in response to wear debris; however, the principal cells associated with periprosthetic osteolysis are macrophages, fibroblasts, and osteoclasts.[44,45] Because the macrophages and fibroblasts are unable to digest most of the inorganic particles that they ingest, the cells synthesize and release a large number of cytokines, growth factors, and proteolytic enzymes. This has been demonstrated by the elevated levels of proinflammatory cytokines in periprosthetic tissues and joint synovial fluid of osteolysis patients. While an inflammatory response by macrophages is central to the development of periprosthetic osteolysis, the nature of this response depends on multiple factors such as prosthetic type, patterns of wear, and host factors. The cellular and molecular regulation of osteoclastogenesis and the influence of wear debris is graphically shown and summarized in Figure 12-3.

The importance of mechanical loading to the maintenance of bone volume or bone density is also well recognized. According to Wolff's law, the structural properties of bone alter to an extent that is determined in large part by the magnitude of change in mechanical stress, which in turn is influenced by the stiffness of the implant. Total joint arthroplasty can dramatically alter the magnitude and direction of load transmission through the joint, so that localized bone remodeling may be expected. Furthermore, implants of different designs or mechanisms of fixation may have different effects on bone remodeling, in which some designs might produce more favorable long-term remodeling patterns than others.

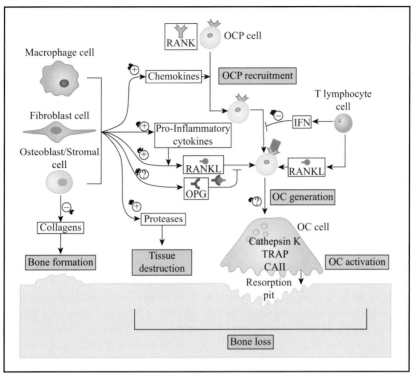

Figure 12-3. Complex network of pathogenesis in the development of periprosthetic osteolysis. Osteoclast precursor cells (OCP) are recruited to the periprosthetic tissues and differentiate into functional osteoclasts (OC), which resorb bone by generation of a resorption pit into which enzymes such as Cathepsin K, tartrate-resistant acid phosphatase (TRAP), and carbonic anhydrase II (CAII) are secreted. Osteoclast maturation and activation is mediated by interaction of receptor activator for nuclear factor kB ligand (RANKL; which can also exist as a cell surface signaling molecule) with the OCP receptor RANK. Osteoprotegerin (OPG), a soluble decoy receptor for RANKL, inhibits this pathway, as does the T lymphocyte cytokine, interferon (IFN) gamma. Various other cell types, including macrophages, fibroblasts, and osteoblasts, can modulate this pathway via production of chemokines and proinflammatory cytokines, and can also contribute directly to tissue destruction and/or formation through expression of proteases and collagens. Positive (+) and negative (–) effects of wear particles on key aspects of this complex regulatory system are shown, as are important steps where possible particles involvement has yet to be established. (Adapted from Purdue PE, Koulouvaris P, Nestor BJ, Sculco TP. The central role of wear debris in periprosthetic osteolysis. *HSS J*. 2006;2(2):102-113.)

Since it is not uncommon to use impaction grafting to replace missing bone during revision hip arthroplasty, the remodeling of the graft can play a critical role in providing structural support and enhancing the longevity of the joint replacement. It is believed that graft remodeling involves a complicated sequence of biological events whereby minimum bone formation may be initiated 1 month after implantation.[46] After 8 to 11 months, the osteoid or bone layer might have a thickness of 3 to 5 mm. After 2 years, bone with hematopoietic marrow is primarily present, except in some locations that likely are not carrying load where the graft will be resorbed and may not be replaced with living bone. The graft particles were usually embedded in dense fibrous tissue, thus forming a supporting composite tissue capable of carrying load.[47]

PREVENTION

Since the underlying mechanism for osteolysis is the inflammatory response to wear debris, strategies for preventing osteolysis should focus on minimizing wear production. This involves the appropriate selection of implant materials and implant designs, as well as careful attention to implant positioning and patient selection. These preventive strategies also apply to minimizing mechanically induced stress shielding.

With regards to implant materials, although the conventional polyethylene has shown excellent physical characteristics and a low coefficient of friction, it has been associated with wear rates of up to 0.55 mm/year.[48] Highly cross-linked polyethylene was introduced in the United States in the late 1990s to reduce the wear rate and accumulation of wear debris. The intent of these second-generation materials is to reduce the potential for material oxidation in the long term while preserving the bulk mechanical properties necessary to use cross-linked polyethylene in higher stress applications, such as thin acetabular liners with larger diameter heads. The improved resistance of highly cross-linked polyethylene to wear and delamination has been shown in hip simulator studies.[49,50] The intermediate clinical results of contemporary highly cross-linked polyethylene have been encouraging, with further follow-up needed to confirm the benefits in long-term patient outcomes. The use of hard-on-hard bearings may also alleviate the incidence of osteolysis, but again, the clinical performance of contemporary designs still requires longer term follow-up.

Surgical considerations such as the choice of implant design may also influence bone remodeling. To maintain bone stock, load must be transferred from the stem to the proximal part of the femur. However, in the revision situation, the proximal femur often has compromised bone tissue. To maintain sufficient stem stability, a long stem may be used, which is designed to provide distal fixation. However, distal fixation decreases proximal load transfer from stem to bone and will increase the risk of proximal stress shielding and proximal bone loss. Most revisions of the femoral component therefore become a compromise between 2 goals, fixation and proximal load transfer with fixation as the highest priority. As an alternative solution, femoral stems with reduced stiffness have the potential of decreasing stress shielding by maintaining physiological loading of the periprosthetic bone and could be an alternative in revision surgery when restoration of bone stock is required. Karrholm et al[51] retrospectively reviewed the bone remodeling around a low stiffness stem in 30 patients (32 hips) with a minimum 2-year follow-up. The stem had a central core of cobalt-chromium surrounded by a polymer and an outer titanium mesh layer containing a proximal coating of hydroxyapatite/tricalcium phosphate. Impacted morselized allografting was used around the stem in 28 of 32 hips. Measurements of bone mineral density at 6 months showed a slight decrease (down to 3%) in zones II to V, no change in zone VII, or a slight increase (up to 5%) in zones I and VI, followed by a further increase up to 2 years in 3 of the regions (2, 3, and 5). Conventional radiography at 2 years demonstrated graft remodeling and incomplete radiolucent lines in 19 hips, mainly in zones I and VII.

Implant positioning is also a critical factor in minimizing wear debris formation,[8,52-55] bone remodeling and osteolysis. On the acetabular side, a high cup angle may lead to the head being constrained by the superior lateral surface and rim of the cup, thus changing the location of the contact zone between the head and the cup and increasing the risk of edge loading. Increases in linear wear of at least 40% have been observed clinically for cups with an abduction angle greater than 45 degrees.[55] Malpositioning of the cup, as well as the femoral component, may also lead to cup-neck impingement,[56,57] providing another mechanism for accelerated wear formation.

The use of grafts treated with bisphosphonates has also been suggested to block resorption of bone during impaction grafting to replace missing bone at revision surgery. Kesteris et al[58] treated 15 patients who were randomized to receive morselized compacted bone allograft which had been rinsed in either an ibandronate solution or in saline. Rinsing the graft in a bisphosphonate solution was found to prevent graft resorption. In the 8 control patients, the grafts were already partially resorbed after 3 months with a decrease in bone density of 9% and then remained constant at this lower level. A large proportion of the mass of the bone graft was lost. In contrast, all 7 patients with grafts treated with bisphosphonate showed a slight (2%) increase in bone density at 3 months and did not change subsequently. The difference between the groups was highly significant at all points in time. However, the safety and efficacy of the widespread use of biphosphonates in impaction grafting still needs to be established.

Periprosthetic osteogenesis may also be promoted by biophysical stimulation, such as electromagnetic fields and low intensity pulsed ultrasound, which were initially developed to accelerate fracture healing. Pulsed electromagnetic field (PEMF) stimulation is one such example and is a noninvasive therapeutic method used to enhance endogenous bone repair and reduce inflammatory events. A randomized, prospective, double-blind study by Dallari et al[59] evaluated the efficacy of PEMF after hip revision surgery to improve bone healing around the prosthesis and reduce the time to functional recovery. Fifteen patients used PEMF at least 6 hours per day from day 7 to day 90, while the remaining 15 patients were placed in a placebo group. The overall increase in BMD was found to be more evident among stimulated subjects. In Gruen zones V and VI, 40% of the control patients demonstrated increase in BMD in both areas, while there was an increase in BMD in 93% and 66% of the stimulated patients, respectively. Due to the short-term follow-up of these patients, it is unclear if the positive effect of PEMF stimulation on BMD will be maintained.

TREATMENT

Acetabulum

Acetabular reconstruction is conducted to provide long-term stability of the acetabular component and restore normal hip mechanics. Surgical modes of treatment are based on the quality, amount, and location of bone loss. Challenging treatment scenarios include defects where the host bone will not support a minimum of 50% of the acetabular component, necessitating reconstruction of surrounding support structures. Treatment of pelvic osteolysis includes treating the osteolytic defect itself in addition to the source of the debris particles. The mode of treatment is based on the stability of the acetabular component and the size and localization of the lesion. For example, revision with a cementless cup is usually warranted in the case of a loose cemented cup because bone grafting is necessary. However, for a well-fixed cementless cup with pelvic osteolysis, there are 2 strategies available:

1. Revision of a cup with or without graft
2. Liner exchange with débridement and/or graft

The use of liner exchange with débridement and graft is limited to patients where the lesion is accessible without implant removal. According to Mallory et al, the cautious mode of treatment is to remove the entire acetabular component to eliminate and avoid the introduction of adverse variables, which may contribute further to the continuation of the osteolytic process.[60]

If liner exchange is opted as the treatment method to remove the source of the debris, access to the osteolytic defect may be limited. Engh et al[61] investigated the quality of osteolysis grafting with cementless cup retention in 13 patients and found that 4 of 22 lesions were neglected at the time of surgery, even with preoperative CT reconstructions and surgical planning. In the 18 lesions that were treated, an average of 49% of the lesion volume was filled. Egawa et al[62] reported similar findings on 10 patients treated with polyethylene liner exchange with débridement and grafting of periacetabular osteolytic lesions using a calcium sulfate bone graft substitute. Relative to the preoperative osteolytic lesion volume, an average of 43% (range: 8% to 72%) of each defect was filled with graft at revision. After resorption of the graft, an average of 24% (range: 9% to 44%) of the original defect volume demonstrated evidence of new mineralization at 1-year follow-up. The amount of new mineralization was directly proportional to the defect filling achieved at revision. In contrast, untreated osteolytic defects showed almost no new bone formation, but demonstrated no enlargement of the preoperative lesion volume. These studies emphasize the need to refine the surgical technique, such as the development of small flexible scopes to improve the visibility of the lesions.[61]

To achieve stable bone ingrowth of acetabular prosthetic components, stable initial interfaces with close contact and an adequate amount of viable host bone is necessary. In cases of acetabular component revision where there is both inadequate and compromised host bone, long-term biologic ingrowth may not be achieved with conventional uncemented porous surfaces. Malkani et al[63] found that in patients with only 50% host bone available for initial fixation, a durable biologic fixation was achieved with at least 2 years follow-up when the initial implant stability was augmented with the use of tantalum wedges . Excellent short-term clinical and radiographic results in patients undergoing acetabular revision with Paprosky type II and type III defects were reported. Implant stability can be achieved also with the use of a cementless hemispherical cup at the anatomic hip center or high hip center, a jumbo cup, an oblong cup, or an uncemented cup initially supported by structural allograft until ingrowth is achieved.[64] Positioning components at a high hip center can provide adequate potential for ingrowth in remaining superior bone stock at a nonanatomic position. However, this method of acetabular reconstruction alters mechanical forces about the hip and is associated with a higher rate of aseptic loosening. In patients with severe medial bone loss, reinforcement rings can be used to place a cemented acetabular component in an anatomic position, which allows stress to be distributed to the remaining periphery of the acetabulum. Antiprotrusio cages remain a useful device in patients with significant acetabular bone loss. They place the hip center near an anatomic location and restore bone stock, while also creating a stable construct for cementing of a polyethylene component to allow for delivery of antibiotics locally and adjustment of version and abduction independent of cage position. The cages bridge the acetabular defect with support from the ilium superiorly and the pubis and ischium inferiorly. This allows for potential bone ingrowth because the cage increases the allograft contact area, acting to decrease the forces across the bone graft. However, if support from the allograft or host bone is not adequate, the use of a cage may provide unacceptable results.

Femoral

The use of cementless femoral components has become predominant for femoral revisions. The commonly used stems include the following:

- Extensively coated cylindrical design
- Proximally coated cylindrical or anatomically shaped designs
- Modular designs

For the treatment of femoral defects, a femoral component, in principal, should be fixed as proximally as possible to prevent stress shielding followed by bone atrophy of the proximal femur. However, for revision surgeries, patients may need distal fixation if the proximal femur has suffered severe bone loss. Based on the extent of bone loss, proximally fixed cementless short stems and fully fixed cementless long stems are used during revision THA. While early cobalt-chrome designs have shown to have a risk of stress shielding and thigh pain,[65] contemporary designs have incorporated refinements such as the use of less rigid material (eg, titanium alloy) and distal tapers, but little published information is available regarding outcomes. Hydroxyapatite coatings have been used as an alternative to porous coating to promote osteoconduction in revision cases.[27-29] Condensation of bone around hydroxyapatite-coated components have been observed, restoring structural integrity to these severely diseased proximal femurs.[29]

Femoral revision with cavitary and segmental bone loss can be facilitated by the use of a modular stem that allows independent metaphyseal/diaphyseal sizing, stem-to-neck length options, and adjustable offset and version. A proximally coated modular stem provides adequate fixation in femurs that have sufficient proximal bone stock such as those in Paprosky class II or IIIA. However, due to cavitary or structural bone loss, metaphyseal/diaphyseal mismatches often exist during revision surgery. The use of a modular stem can provide reliable fixation with relative preservation of proximal bone stock in complex revisions.[31]

Impaction grafting is an alternative technique to maintain or improve proximal femoral bone stock but results from this technique have been variable. If bony fixation can be achieved reliably using a proximal ingrowth stem, it appears desirable to use such stems in revision cases. Using impaction grafting in lieu of long stem distal ingrown prostheses prevents violation of the femoral canal distally and can reduce proximal bone loss caused by stress shielding.

The use of biological factors and stem cells to aid in the longevity of the revision stem has also been investigated. Korda et al[66] explored the use of allograft impaction with mesenchymal stem cells in an ovine hip hemiarthroplasty model. Their study showed that the use of stem cells generated significantly more new bone at the implant-allograft interface and within the graft than the control group. These results indicate that stem cells on an allograft scaffold increases bone formation and suggest that its use may be beneficial for patients undergoing revision surgery where the bone stock is compromised.

Another biological approach for therapeutic treatment is the use of anti-inflammatory agents and suppressors of bone resorption.[44] Anti-inflammatory agents, such as COX-2 inhibitors and tumor necrosis factor antagonists, have yielded encouraging results, demonstrating diminished particle induced osteolysis in animal models.[67,68] The bisphosphonate class of osteoclast inhibitors also holds promise for the prevention and treatment of osteolysis, but it has yet to be determined how well these agents will perform in a clinical setting. Alendronate and zoledronic acid have been shown to inhibit wear debris-induced osteolysis in various animal models,[69,70] but there is presently little or no clinical evidence supporting the effectiveness of these drugs in the treatment of osteolysis patients.

SUMMARY

Revision prostheses have poorer outcomes compared with primary joint replacement because the bone quality where the revision prosthesis is to be implanted is usually compromised with loss of bone mass, osteoporosis, bone defects, and lack of structural integrity. Poorer implant bed quality compared to primary arthroplasty impairs reparative osteogenesis around revision implants. Favorable bone remodeling is further complicated when wide areas of osteolysis are present. Lack of stability may contribute to fixation failure, leading to further loss of structural support, further ingress of wear debris, and increased risk of osteolysis. All of these factors weigh against the survivorship of the revision femur and acetabular component. Analysis of the Medicare database shows that patients that undergo revision hip surgery are almost 5 times more likely to undergo a subsequent rerevision surgery compared with primary THA patients.

REFERENCES

1. Agency for Healthcare Research and Quality. *HCUP Databases.* Healthcare Cost and Utilization Project (HCUP) Web site. http://www.hcup-us.ahrq.gov/nisoverview.jsp. Accessed January 9, 2009.

2. Ong KL, Lau E, Suggs J, Kurtz SM, Manley MT. *Clin Orthop Relat Res.* 2010;468(11):3070-3076.

3. Bozic KJ, Durbhakula S, Berry DJ, et al. Differences in patient and procedure characteristics and hospital resource use in primary and revision total joint arthroplasty: a multicenter study. *J Arthroplasty.* 2005;20 (7 Suppl 3):17-25.

4. Bozic KJ, Katz P, Cisternas M, Ono L, Ries MD, Showstack J. Hospital resource utilization for primary and revision total hip arthroplasty. *J Bone Joint Surg Am.* 2005;87(3):570-576.

5. Bozic KJ, Kurtz SM, Lau E, Ong K, Vail TP, Berry DJ. The epidemiology of revision total hip arthroplasty in the United States. *J Bone Joint Surg Am.* 2009;91(1):128-133.

6. Springer BD, Fehring TK, Griffin WL, Odum SM, Masonis JL. Why revision total hip arthroplasty fails. *Clin Orthop Relat Res.* 2009;467(1):166-173.

7. Zicat B, Engh CA, Gokcen E. Patterns of osteolysis around total hip components inserted with and without cement. *J Bone Joint Surg Am.* 1995;77(3):432-439.

8. Schmalzried TP, Guttmann D, Grecula M, Amstutz HC. The relationship between the design, position, and articular wear of acetabular components inserted without cement and the development of pelvic osteolysis. *J Bone Joint Surg Am.* 1994;76(5):677-688.

9. Hellman EJ, Capello WN, Feinberg JR. Omnifit cementless total hip arthroplasty. A 10-year average followup. *Clin Orthop Relat Res.* 1999;(364):164-174.

10. D'Antonio JA, Capello WN, Manley MT, Geesink R. Hydroxyapatite femoral stems for total hip arthroplasty: 10- to 13-year followup. *Clin Orthop Relat Res.* 2001;(393):101-111.

11. Dorr LD, Wan Z, Shahrdar C, Sirianni L, Boutary M, Yun A. Clinical performance of a Durasul highly cross-linked polyethylene acetabular liner for total hip arthroplasty at five years. *J Bone Joint Surg Am.* 2005;87(8):1816-1821.

12. Leung SB, Egawa H, Stepniewski A, Beykirch S, Engh CA Jr, Engh CA Sr. Incidence and volume of pelvic osteolysis at early follow-up with highly cross-linked and noncross-linked polyethylene. *J Arthroplasty.* 2007;22(6 Suppl 2):134-139.

13. Geller JA, Malchau H, Bragdon C, Greene M, Harris WH, Freiberg AA. Large diameter femoral heads on highly cross-linked polyethylene: minimum 3-year results. *Clin Orthop Relat Res.* 2006;447:53-59.

14. Lachiewicz PF, Heckman DS, Soileau ES, Mangla J, Martell JM. Femoral head size and wear of highly cross-linked polyethylene at 5 to 8 years. *Clin Orthop Relat Res.* 2009;467(12):3290-3296.

15. Bozic KJ, Kurtz S, Lau E, et al. The epidemiology of bearing surface usage in total hip arthroplasty in the United States. *J Bone Joint Surg Am.* 2009;91(7):1614-1620.

16. Silva M, Heisel C, Schmalzried TP. Metal-on-metal total hip replacement. *Clin Orthop Relat Res.* 2005;(430):53-61.

17. Willert HG, Buchhorn GH, Fayyazi A, et al. Metal-on-metal bearings and hypersensitivity in patients with artificial hip joints. A clinical and histomorphological study. *J Bone Joint Surg Am.* 2005;87(1):28-36.

18. Mai K, Verioti C, Ezzet KA, Copp SN, Walker RH, Colwell CW Jr. Incidence of "squeaking" after ceramic-on-ceramic total hip arthroplasty. *Clin Orthop Relat Res.* 2010;468(2):413-417.

19. Jarrett CA, Ranawat AS, Bruzzone M, Blum YC, Rodriguez JA, Ranawat CS. The squeaking hip: a phenomenon of ceramic-on-ceramic total hip arthroplasty. *J Bone Joint Surg Am.* 2009;91(6):1344-1349.

20. Park YS, Moon YW, Lim SJ, Yang JM, Ahn G, Choi YL. Early osteolysis following second-generation metal-on-metal hip replacement. *J Bone Joint Surg Am.* 2005;87(7):1515-1521.

21. Mahendra G, Pandit H, Kliskey K, Murray D, Gill HS, Athanasou N. Necrotic and inflammatory changes in metal-on-metal resurfacing hip arthroplasties. *Acta Orthop.* 2009;80(6):653-659.

22. Kwon YM, Thomas P, Summer B, et al. Lymphocyte proliferation responses in patients with pseudotumors following metal-on-metal hip resurfacing arthroplasty. *J Orthop Res.* 2010;28(4):444-450.

23. Clayton RA, Beggs I, Salter DM, Grant MH, Patton JT, Porter DE. Inflammatory pseudotumor associated with femoral nerve palsy following metal-on-metal resurfacing of the hip. A case report. *J Bone Joint Surg Am.* 2008;90(9):1988-1993.

24. Grammatopoulos G, Pandit H, Glyn-Jones S, et al. Optimal acetabular orientation for hip resurfacing. *J Bone Joint Surg Br.* 2010;92(8):1072-1078.

25. Glyn-Jones S, Pandit H, Kwon YM, Doll H, Gill HS, Murray DW. Risk factors for inflammatory pseudotumor formation following hip resurfacing. *J Bone Joint Surg Br.* 2009;91(12):1566-1574.

26. Grammatopolous G, Pandit H, Kwon YM, et al. Hip resurfacings revised for inflammatory pseudotumor have a poor outcome. *J Bone Joint Surg Br.* 2009;91(8):1019-1024.

27. Adolphson PY, Salemyr MO, Sköldenberg OG, Bodén HS. Large femoral bone loss after hip revision using the uncemented proximally porous-coated Bi-Metric prosthesis: 22 hips followed for a mean of 6 years. *Acta Orthop.* 2009;80(1):14-19.

28. Raman R, Kamath RP, Parikh A, Angus PD. Revision of cemented hip arthroplasty using a hydroxyapatite-ceramic-coated femoral component. *J Bone Joint Surg Br.* 2005;87(8):1061-1067.

29. Mahoney OM, Kinsey TL, Asayama I. Durable fixation with a modern fully hydroxylapatite-coated long stem in complex revision total hip arthroplasty. *J Arthroplasty.* 2010;25(3):355-562.

30. Kimura H, Kaneuji A, Sugimori T, Matsumoto T. Revision total hip arthroplasty by nonmodular short and long cementless stems. *J Orthop Sci.* 2008;13(4):335-340.

31. McCarthy JC, Lee JA. Complex revision total hip arthroplasty with modular stems at a mean of 14 years. *Clin Orthop Relat Res.* 2007;465:166-169.

32. Koster G, Walde TA, Willert HG. Five- to 10-year results using a noncemented modular revision stem without bone grafting. *J Arthroplasty.* 2008;23(7):964-970.

33. Pitto RP, Bhargava A, Pandit S, Munro JT. Retroacetabular stress-shielding in THA. *Clin Orthop Relat Res.* 2008;466(2):353-358.

34. Schmidt R, Muller L, Kress A, Hirschfelder H, Aplas A, Pitto RP. A computed tomography assessment of femoral and acetabular bone changes after total hip arthroplasty. *Int Orthop.* 2002;26(5):299-302.

35. Wright JM, Pellicci PM, Salvati EA, Ghelman B, Roberts MM, Koh JL. Bone density adjacent to press-fit acetabular components. A prospective analysis with quantitative computed tomography. *J Bone Joint Surg.* 2001;83-A(4):529-536.

36. Mueller LA, Voelk M, Kress A, Pitto RP, Schmidt R. An ABJS best paper: progressive cancellous and cortical bone remodeling after press-fit cup fixation: a 3-year followup. *Clin Orthop Relat Res.* 2007;463:213-220.

37. Korovessis P, Piperos G, Michael A. Periprosthetic bone mineral density after Mueller and Zweymueller total hip arthroplasties. *Clin Orthop Relat Res.* 1994;(309):214-221.

38. Kim YH, Yoon SH, Kim JS. Changes in the bone mineral density in the acetabulum and proximal femur after cementless total hip replacement: alumina-on-alumina versus alumina-on-polyethylene articulation. *J Bone Joint Surg Br.* 2007;89(2):174-179.

39. Mueller LA, Nowak TE, Mueller LP, et al. Acetabular cortical and cancellous bone density and radiolucent lines after cemented total hip arthroplasty: a prospective study using computed tomography and plain radiography. *Arch Orthop Trauma Surg.* 2007;127(10):909-917.

40. Digas G, Karrholm J, Thanner J. Different loss of BMD using uncemented press-fit and whole polyethylene cups fixed with cement: repeated DXA studies in 96 hips randomized to 3 types of fixation. *Acta Orthop.* 2006;77(2):218-226.

41. Digas G, Kärrholm J, Thanner J, Malchau H, Herberts P. Highly cross-linked polyethylene in cemented THA: randomized study of 61 hips. *Clin Orthop Relat Res.* 2003;(417):126-138.

42. Jones LC, Hungerford DS. Cement disease. *Clin Orthop Relat Res.* 1987;(225):192-206.

43. Maloney WJ, Jasty M, Harris WH, Galante JO, Callaghan JJ. Endosteal erosion in association with stable uncemented femoral components. *J Bone Joint Surg Am.* 1990;72(7):1025-1034.

44. Purdue PE, Koulouvaris P, Nestor BJ, Sculco TP. The central role of wear debris in periprosthetic osteolysis. *HSS J.* 2006;2(2):102-113.

45. Rubash HE, Sinha RK, Shanbhag AS, Kim SY. Pathogenesis of bone loss after total hip arthroplasty. *Orthop Clin North Am.* 1998;29(2):173-186.

46. Ullmark G, Obrant KJ. Histology of impacted bone-graft incorporation. *J Arthroplasty.* 2002;17(2):150-157.

47. Linder L. Cancellous impaction grafting in the human femur: histological and radiographic observations in 6 autopsy femurs and 8 biopsies. *Acta Orthop Scand.* 2000;71(6):543-552.

48. Sochart DH. Relationship of acetabular wear to osteolysis and loosening in total hip arthroplasty. *Clin Orthop Relat Res.* 1999;(363):135-150.

49. Muratoglu OK, Bragdon CR, O'Connor DO, Jasty M, Harris WH. A novel method of cross-linking ultra-high-molecular-weight polyethylene to improve wear, reduce oxidation, and retain mechanical properties. Recipient of the 1999 HAP Paul Award. *J Arthroplasty.* 2001;16(2):149-160.

50. Dumbleton JH, D'Antonio JA, Manley MT, Capello WN, Wang A. The basis for a second-generation highly cross-linked UHMWPE. *Clin Orthop Relat Res.* 2006;453:265-271.

51. Karrholm J, Razaznejad R. Fixation and bone remodeling around a low stiffness stem in revision surgery. *Clin Orthop Relat Res.* 2008;466(2):380-388.

52. Gallo J, Havranek V, Zapletalova J. Risk factors for accelerated polyethylene wear and osteolysis in ABG I total hip arthroplasty. *Int Orthop.* 2010;34(1):19-26.

53. Williams S, Leslie I, Isaac G, Jin Z, Ingham E, Fisher J. Tribology and wear of metal-on-metal hip prostheses: influence of cup angle and head position. *J Bone Joint Surg Am.* 2008;90(Suppl 3):111-117.

54. Wan Z, Boutary M, Dorr LD. The influence of acetabular component position on wear in total hip arthroplasty. *J Arthroplasty*. 2008;23(1):51-56.

55. Patil S, Bergula A, Chen PC, Colwell CW Jr, D'Lima DD. Polyethylene wear and acetabular component orientation. *J Bone Joint Surg Am*. 2003;85-A(Suppl 4):56-63.

56. Onda K, Nagoya S, Kaya M, Yamashita T. Cup-neck impingement due to the malposition of the implant as a possible mechanism for metallosis in metal-on-metal total hip arthroplasty. *Orthopedics*. 2008;31(4):396.

57. Malik A, Maheshwari A, Dorr LD. Impingement with total hip replacement. *J Bone Joint Surg Am*. 2007;89(8):1832-1842.

58. Kesteris U, Aspenberg P. Rinsing morcellised bone grafts with bisphosphonate solution prevents their resorption. A prospective randomised double-blinded study. *J Bone Joint Surg Br*. 2006;88(8):993-996.

59. Dallari D, Fini M, Giavaresi G, et al. Effects of pulsed electromagnetic stimulation on patients undergoing hip revision prostheses: a randomized prospective double-blind study. *Bioelectromagnetics*. 2009;30(6):423-430.

60. Mallory TH, Lombardi AV Jr, Fada RA, Adams JB, Kefauver CA, Eberle RW. Noncemented acetabular component removal in the presence of osteolysis: the affirmative. *Clin Orthop Relat Res*. 2000;(381):120-128.

61. Engh CA Jr, Egawa H, Beykirch SE, Hopper RH Jr, Engh CA. The quality of osteolysis grafting with cementless acetabular component retention. *Clin Orthop Relat Res*. 2007;465:150-154.

62. Egawa H, Ho H, Huynh C, Hopper RH Jr, Engh CA Jr, Engh CA. A three-dimensional method for evaluating changes in acetabular osteolytic lesions in response to treatment. *Clin Orthop Relat Res*. 2010;468(2):480-490.

63. Malkani AL, Price MR, Crawford CH 3rd, Baker DL. Acetabular component revision using a porous tantalum biomaterial: a case series. *J Arthroplasty*. 2009;24(7):1068-1073.

64. Paprosky WG, Sporer SS, Murphy BP. Addressing severe bone deficiency: what a cage will not do. *J Arthroplasty*. 2007;22(4 Suppl 1):111-115.

65. Paprosky WG, Greidanus NV, Antoniou J. Minimum 10-year-results of extensively porous-coated stems in revision hip arthroplasty. *Clin Orthop Relat Res*. 1999;(369):230-242.

66. Korda M, Blunn G, Goodship A, Hua J. Use of mesenchymal stem cells to enhance bone formation around revision hip replacements. *J Orthop Res*. 2008;26(6):880-885.

67. Childs LM, Goater JJ, O'Keefe RJ, Schwarz EM. Efficacy of etanercept for wear debris-induced osteolysis. *J Bone Miner Res*. 2001;16(2):338-347.

68. Zhang X, Morham SG, Langenbach R, et al. Evidence for a direct role of cyclo-oxygenase 2 in implant wear debris-induced osteolysis. *J Bone Miner Res*. 2001;16(4):660-670.

69. Millett PJ, Allen MJ, Bostrom MP. Effects of alendronate on particle-induced osteolysis in a rat model. *J Bone Joint Surg Am*. 2002;84-A(2):236-249.

70. von Knoch M, Wedemeyer C, Pingsmann A, et al. The decrease of particle-induced osteolysis after a single dose of bisphosphonate. *Biomaterials*. 2005;26(14):1803-1808.

13

Periprosthetic Hip Fractures

Adam J. Schwartz, MD and Christopher P. Beauchamp, MD

INCIDENCE AND ETIOLOGY

Periprosthetic fracture is estimated to occur in 1% to 18% of primary and revision total hip procedures.[1,2] As the number of total hip arthroplasties (THAs) performed in the United States is estimated to increase by over 150% by the year 2030,[3] one would expect a concomitant increase in this catastrophic postoperative event. Additionally, as the number of primary THA increases, the prevalence of implant failure and the need for revision hip surgery, which carries a higher risk of periprosthetic fracture, will also likely rise.[3] Commonly accepted risk factors for periprosthetic fracture following THA include the use of cementless implants, advanced age, osteoporotic bone, female gender, index diagnosis at the time of the primary surgery, and the need for revision surgery.[4] Additionally, surgical technique and implant geometry are likely to play a role intraoperatively.

Although cementless femoral and acetabular implants are associated with excellent long-term clinical results, the surgical technique and implant geometry are less forgiving than with cemented components. Bony integration of both the femoral and acetabular implant relies upon immediate rotational and axial stability.[5-7] To achieve such stability, press-fit techniques and implant modifications (including tapered, tapered flat wedge, square tapered, anatomic designs, among others) have been made that place significant stresses on the host bone during implantation.[8-10] The press-fit technique attempts to reduce micromotion by underreaming the acetabular component relative to the native acetabulum to achieve tight interference fit. The result is a secure rim-fit which has been demonstrated to be superior to line-to-line reaming and screw fixation. The disadvantage of this technique is an increased risk of periprosthetic fracture and subsequent loosening of the acetabular component. In a series of more than 20,000 primary THAs, Berry reported an incidence of periprosthetic fracture in 0.3% of cemented and 5.4% of uncemented primary THAs.[1]

Patient demographics, particularly advanced age, female gender, and poor bone quality are also risk factors for intraoperative and postoperative periprosthetic THA fracture.[4,11,12] Elderly patients, particularly those who present for prosthetic replacement due to insufficiency fracture, frequently have poor bone quality, a capacious femoral canal, and thin cortices. In their review of

Jacofsky DJ, Hedley AK.
Fundamentals of Revision Hip Arthroplasty:
Diagnosis, Evaluation, and Treatment (pp 189-200).
© 2013 SLACK Incorporated.

454 consecutive THA, Wu et al[13] found that among 16 periprosthetic fractures, osteoporosis at the time of index arthroplasty was an independent predictor of periprosthetic fracture following THA. Another study found that 38% of 93 patients with periprosthetic hip fractures demonstrated a history of at least one other insufficiency fracture.[11] Patients who are suspected of having poor bone quality preoperatively should undergo evaluation with dual energy x-ray absorptiometry (DEXA) scanning. If osteoporosis is suspected, the use of cemented implants should be considered. In addition to advanced age, younger age at the time of index arthroplasty may confer a higher long-term risk of fracture,[14] potentially a result of higher activity levels and greater demand placed on the implant.

The diagnosis at the time of the index arthroplasty is an important factor that may contribute to periprosthetic fracture. Rheumatoid arthritis, metabolic bone disease, and other underlying disorders leading to bone loss, including periprosthetic infection, have been shown to be independent risk factors for periprosthetic fracture.[12] Additionally, the presence of severe deformity of the acetabulum and/or femoral canal, as can be seen in hip dysplasia, can lead to intraoperative periprosthetic fracture if appropriate implants and bone preparation equipment are not available. Aseptic loosening of the femoral stem is considered to predispose patients to periprosthetic fracture. In their review of 93 periprosthetic hip fractures, Beals and Tower found that 23 patients (24.7%) had evidence of stem loosening at the time of fracture.[11] In the setting of hip resurfacing, many authors believe that an index diagnosis of osteonecrosis may place the patient at elevated risk for femoral neck fracture. In a retrieval study of 123 failed hip resurfacing procedures, osteonecrosis was associated with 60% of failures due to periprosthetic fracture.[15] Lindahl et al found that 75% of postoperative late periprosthetic fractures occur from low-energy trauma.[12] As a result, most of these injuries result in simple fracture patterns.[11]

Revision THA is frequently complicated by severe bone loss, the presence of previous hardware, cortical perforations, and osteolysis. As a result, the incidence of periprosthetic fracture is significantly elevated during revision surgery. In a review of the Mayo Clinic database, Berry reported a 20.9% incidence of intraoperative periprosthetic fracture in uncemented revision THA.[1] Kavanagh et al reported an almost 4-fold increase in the risk of periprosthetic fracture during revision THA when compared to the primary setting.[16] As the number of primary joint arthroplasties performed in the United States continue to increase, it is likely that joint arthroplasty surgeons will face an increasing burden of periprosthetic fractures in the future.[2]

CLASSIFICATION

Periprosthetic total hip fractures can occur around either the femoral or acetabular implants, and can further be subclassified as those that occur either intraoperatively or postoperatively. Inherent to all classification systems are 2 underlying issues:

1. The quality of the host bone that remains despite the fracture
2. The stability of the femoral and/or acetabular components

In general, the classification of periprosthetic fracture should guide the surgeon toward one of 3 potential treatment options:

1. Nonoperative management
2. Fixation of the fracture alone
3. Revision of the femoral and/or acetabular components and fixation of the fracture

Intraoperative Femoral Fractures

Fractures that occur intraoperatively around a femoral implant are classified into 3 types by the Vancouver system depending on the location of the fracture.[17] Type A fractures involve the proximal metaphysis, type B fractures involve the diaphysis, and type C fractures are those that are distal to the isthmus. Each fracture type is further subclassified into the following:

1. Cortical perforation
2. Nondisplaced crack
3. Unstable fracture pattern

Postoperative Femoral Fractures

The most widely studied periprosthetic hip fractures in the literature are those that occur postoperatively around a femoral implant. While a variety of classification systems are reported, the most commonly used classification scheme for periprosthetic femoral fractures following THA is the Vancouver system.[18] Two fracture classification systems are described for intraoperative and/or postoperative fractures.

Type A fractures are those involving the proximal aspect of the femur, and are subclassified as greater trochanteric or lesser trochanteric fractures. Type A fractures typically do not compromise implant stability unless they occur intraoperatively during placement of a proximally coated cementless stem. In this case, the surgeon should consider the use of a stem that relies on distal fixation as the stability of a proximally engaging stem could be compromised.

Type B fractures are located at or just below the femoral stem. These fractures are further subclassified into those with a stable femoral stem (type IB fractures), and those with an unstable femoral stem (type IIB and IIIB fractures). Type IIIB fractures are those with poor femoral bone stock proximally.

Type C fractures are well below the tip of the femoral stem, and typically do not compromise implant stability. In practice, there is some overlap among fracture types. For example, long spiral fractures that occur distal to the tip of a well-fixed cementless implant but exit in the supracondylar portion of the femur are best classified as type IB fractures, although the fracture obviously extends to a level very distal to the stem (type C). The critical aspect of this classification scheme is whether or not the femoral component is loose at the time of fracture.

Acetabular Fractures

Acetabular fractures are classified into 5 subtypes, depending on the timing of the fracture and fracture pattern.[19] Type I fractures occur intraoperatively secondary to component insertion. These fractures are further subclassified into nondisplaced with a stable implant (IA), displaced (IB), and those that are not recognized intraoperatively (IC). Type II fractures occur secondary to component removal at the time of revision arthroplasty. Type IIA fractures are associated with less than 50% loss of acetabular bone stock. Type IIB are those with greater than 50% bone loss. Type III acetabular fractures occur traumatically following THA. Type IIIA fractures are those that maintain a stable acetabular component, and type IIIB have lost component stability. Type IV fractures, those that occur spontaneously following THA, are typically the result of large osteolytic defects. As in the type II fracture, these fractures are further subclassified into those with greater than (type IVA) or less than (type IVB) 50% bone stock remaining. Type V periprosthetic acetabular fractures are also known as a pelvic discontinuity, as they typically involve the major columns of the acetabulum. Again, these fractures are further subclassified into those with greater than (type VA) or less than (type VB) 50% bone stock remaining. These fractures also may present in the setting of prior radiation to the hemipelvis (type VC).

TREATMENT

Treatment of periprosthetic hip fractures depends upon 3 major factors:
1. The stability of the femoral and/or acetabular component
2. The quality of the host bone
3. The location and pattern of fracture

In general, fractures that compromise the stability of either the femoral or acetabular component require revision to a construct that bypasses the fracture site.

Preoperative Evaluation

Treatment begins with a thorough history and physical examination. Factors should be identified that may predispose the patient to poor bone healing, such as underlying metabolic bone disease, history of radiation, and osteoporosis, among others. Implant records from the patient's previous surgery should be readily available, in the event that modular components need to be changed intraoperatively. Knowledge of the previous surgical approach is also useful, particularly if the acetabular component or liner will be addressed.

Examination of the patient's skin may reveal previous incisions, areas of radiation necrosis, or scars that may complicate wound healing; in this case, it is useful to have a plastic surgeon available to help obtain adequate soft tissue coverage. Laboratory evaluation following periprosthetic fracture can be difficult to interpret.[20] In their study of 204 patients with periprosthetic hip fracture, Chevillotte et al[20] showed that more than 50% of patients can have an elevated C-reactive protein. There was very poor correlation between these laboratory markers and the presence or absence of infection. False-positive elevation of inflammatory markers which are typically normal in the absence of infection is common in the setting of periprosthetic fracture, and if infection is suspected based on clinical findings, hip aspiration and intraoperative frozen section analysis of periprosthetic tissue may be useful.

Good quality radiographs should be obtained of the pelvis, hip, and entire femur. If adequate radiographs cannot be obtained (typically due to patient body habitus) and the implant interfaces cannot be adequately assessed, a computed tomography (CT) scan may be useful. Comparison to any available previous x-rays of the implant prior to fracture can also help establish implant stability.

Intraoperative Fractures

Fractures of the femur or acetabulum that occur intraoperatively are best treated when recognized immediately and should be addressed according to implant stability. Intraoperative femoral fractures typically occur during placement of a cementless femoral component. Fractures may also occur with forceful leg manipulation, poor visualization, or overly vigorous retraction. Type IA and IIA intraoperative fractures that involve a cortical split or crack in the proximal metaphysis can be managed with cerclage wiring and placement of the same implant. If displaced and compromising the stability of a proximally engaging stem (type IIIA), the fracture may be bypassed with a stem that relies upon distal fixation. In this case, a cerclage wire should be placed prior to implantation of the distally based implant so as to avoid fracture propagation. The treatment of nondisplaced intraoperative diaphyseal fractures (types IB and IIB) depends upon implant stability. If the surgeon believes that the cortical perforation or nondisplaced crack will compromise the stability of the femoral implant, then the site may be fixed with a cerclage plate or allograft strut with or without morselized cancellous bone graft for cortical perforations. Displaced intraoperative diaphyseal fractures (type IIIB) should be treated with open reduction and internal fixation using cerclage wiring alone or cerclage wiring and plating. Allograft struts can be used to supplement the fixation construct, particularly in cases of poor host bone.

Acetabular fractures that occur intraoperatively are best managed when recognized immediately.[19] For stable nondisplaced fractures that occur following insertion of a press-fit component, the implant may be safely left in place. If the fracture compromises the stability of the acetabular component, the implant should be removed, and the fracture allowed to reduce spontaneously. At this point, the fracture should be assessed for stability and remaining bone quality. In cases of nondisplaced intra-articular fractures where the bone quality will allow for good circumferential screw purchase, the native socket may be reamed line to line and a component with multiple screw holes placed. A displaced fracture that involves the major columns of the acetabulum has a high risk of nonunion and early component loosening. Depending on the amount and quality of host bone remaining, this scenario is best addressed with either anterior/posterior column plating or an acetabular cage that will obtain bridging fixation. The use of a multihole, highly porous metal revision acetabular component may be helpful to achieve initial fixation.

Postoperative Femoral Fractures

Femoral fractures that occur postoperatively are best managed according to the Vancouver classification system, based on implant stability and the quality of the remaining host bone. Type A fractures of the greater and lesser trochanter typically result from progressive osteolysis due to polyethylene wear or cement debris. Nondisplaced fractures are typically managed nonoperatively, with limited weightbearing and activity modification (ie, limited active abduction for fractures of the greater trochanter). A hip abduction brace may be helpful to prevent adduction and resultant displacement of the fracture. For displaced fractures (generally more than 1 cm) of the greater trochanter, surgical management is typically preferred due to the risk of nonunion, abductor weakness, and gait disturbance. Various techniques of cerclage wiring have been advocated.[21,22] One effective method calls for the placement of a looped 16- or 18-gauge sternal wire into the lateral cortex of the distal fragment that is then brought out through the superior tendinous insertion site of the gluteus medius muscle.[22] This wire is then brought back through the lateral loop and tightened over 2 separate transverse wires.

Another option for fixation is the use of various types of laterally based claw plates that engage into the superior tip of the trochanter, and are fixed distally with either unicortical locking screws or cerclage wires.[23] Fractures of the lesser trochanter are typically managed nonoperatively. Surgical fixation of displaced fractures is recommended only in the case of an associated loose femoral component, generally seen with proximally coated femoral components.

Type B fractures are those that involve the femoral diaphysis at the level of or just distal to the tip of the femoral implant. Nonoperative management is reserved for nondisplaced fractures or cracks that do not compromise implant stability. Patients should be treated with protected weightbearing for a period of 6 to 8 weeks, and serial radiographs are performed to document maintenance of fracture alignment and implant stability. Type B fractures frequently involve a loose femoral component (type IIB and IIIB fractures). These fractures are best addressed with removal of the loose implant along with any retained cement or debris, fixation of the fracture, and revision to a long-stemmed diaphyseal engaging or tapered-conical modular implant, depending on the quality of the remaining bone. An extensive lateral approach is the workhorse for all periprosthetic fractures around a femoral implant that will require revision. Distally, the approach may split the fascia lata, and either proceeds by splitting the fibers of the vastus lateralis or elevating the entire muscle off the intermuscular septum. Perforating vessels of the deep femoral artery are encountered along the lateral aspect of the femur and are ligated. An extended trochanteric osteotomy of the proximal fracture fragment is occasionally useful to allow for implant removal, cement extraction, and placement of the final implant into the distal fragment, particularly if there has been significant varus remodeling. However, often the fracture itself will dictate the location of an osteotomy, as the fracture may easily act as one or both longitudinal limbs of the osteotomy. In more severe fractures, where a transverse component exists as well, the proximal fracture fragment may be separated for exposure of the stem to be removed and later cabled around the proximal aspect of the new implant. If based on the preoperatively templated radiographs, the host bone will allow for placement of a fully coated diaphyseal engaging stem, and the fracture may be reduced initially, followed by placement of a cementless stem. The use of a fully coated cylindrical stem is reserved for cases where the diaphysis will allow for at least 4 cm of contact between the bone and the implant surface. In patients with more osteopenic bone, or more distal fractures, modular tapered stems are gaining popularity due to the stable nature of the conical shape and the versatility afforded by the ability to choose body length and version after seating the distal stem. With either stem choice, the distal canal is reamed antegrade. A trial implant is placed to help obtain provisional fracture alignment. Reduction of the fracture is obtained with gentle traction on the extremity and provisional fixation with either 16-gauge cerclage wire or a large bone holding reduction clamp. Provisional cerclage wires should be low profile if the fracture pattern mandates to allow a lateral plate and/or allograft strut to be placed against the host bone. A femoral distractor is useful in the presence of limited surgical assistants. Two pins are placed anteriorly, one in the area of dense bone of the medial calcar, and another in the anterior or anterolateral femoral cortex to avoid any laterally placed implants. Once a satisfactory reduction of the fracture is obtained, plate application proceeds in the usual fashion.

In cases of severe proximal bone loss, the proximal fragment provides limited fixation. In this instance, acceptable results have been obtained with the use of cementless tapered cone-shaped implants that can obtain fixation over very short distal segments. Essentially, the proximal fragment and the fracture itself is largely bypassed, and the implant is wedged into the distal fragment. The abductor mechanism may be wired to the lateral shoulder of the implant, or supplemental fixation may be obtained with the use of a hernia mesh or Dacron aortic graft wrapped around the implant. Preoperative templating and comparison to the opposite leg intraoperatively help to achieve equalized leg lengths as most other landmarks are absent.

For displaced fractures around a well-fixed implant (type IB or C), open reduction and internal fixation is warranted (Figure 13-1). Good quality preoperative radiographs are necessary to document the stability of the femoral component that will be retained. A lateral vastus-splitting or vastus-elevating approach as described previously is utilized. The fracture is reduced with gentle traction and provisionally fixed with a low-profile cerclage wire. In spiral Vancouver type C fractures that are well distal to the tip of the implant, multiple compression lag screws are placed. Once provisional fixation is achieved, a laterally based plate is placed that will allow for purchase of a minimum of 6 cortices (preferably 8 cortices) on either side of the fracture.[24] Proximal screw fixation is hindered by the retained intramedullary implant, which can either be addressed with large-diameter cerclage cables or unicortical locking screws.[25-29] Adequate fixation can also be achieved with cortical onlay struts, either alone or supplemented with plate fixation.[30,31]

Postoperative Acetabular Fractures

Acetabular fractures that occur postoperatively are most frequently the result of periprosthetic osteolysis due to cement or wear debris. The degree of bone loss typically dictates the surgical management of these fractures. Preoperative x-rays are critically evaluated, along with CT scan of the hemipelvis, if necessary. Severe bone loss and the need for supplemental fixation is indicated by greater than 2 to 3 cm of superior migration of the acetabular component, the presence of severe ischial osteolysis, or a break in the ilioischial (Kohler's) line.[32] If none of these finding are present, and greater than 50% of host bone remains at the time of surgery, revision to a hemispherical socket with multiple screws will likely provide adequate fixation. For cases involving greater than 50% bone loss, acetabular component fixation can be greatly enhanced with metallic augments or structural allografting. A pelvic discontinuity represents a transverse fracture through both anterior and posterior columns. If an adequate reduction can be obtained and the remaining bone will allow for compression at the fracture site, a posterior column plate may be placed along with a porous hemispherical socket.[33] A pelvic discontinuity that occurs years following THA is frequently associated with poor bone quality, large lytic defects, and lacks healing potential. In the last case, the fracture is either bridged with a cage or cup-cage construct,[34] or further distracted and allowed to compress around a porous acetabular implant.[35]

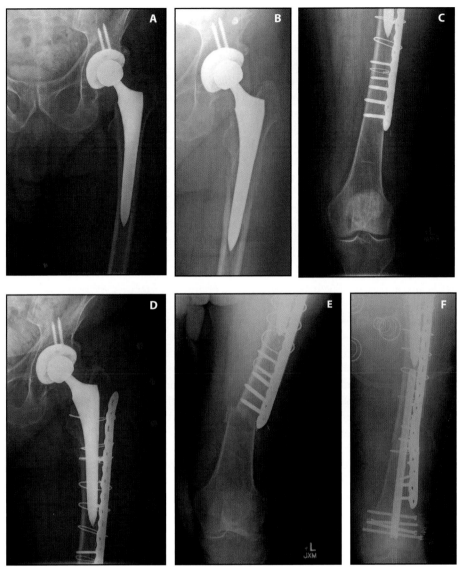

Figure 13-1. Case example. (A) A 70-year-old male underwent left total hip arthroplasty. Approximately 2 years postoperatively, the patient sustained a low-energy fall from a standing height. He was noted to have a Vancouver B1 fracture with a well-fixed cementless femoral stem (B). The patient underwent open reduction and internal fixation of the periprosthetic fracture using a broad cerclage plate supplemented by an anterior allograft strut (C). Eight weeks postoperatively, the patient sustained another low-energy fall and fractured below the tip of the cerclage plate (Vancouver Type C fracture), maintaining a well-fixed femoral implant (D, E). Fixation was achieved with a retrograde femoral nail along with an additional cerclage plate that allowed for supplementary screw fixation (F).

OUTCOMES

The outcomes following surgical fixation of periprosthetic hip fracture are varied. Beals and Tower reviewed the results of 93 periprosthetic femoral fractures treated with a range of techniques, including plating, cemented revision, uncemented revision, and conservative treatment.[11] At a mean of 2.4 years postoperatively, 32% of patients demonstrated excellent, 16% good, and 52% poor results. As expected, the lowest number of arthroplasty-related complications was seen in those patients treated with plating, while the lowest number of fracture-related complications was those who underwent cementless revision. Similarly, Jukkala-Partio and colleagues reviewed the results of 75 type B fractures treated with either stem revision (11 cemented and 29 uncemented) or plate fixation (35 cases).[36] A total of 47 reoperations were necessary, including 20 among stem revisions, and 27 among those who underwent plate fixation.

Fractures that do not compromise implant stability are typically treated with implant retention and fracture fixation. Cerclage plating with or without cortical strut allograft has demonstrated good results. Haddad et al[31] reviewed the results of 40 patients with periprosthetic fracture around a stable femoral implant. Nineteen patients were treated with allograft struts alone, and the remaining 21 patients treated with a combined plate and strut construct. Ninety-eight percent of fractures healed and all but one patient returned to prefracture function. Wilson et al[29] performed a biomechanical study to compare the strength of constructs that employed various combinations of plating and allograft cortical struts. The authors concluded that a combination that employs both plating and allograft strut was superior to 2 struts alone or a plate alone.

While most fractures around a well-fixed implant can be addressed adequately with implant retention and fracture fixation, femoral revision should be considered for fractures that occur around a poorly positioned implant. In particular, a femoral component that is in varus may predispose to fracture nonunion. Tadross et al[37] reported the results of 7 patients with type IB fractures treated with open reduction and plating, 6 of which demonstrated prefracture varus implant positioning. At a mean 1.2 years postoperatively, all 6 patients with a varus femoral stem demonstrated evidence of varus collapse of the fracture.

Locked plating constructs may improve upon conventional cable plate systems by making use of the internal fixator concept. This type of fixed-angle device may help decrease the incidence of fracture displacement and varus collapse as a result of mechanical forces on the limb. Sah et al reported the results of 22 patients with interprosthetic fracture between well-fixed hip and knee implants treated with single locked plating with or without cerclage cables.[24] At a mean follow-up of 17.7 months, all fractures united and all patients regained prefracture function.

For fractures associated with a loose femoral component, the results of cementless revision using a tapered fluted stem have been encouraging. Berry reported on 8 patients who sustained a type IIIB fracture. At a mean of 1.5 years, all patients demonstrated evidence of complete fracture healing and implant stability.[38] In a study of 12 patients with Vancouver B2 fractures, Ko et al[39] reported 100% union and excellent clinical results following revision arthroplasty using a tapered fluted implant. MacDonald et al[40] reported excellent results following revision THA combined with cable plate and/or cortical strut grafting for 14 periprosthetic fractures associated with a loose implant. All fractures were treated with a long-stem extensively coated implant. At mean follow-up of 8.2 years, all fractures united, and there were no revisions required among femoral implants.

PEARLS FOR PREVENTION

Prevention of periprosthetic fracture around a THA is an ongoing concern from the patient's initial evaluation to the long-term postoperative follow-up. At the outset, patients should undergo a thorough history and physical examination to reveal any particular risk factors for periprosthetic fracture, particularly the underlying diagnosis, history of any previous fractures, or other medical comorbidities that can result in poor bone quality (previous radiation, malnutrition, osteoporosis, among others). High-quality radiographs should be obtained and used along with overlay or digital templates to help plan the surgical procedure and guide implant selection. The presence of hardware or implants already removed should alert the surgeon to the possible need for supplemental fixation or a construct that will sufficiently bypass cortical defects. In patients with capacious femoral canals, prior hip or pelvic radiation, or thinned cortices, consideration should be given to cemented primary THA. For surgeons who typically rely on cementless implants alone, it is useful to become familiar with an alternative system that allows for both cemented femoral and acetabular components.

Intraoperative periprosthetic fractures are best avoided by meticulous preoperative templating and anticipation of poor bone quality or the need for alternative fixation techniques. When intraoperative fractures do occur, they are typically the result of an excessive press-fit technique that exceeds the strain limits of the host bone. During acetabular preparation, such a scenario is typically encountered when attempting to implant a small (50-mm or less) socket into a native acetabulum that is underreamed by 2 mm. Smaller acetabular sizes are associated with columnar fracture patterns that essentially represent pelvic discontinuity, and may lead to early implant failure. To avoid such a scenario, the surgeon should either ream to a larger size (resulting in a decreased press-fit) or ream line to line and rely on screw fixation for immediate stability. Rim fractures of the acetabulum occur with poor circumferential visualization of the bone. Thorough débridement of peripheral labrum along with accurate retractor placement helps to optimize cup positioning and minimize the risk of acetabular rim fracture.

Underpreparation of the femur can lead to an overzealous press-fit and cortical fracture. Options to minimize this problem include decreasing the amount of press-fit, employing a pneumatic broach, or abandoning cementless fixation altogether in favor of a cemented implant. For cylindrical stems that employ distal fixation, a press-fit of 0.25 to 0.5 mm over a length of 4 cm is typically recommended for immediate axial and rotational stability. Proximally based stems, prepared using a cutting-type or toothed broach, maintain axial and rotational stability by a wedged tapered fit into the metaphyseal cortical bone. Recently, a pneumatic broaching device has been introduced to help reduce the incidence of intraoperative cortical disruption caused by variation in manual force applied while broaching the femoral metaphysis or diaphysis. The device allows for slight variation in axial compression, providing 0.8 to 1 Newton of axial force on the bone at a pneumatic pressure of 100 PSI. For patients with a wide femoral canal, thinned cortices, or history of prior insufficiency fracture, a cemented femoral implant is indicated. Advantages of a cemented component include immediate fixation and weightbearing status, decreased need for vigorous broaching, and virtually limitless ability to modulate implant version and leg lengths intraoperatively.

Periprosthetic fracture during revision THA is commonly encountered due to large osteolytic defects, cortical defects, and bone deficiencies caused by removal of pre-existing hardware. Multiple classification systems exist to help the surgeon preoperatively identify patterns of bone loss, and predict the need for special equipment.[32,35,41,42] Prevention of periprosthetic fracture during revision THA is best accomplished with good preoperative planning, anticipation of bone defects following implant removal, and meticulous surgical technique. Prophylactic cerclage wiring should be considered when preparing a femur with significant bone loss.

Prevention of late periprosthetic fracture is best accomplished with routine serial radiographs, patient education, and preemptive surgical intervention for large rapidly progressive osteolytic lesions that threaten bone or implant stability. Vancouver A fractures that involve large osteolytic defects are frequently associated with acetabular defects, liner wear, and cement debris that may reflect a secondary indication for revision arthroplasty. Likewise, in fractures that are classified as Vancouver B1 or C fractures, the femoral stem should be thoroughly evaluated for evidence of periprosthetic osteolysis, cement mantle fractures, or impending loosening. Serial radiographs are invaluable to help determine implant stability over time. If question exists regarding stem stability, the implant should be tested manually during surgery, and revision performed as necessary.

REFERENCES

1. Berry DJ. Epidemiology: hip and knee. *Orthop Clin North Am.* 1999;30(2):183-190.
2. Berry DJ. Periprosthetic fractures associated with osteolysis: a problem on the rise. *J Arthroplasty.* 2003;18 (3, Part 2):107-111.
3. Kurtz S, Ong K, Lau E, Mowat F, Halpern M. Projections of primary and revision hip and knee arthroplasty in the United States from 2005 to 2030. *J Bone Joint Surg Am.* 2007;89(4):780-785.
4. Franklin J, Malchau H. Risk factors for periprosthetic femoral fracture. *Injury.* 2007;38(6):655-660.
5. Bobyn JD, Pilliar RM, Cameron HU, Weatherly GC. The optimum pore size for the fixation of porous-surfaced metal implants by the ingrowth of bone. *Clin Orthop Relat Res.* 1980;(150):263-270.
6. Pilliar RM, Lee JM, Maniatopoulos C. Observations on the effect of movement on bone ingrowth into porous-surfaced implants. *Clin Orthop Relat Res.* 1986;(208):108-113.
7. Kuhn A, Scheller G, Schwarz M. [Primary stability of cement-free press-fit acetabulum cups. In vitro displacement studies]. *Biomed Tech (Berl).* 1999;44(12):356-359.
8. Mallory TH, Lombardi AV, Leith JR, et al. Why a taper? *J Bone Joint Surg Am.* 2002;84-A(Suppl 2):81-89.
9. Mallory TH, Lombardi AV, Leith JR, et al. Minimal 10-year results of a tapered cementless femoral component in total hip arthroplasty. *J Arthroplasty.* 2001;16(8 Suppl 1):49-54.
10. Grübl A, Chiari C, Gruber M, Kaider A, Gottsauner-Wolf F. Cementless total hip arthroplasty with a tapered, rectangular titanium stem and a threaded cup: a minimum ten-year follow-up. *J Bone Joint Surg Am.* 2002;84-A(3):425-431.
11. Beals RK, Tower SS. Periprosthetic fractures of the femur. An analysis of 93 fractures. *Clin Orthop Relat Res.* 1996;(327):238-246.
12. Lindahl H, Malchau H, Herberts P, Garellick G. Periprosthetic femoral fractures classification and demographics of 1049 periprosthetic femoral fractures from the Swedish National Hip Arthroplasty Register. *J Arthroplasty.* 2005;20(7):857-865.
13. Wu CC, Au MK, Wu SS, Lin LC. Risk factors for postoperative femoral fracture in cementless hip arthroplasty. *J Formos Med Assoc.* 1999;98(3):190-194.
14. Lindahl H, Garellick G, Regnér H, Herberts P, Malchau H. Three hundred and twenty-one periprosthetic femoral fractures. *J Bone Joint Surg Am.* 2006;88(6):1215-1222.
15. Zustin J, Sauter G, Morlock MM, Rüther W, Amling M. Association of osteonecrosis and failure of hip resurfacing arthroplasty. *Clin Orthop Relat Res.* 2010;468(3):756-761.
16. Kavanagh BF. Femoral fractures associated with total hip arthroplasty. *Orthop Clin North Am.* 1992;23(2): 249-257.
17. Greidanus NV, Mitchell PA, Masri BA, Garbuz DS, Duncan CP. Principles of management and results of treating the fractured femur during and after total hip arthroplasty. *Instr Course Lect.* 2003;52:309-322.
18. Brady OH, Garbuz DS, Masri BA, Duncan CP. Classification of the hip. *Orthop Clin North Am.* 1999;30(2):215-220.
19. Della Valle CJ, Momberger NG, Paprosky WG. Periprosthetic fractures of the acetabulum associated with a total hip arthroplasty. *Instr Course Lect.* 2003;52:281-290.
20. Chevillotte CJ, Ali MH, Trousdale RT, et al. Inflammatory laboratory markers in periprosthetic hip fractures. *J Arthroplasty.* 2009;24(5):722-727.
21. Jensen NF, Harris WH. A system for trochanteric osteotomy and reattachment for total hip arthroplasty with a ninety-nine percent union rate. *Clin Orthop Relat Res.* 1986;(208):174-181.
22. Wroblewski BM, Shelley P. Reattachment of the greater trochanter after hip replacement. *J Bone Joint Surg Br.* 1985;67(5):736-740.
23. McGrory BJ, Lucas R. The use of locking plates for greater trochanteric fixation. *Orthopedics.* 2009;32(12): 917-920.
24. Sah AP, Marshall A, Virkus WV, Estok DM, Della Valle CJ. Interprosthetic fractures of the femur: treatment with a single-locked plate. *J Arthroplasty.* 2010;25(2):280-286.
25. Buttaro M, Farfalli G, Nunez MP, Comba F, Piccaluga F. Locking compression plate fixation of Vancouver type-B1 periprosthetic femoral fractures. *J Bone Joint Surg Am.* 2007;89(9):1964-1969.
26. Schütz M, Müller M, Krettek C, et al. Minimally invasive fracture stabilization of distal femoral fractures with the LISS: a prospective multicenter study. Results of a clinical study with special emphasis on difficult cases. *Injury.* 2001;32(Suppl 3):SC48-SC54.
27. Ricci WM, Bolhofner BR, Loftus T, et al. Indirect reduction and plate fixation, without grafting, for periprosthetic femoral shaft fractures about a stable intramedullary implant. *J Bone Joint Surg Am.* 2005;87(10):2240-2245.

28. Dennis MG, Simon JA, Kummer FJ, Koval KJ, Di Cesare PE. Fixation of periprosthetic femoral shaft fractures: a biomechanical comparison of two techniques. *J Orthop Trauma*. 2001;15(3):177-180.

29. Wilson D, Frei H, Masri BA, Oxland TR, Duncan CP. A biomechanical study comparing cortical onlay allograft struts and plates in the treatment of periprosthetic femoral fractures. *Clin Biomech (Bristol, Avon)*. 2005;20(1):70-76.

30. Emerson RH, Malinin TI, Cuellar AD, Head WC, Peters PC. Cortical strut allografts in the reconstruction of the femur in revision total hip arthroplasty. A basic science and clinical study. *Clin Orthop Relat Res*. 1992;(285):35-44.

31. Haddad FS, Duncan CP, Berry DJ, et al. Periprosthetic femoral fractures around well-fixed implants: use of cortical onlay allografts with or without a plate. *J Bone Joint Surg Am*. 2002;84-A(6):945-950.

32. Paprosky WG, Perona PG, Lawrence JM. Acetabular defect classification and surgical reconstruction in revision arthroplasty. A 6-year follow-up evaluation. *J Arthroplasty*. 1994;9(1):33-44.

33. Berry DJ, Lewallen DG, Hanssen AD, Cabanela ME. Pelvic discontinuity in revision total hip arthroplasty. *J Bone Joint Surg Am*. 1999;81(12):1692-1702.

34. Noordin S, Duncan CP, Masri BA, Garbuz DS. Pelvic dissociation in revision total hip arthroplasty: diagnosis and treatment. *Instr Course Lect*. 2010;59:37-43.

35. Paprosky WG, O'Rourke M, Sporer SM. The treatment of acetabular bone defects with an associated pelvic discontinuity. *Clin Orthop Relat Res*. 2005;441:216-220.

36. Jukkala-Partio K, Partio EK, Solovieva S, et al. Treatment of periprosthetic fractures in association with total hip arthroplasty: a retrospective comparison between revision stem and plate fixation. *Ann Chir Gynaecol*. 1998;87(3):229-235.

37. Tadross TS, Nanu AM, Buchanan MJ, Checketts RG. Dall-Miles plating for periprosthetic B1 fractures of the femur. *J Arthroplasty*. 2000;15(1):47-51.

38. Berry DJ. Treatment of Vancouver B3 periprosthetic femur fractures with a fluted tapered stem. *Clin Orthop Relat Res*. 2003;(417):224-231.

39. Ko PS, Lam JJ, Tio MK, Lee OB, Ip FK. Distal fixation with Wagner revision stem in treating Vancouver type B2 periprosthetic femur fractures in geriatric patients. *J Arthroplasty*. 2003;18(4):446-452.

40. Macdonald SJ, Paprosky WG, Jablonsky WS, Magnus RG. Periprosthetic femoral fractures treated with a long-stem cementless component. *J Arthroplasty*. 2001;16(3):379-383.

41. Sporer SM, Paprosky WG. Femoral fixation in the face of considerable bone loss: the use of modular stems. *Clin Orthop Relat Res*. 2004;(429):227-231.

42. Noordin S, Masri BA, Duncan CP, Garbuz DS. Acetabular bone loss in revision total hip arthroplasty: principles and techniques. *Instr Course Lect*. 2010;59:27-36.

Financial Disclosures

Dr. *Wael K. Barsoum* receives grant or research support from Stryker Orthopaedics; Zimmer, Inc; CoolSystems; Orthovita; DJO; Active Implants; Recothrom; and the Orthopaedic Research and Education Foundation. Dr. Barsoum receives royalties from Stryker Orthopaedics; Zimmer, Inc; Exactech; Wright Medical Technology; and Shukla Medical. He is a consultant for Stryker Orthopaedics and Shukla Medical; and has stock options in OtisMed Corporation, Custom Arthroplasty Solutions, Custom Orthopaedic Solutions, and iVHR. Dr. Barsoum has 2 issued patents and 30 applications.

Dr. *Christopher P. Beauchamp* has no financial or proprietary interest in the materials presented herein.

Dr. *Michael R. Bloomfield* has no financial or proprietary interest in the materials presented herein.

Dr. *Justin Brothers* has not disclosed any relevant financial relationships.

Dr. *James Cashman* has no financial or proprietary interest in the materials presented herein.

Dr. *Robert M. Cercek* has no financial or proprietary interest in the materials presented herein.

Dr. *Craig J. Della Valle* is a consultant for Biomet and Smith & Nephew. Dr. Della Valle receives research support from Smith & Nephew and Stryker Orthopaedics, and institutional research support from Zimmer, Inc. He holds stock options in CD Diagnostics.

Dr. *Douglas A. Dennis* receives royalties from the transfer of intellectual property from Depuy, Inc and Innomed. Dr. Dennis is a consultant for Depuy, Inc and receives laboratory research support from Depuy, Inc and Porter Adventist Hospital.

Dr. *Jared R. H. Foran* gives paid presentations for Conmed Corporation, and is on the editorial/governing board for the AAOS publication *OrthoInfo*.

Dr. Gregory J. Golladay is a consultant for Zimmer, Inc and OrthoSensor. Dr. Golladay also receives research support from OrthoSensor.

Dr. Ian M. Gradisar has no financial or proprietary interest in the materials presented herein.

Dr. Kenneth A. Greene is a consultant for and receives royalties from Stryker Orthopaedics.

Dr. Anthony K. Hedley has several patents with Synvasive Technology Inc and Stryker Orthopaedics and receives financial compensation for his work as a consultant with Stryker Orthopaedics.

Dr. Carlos A. Higuera has no financial or proprietary interest in the materials presented herein.

Dr. David J. Jacofsky is a consultant for Bacterin, Comprehensive Care Solutions, Safe Independence, Stryker Orthopaedics, Smith & Nephew, and Technology Capital Investors. He receives research support from Biomet, DePuy, Stryker Orthopaedics, Smith & Nephew, and VQ Ortho Care. Dr. Jacofsky receives royalties from Stryker Orthopaedics.

Dr. David E. Jaffe has no financial or proprietary interest in the materials presented herein.

Dr. Aaron J. Johnson has no financial or proprietary interest in the materials presented herein.

Dr. Raymond H. Kim is a consultant for Stryker Orthopaedics and receives royalties from Innomed, Inc and institutional research support from DePuy.

Dr. Viktor E. Krebs has not disclosed any relevant financial relationships.

Dr. Steven M. Kurtz works for an institution that receives grants from Stryker Orthopaedics.

Dr. Michael T. Manley has not disclosed any relevant financial relationships.

Dr. David C. Markel is a consultant for Stryker Orthopaedics. He receives institutional resarch support from Stryker Orthopaedics and OREF; and royalties from Stryker Orthopaedics, Arboretum Ventures, and the Bone and Joint Surgery Center of Novi. Dr. Markel is on the board of the American Association of Hip and Knee Surgeons and the Michigan Orthopedic Society.

Dr. Andrew Michael has not disclosed any relevant financial relationships.

Dr. Michael A. Mont has no financial or proprietary interest in the materials presented herein.

Dr. Steven L. Myerthall is a consultant for Stryker Orthopaedics and Stryker Instruments.

Dr. Kevin L. Ong has received a research grant from Biomet and Stryker Orthopaedics.

Dr. Javad Parvizi is on the speaker's bureau for Elsevier, Wolters Kluwer, and SLACK Incorporated. Dr. Parvizi is a consultant for Biomet; Smith & Nephew; Zimmer, Inc; Convatech; Covidien; TissueGene; Ceramtec; OsteoMEM; and Pfizer. He holds stock options in SmarTech, and is a board member for Philadelphia Orthopaedics, Eastern Orthopaedics, CD Diagnostics, United Healthcare, Magnifi Group (Publishers), and 3M.

Dr. Michael D. Ries is a consultant for Stryker Orthopaedics.

Dr. Adam J. Schwartz has no financial or proprietary interest in the materials presented herein.

Dr. Scott Sporer is a consultant for Zimmer, Inc and Smith & Nephew. Dr. Sporer receives research support from Zimmer, Inc.

Dr. Bryan D. Springer is a consultant for Depuy, Inc and Convatec. Dr. Springer also receives educational honoraria from Depuy, Inc.

Dr. Creighton C. Tubb has no financial or proprietary interest in the materials presented herein.

Dr. Jonathan M. Vigdorchik has no financial or proprietary interest in the materials presented herein.

Dr. Antonia Woehnl has no financial or proprietary interest in the materials presented herein.

Index